Imaging of the
INFERTILE
COUPLE

Imaging of the
INFERTILE COUPLE

Edited by

Steven R Goldstein MD
Professor of Obstetrics & Gynecology, and
Director of Gynecologic Ultrasound
New York University School of Medicine
NYU Medical Center
New York NY 10016
USA

and

Carol B Benson MD
Associate Professor of Radiology
Harvard Medical School, and
Director of Ultrasound and
Co-Director of High Risk Obstetrical Ultrasound
Brigham & Women's Hospital
Department of Radiology
Boston MA 02115
USA

MARTIN DUNITZ

First published in the United Kingdom in 2001 by
Martin Dunitz Ltd
The Livery House
7–9 Pratt Street
London NW1 0AE

Tel: +44-(0)20-7482-2202
Fax: +44-(0)20-7267-0159
E-mail: info.dunitz@tandf.co.uk
Website: http://www.dunitz.co.uk

A CIP record for this book is available from the British Library

ISBN 1-85317-514-5

Distributed in the United States by:
Blackwell Science Inc.
Commerce Place, 350 Main Street
Malden MA 02148, USA
Tel: 1-800-215-1000

Distributed in Canada by:
Login Brothers Book Company
324 Salteaux Crescent
Winnipeg, Manitoba R3J 3T2
Canada
Tel: 1-204-224-4068

Distributed in Brazil by:
Ernesto Reichmann Distribuidora de Livros, Ltda
Rua Coronel Marques 335, Tatuape 03440-000
Sao Paulo
Brazil

Composition by Scribe Design, Gillingham, Kent
Printed and bound in Hong Kong by Imago

Contents

Contributors

Carol B Benson MD
Associate Professor of Radiology, Harvard Medical School, and Director of Ultrasound and Co-Director of High Risk Obstetrical Ultrasound, Brigham & Women's Hospital, Department of Radiology, 75 Francis Street, Boston MA 02115-6195, USA

Douglas L Brown MD
Associate Professor of Radiology, Harvard Medical School, 75 Francis Street, Boston, MA 02115-6195, USA

Jeanne A Cullinan MD
803 Wickfield Road, Wynnewood, PA 19096, USA

Donald N Di Salvo MD
Assistant Professor of Radiology, Harvard Medical School, Brigham & Women's Hospital, 75 Francis Street, Boston, MA 02115-6195, USA

Helen M Fenlon MD
Assistant Professor of Radiology, Boston University School of Medicine, BU Medical Center, 88 East Newton Street, Boston, MA 02118-2393, USA

Arthur C Fleischer MD
Professor of Radiology and Radiological Sciences, Professor of Obstetrics and Gynecology, and Chief, Diagnostic Sonography, Department of Radiology and Radiological Sciences, School of Medicine, Vanderbilt University Medical Center, Nashville, TN 37232-2675, USA

Mary C Frates MD
Assistant Professor of Radiology, Harvard Medical School, Department of Radiology, Brigham & Women's Hospital, 75 Francis Street, Boston, MA 02115-6195, USA

Antonio R Gargiulo MD
Instructor of Obstetrics, Gynecology and Reproductive Biology, Division of Reproductive Medicine, Brigham & Women's Hospital, Harvard Medical School, 75 Francis Street, Boston, MA 02115-6195, USA

Steven R Goldstein MD
Professor of Obstetrics and Gynecology, New York University School of Medicine, New York Medical Center, 550 First Avenue, New York, NY 10016, USA

Lawrence Grunfeld MD
Clinical Associate Professor, Department of Obstetrics & Gynecology, Mount Sinai Medical Center, New York, NY 10029, USA

Robert S Howe MD, FACOG
Medical Director, Reproductive Medicine Center of Western Massachusetts, 281 Maple Street, East Longmeadows, MA 01028, USA

Howard W Jones Jr MD
The Howard and Georgeanna Jones Institute for Reproductive Medicine, 601 Colley Avenue, Norfolk, VA 23507-1627, USA

Ewa Kuligowska MD
Professor of Radiology, Boston University School of Medicine, and Head, Body Imaging, BU Medical Center, 88 East Newton Street, Boston, MA 02118-2393, USA

Faye C Laing MD
Professor of Radiology, Harvard Medical School, Director of Resident Education & Training, Department of Radiology, Brigham & Women's Hospital, 75 Francis Street, Boston, MA 02115-6195, USA

Jodi P Lerner MD
Assistant Professor of Clinical Obstetrics and Gynecology, Columbia-Presbyterian Medical Center, 622 W 168 Street, New York, NY 10032, USA

Ana Monteagudo MD
Associate Professor of Obstetrics and Gynecology,
Director of Obstetrics and Obstetrics/Gynecology
Ultrasound, Bellevue Hospital Center, and
Department of Obstetrics and Gynecology, New
York University School of Medicine, New York
University Medical Center, 550 First Avenue, New
York, NY 10016, USA

Jeffrey Nelson DO
Huntington Reproductive Center, 301 South Fair
Oaks Street, #401, Pasadena, CA 91105, USA

Anna K Parsons MD
Harborside Medical Tower, 4 Columbia Drive Suite
440, Tampa, FL 33606, USA

John A Richmond MD
Associate Clinical Professor of Radiology, Los
Angeles County – University of Southern
California Medical Center, Los Angeles, CA 90033,
USA

Paulo Serafini MD
Department of Obstetrics and Gynecology, Division
of Reproductive Endocrinology, Yale University
School of Medicine, 333 Cedar Street, PO Box
208063, New Haven, CT 06520-8063, USA

James M Shwayder MD
Director of Gynecology and Gynecologic
Ultrasound, Denver Health Medical Center, 777
Bannock Street, MC 0660, Denver, CO 80220, USA

Clare M C Tempany MD
Professor of Radiology, Harvard Medical School,
Director of Body MRI, Department of Radiology,
Brigham & Women's Hospital, 75 Francis Street,
Boston, MA 02115-6195, USA

Ilan E Timor-Tritsch MD
Professor of Obstetrics and Gynecology, and
Director, Division of Obstetrics and Gynecology,
Bellevue Hospital Center, and Department of
Obstetrics and Gynecology, New York University
School of Medicine, New York University Medical
Center, 550 First Avenue, New York, NY 10016,
USA

Jaime M Vasquez MD
Director, Center for Reproductive Health, 326 21st
Avenue North, Nashville, TN 37203, USA

Preface

The field of infertility has undergone an absolute revolution in the last quarter century, both in terms of diagnostic capabilities to evaluate the infertile couple as well as incredible advances in overcoming the multitude of reasons why the process of conception fails to take place. Nothing has been more central to this revolution than diagnostic ultrasound.

This book grew out of a categorical course of the same title that I was asked to organize for the annual meeting of The American Institute of Ultrasound in Medicine. I was fortunate enough to cajole Dr Carol Benson of Harvard's Radiology Department at Brigham and Women's Hospital in Boston to co-edit this volume. We have attempted to systematically include all aspects of diagnostic imaging in the infertile couple.

The broad range of topics covered in this volume goes from the old and proven, like hysterosalpingography, to the latest and cutting edge, such as sonohysterography and sonosalpingography. The dysfunctional pelvis and male infertility parts cover standard issues as well as the contribution of imaging to various sources of infertility (endometriosis, inflammatory disease, scrotal abnormalities), while also exploring the use of imaging in newer areas such as impotence and various forms of the assisted reproductive technologies. The role of ultrasound when conception finally does take place, the understanding of what early pregnancy looks like, and why and how to differentiate normal early pregnancy from those pregnancies destined to fail are also considered, as are new concepts in extrauterine pregnancies. Doppler ultrasound and ultrasound-guided multifetal pregnancy reduction.

In summary we believe this monograph will be clinically relevant to many health care providers who pick up an ultrasound transducer in the evaluation of men, women, or both, who may present with infertility. This will be regardless of what the medical specialty (obstetrician/gynecologist, radiologist, urologist, neurologist, family physician) or professional degree (physician, sonographer, nurse) of that health care provider actually is.

Steven R Goldstein MD
New York, NY

Carol B Benson MD
Boston, MA

Acknowledgments

This book is dedicated to The American Institute of Ultrasound in Medicine, an organization whose sole interest in diagnostic ultrasound brings together diverse physicians like ourselves, and thus enables collaborations that culminate in a monograph like this one.

1 Overview of infertility: the scope of the problem

Howard W Jones Jr

An overview of the ever-changing vista of fertility can conveniently be seen from three vantage points: (a) from that of estimating the prevalence of infertility and whether it is changing with time, (b) from that of the ever-changing medical capability of treating infertility, and (c) from the view of the changing attitude of society in general and the individuals thereof toward infertility. While these are intimately interrelated, a section will be devoted to each.

Estimates of the prevalence of infertility

Because of the many variables involved, prevalence, i.e. the number of cases occurring in a particular population at a point in time, is not easy to determine. For the USA, the most comprehensive estimates have come from face-to-face interviews of about 8000 women conducted by the National Center for Health Statistics of the US Department of Health and Human Services in 1965, 1976, and 1988.[1,2] The data are extensive and complex, but about 8.4% of women aged 15–44 years were found to have unresolved impaired ability to have children. The 8.4% figure was true for the surveys of 1965, 1976, and 1988. However, the actual number of women in the age category 15–44 is different for each of these years. For example, in 1965 it was 38.9 million, in 1976 it was 46.9 million, and in 1988 it was 58.7 million. Thus, the number of involuntarily infertile women was actually 3.3 million in 1965, 4.0 million in 1976, and 4.9 million in 1988. If the prevalence figure continues as experience suggests, the number of women aged 15–44 with uncured infertility in 1997, that is the latest year for which figures are available, should be about 5.1 million with primary infertility and with secondary infertility as defined by the study. The study defined infertility as individuals who had not had one term birth.[3]

Unfortunately, the prevalence study referred to did not give consideration to 'cured' cases of infertility. Furthermore, the definition of secondary infertility is problematic in that it required a full term delivery. There seems to have been no study of those individuals who had a pregnancy which did not carry to term and became infertile subsequent to that. Thus, the stated prevalence rates for both primary and secondary infertility seem likely to underestimate the actual original rate.

A British study addressed the infertility prevalence difficulties described above.[4] The authors of this study took advantage of the captive defined population of a general practice group in Oxford, UK. Such practice groups are thought to give a good approximation of the general population.

The authors recognized four types of subfertility as follows: unresolved primary subfertility, resolved primary subfertility, unresolved secondary subfertility, and resolved secondary subfertility. In the UK study, secondary subfertility seems to refer to failure to get pregnant after a previous conception, i.e. a term delivery did not seem to be required. The general practice arm of this fine study concluded that 20.5% of the population studied had had an episode of subfertility at some time. The details of the patient population are shown in *Table 1.1* and the prevalence figures for the various types of infertility are shown in *Table 1.2*.

It should be noted that the British study considered women between the ages of 25 and 44, while the American study used ages 15–44. This would seem to make the British figures higher by decreasing the number of patients in the numerator. On the other hand, of course, it eliminates infertility in patients < 25 years of age from the numerator.

On balance, it seems that the British figure is more apt to be reality for the study of the occurrence of

Table 1.1 General practice study.[4]

Category	Number of women
Total sample	872
Numerators	
(1) Unresolved primary subfertility	23
(2) Resolved primary subfertility	49
(3) Unresolved secondary subfertility	43
(4) Resolved secondary subfertility	55
(5) Any primary subfertility	72
(6) Any secondary subfertility	91
(7) Any episode of subfertility	138
Denominators	
(A) Having or attempting to have at least one child	674
(B) Having or attempting to have more than one child	561

It is, therefore, possible to conclude that in a cross-sectional population an infertility problem has affected about 20% of women up to the age of 44 years. The US study found about half this prevalence in the population, but did not consider resolved fertility problems. The two studies taken together suggest that about 50% of the infertility problems in a given population can be solved with informed attention.

In an ideal situation, therefore, in calculating medical needs to provide for infertility, it seems likely, according to the British study, that about 20 of 100 couples will at some time require medical help. Also, according to the US study, about half of the couples with a problem will have found a solution by means that do not reflect the contribution of assisted reproductive technology, as the surveys were made only when assisted reproductive technology was coming into vogue and was not widely used.

There are more footnotes to the above conclusion. The US study showed no change in prevalence over time and the authors of this study concluded that there was no 'epidemic' of infertility. However, tubal disease has surely increased with sexual promiscuity and the therapy of infertility has improved remarkably from the interval of 1965 when the first survey was done until 1988 when the last survey was done. If these statements are accurate, it must mean that the increase in incidence

infertility in a given population if for no other reason than that it includes resolved infertility. When it is realized that about one-half of the British prevalence figure of 20.5% is actually accounted for by resolved fertility problems, the discrepancy between the US and British studies tends to disappear.

Table 1.2 Subfertility rates.[4]

Category of subfertility	Prevalence rates* (general practice study)
Unresolved primary subfertility in those women having or attempting to have at least one child	3.4 (2.3,5.1)
Resolved primary subfertility in those women having or attempting to have at least one child	7.3 (5.5,9.5)
Unresolved secondary subfertility in those women having or attempting to have more than one child	7.7 (5.7,10.2)
Resolved secondary subfertility in those women having or attempting to have more than one child	9.8 (7.6,12.5)
Any episode of primary subfertility in those women having or attempting to have at least one child	10.7 (8.6,13.2)
Any episode of secondary subfertility in those women having or attempting to have more than one child	16.2 (13.4,19.5)
Any episode of subfertility in all women having or attempting to have at least one child	20.5 (17.6,23.7)

*95% confidence limits in parentheses.

Table 1.3 Number of women per 100 women who had not given birth during the specified age interval.[5]

Duration of interval	Number of intervals	% women without birth
< 12	14	1.2
12–17	198	16.9
18–23	442	37.7
24–29	285	24.3
30–35	108	9.2
36–41	49	4.2
42–47	32	2.7
48–59	28	2.4
⩾ 60	16	1.4
Total	1172	100.0

Average age of marriage = 20.7 years.

(that is the new cases entering the infertility population) has been balanced by the augmentation in therapy.

In addition, population studies are not age specific. The classic study of Tietze among the Hutterites[5] is still relevant. Maximum fertility occurred early and declined steadily thereafter (*Table 1.3*). Age is surely the greatest enemy of fertility as it cannot be overcome.

Finally, the cross-sectional studies are just that. There are numerous studies which show a very high infertility rate among the lower socioeconomic groups, probably owing to a high incidence of sexually transmitted disease affecting the tubes among this group. Therefore, the cross-sectional figure given above must be modulated according to the population group under consideration.

The medical capability of treating infertility

It is astonishing to realize that immediately after World War II, i.e. in the late 1940s, the standard work-up for infertility consisted of a history, a physical examination, a semen analysis, a post-coital test, a basal body temperature examination charted by the patient, a timed endometrial biopsy, a maturation index of the vaginal epithelium as an index to the hormonal status, a Rubin's test (i.e. the transmission of carbon dioxide through the fallopian tubes as a test for tubal patency), and an exploratory laparotomy on suspicion of a peritoneal factor.

Therapy was limited to the surgical treatment of anything found on exploratory laparotomy, but principally to endometriosis and adhesions, as the surgical therapy of tubal disease was very problematic. For example, Richard TeLinde, Chairman of the Department of Gynecology at Johns Hopkins, immediately after World War II, did not operate on diseased fallopian tubes himself, and recommended that younger members of the staff not waste their time operating on fallopian tubes because the results were so dismal. Cauterization of the cervix was used if there was a poor post-coital test on the theory that there was probably some disease in the cervix causing this. Donor insemination was available and used when there was a sperm count below 20 million in the male partner. Therapy for anovulation, which was established by the basal temperature chart and endometrial biopsy, was limited to radiation therapy to the pituitary or to the ovaries, or to both, and was widely used. Weight reduction for obesity and weight gain for asthenic individuals was advocated where this seemed to apply.

Hysterosalpingography, culdoscopy, laparoscopy, hysteroscopy, or any other '-oscopy' were not known and not used. Ultrasound was not yet invented. Urinary assays to be followed by serum assays for steroid and protein hormones were not yet available. The therapeutic availability of endocrine products was non-existent and surgical therapies for peritoneal difficulties were limited to those done by open laparotomy.

It would be superfluous to list here the diagnostic and therapeutic modalities now at the disposal of the specialist. The sweeping changes that have occurred are well illustrated by the requirement that an entire book be devoted to the imaging of the infertile couple.

The sweeping changes in diagnosis and therapy which have been seen in the last half of the 20th century, especially since the introduction of assisted reproductive technology, have been accompanied by a greater expectancy for relief on the part of the infertile couple. This in turn has encouraged more couples to seek help than was the case at mid-century.

Finally, there is certainly no reason to believe that the dynamic changes which have occurred in the latter half of the century will come to an end in the immediate future. We seem to be in the midst of an evolving process.

The attitude of society and the members thereof toward infertility

It seems that society has not accepted infertility, even now, as a legitimate health problem. One need not look further than the insurance industry to illustrate this particular point. In the competition by the insurance industry to offer low premium rates to other industries who buy bulk insurance, benefits are often cut. Infertility is among those areas that may not be covered. If infertility is covered in its diagnostic aspects and in some therapeutic aspects, it is very unusual for therapy by assisted reproductive technology to be included. However, some states, for example, Arkansas, California, Connecticut, Hawaii, Illinois, Maryland, Massachusetts, Montana, New York, Ohio, Rhode Island, and Texas, have passed legislation to mandate coverage of assisted reproductive technology, if the insurance company in that state offers health coverage for infertility. However, the details of the coverage are often patchy and inadequate, as the legislatures seldom specify the required detail (*Table 1.4*). Furthermore, insurance coverage in general for

Table 1.4 American Society for Reproductive Medicine: tabulation of state mandates as at October 1997.

State	Date enacted	Mandate to cover	Mandate to offer	Includes IVF coverage	Excludes IVF coverage	IVF coverage only
Arkansas	1987					X(1)
California	1989		X		X(2)	
Connecticut	1989		X	X		
Hawaii	1987	X				X(3)
Illinois	1991	X		X(4)		
Maryland	1985	X				X(5)
Massachusetts	1987	X		X		
Montana	1987	X(6)				
New York	1990				X(7)	
Ohio	1991	X(8)				
Rhode Island	1989	X		X		
Texas	1987		X			X

(1) Includes a lifetime maximum benefit of not less than 15 000.
(2) Excludes IVF, but covers gamete intrafallopian transfer (GIFT).
(3) Provides a one-time only benefit covering all outpatient expenses arising from IVF.
(4) Limits first-time attempts to four oocyte retrievals. If a child is born, two complete oocyte retrievals for a second birth are covered. Businesses with ≤ 25 employees are exempt from having to provide the coverage specified by the law.
(5) Businesses with ≤ 50 employees do not have to provide coverage specified by law.
(6) Applies to health maintenance organizations (HMOs) only; other insurers specifically are exempted from having to provide the coverage.
(7) Provides coverage for the 'diagnosis and treatment of correctable medical conditions'. Does not cover IVF as a corrective treatment.
(8) Applies to HMOs only.

infertility, and perhaps even other diseases, is apt to be bureaucratic. For example, tests may be required to be carried out at particular laboratories. Often when there are endocrine tests involved, the interpretation of these tests becomes very difficult. The insurance industry seems deaf and blind to studies which have shown that the treatment of infertility by assisted reproductive technology may well be less expensive than treatment by more traditional modalities which have very low success rates.[6,7]

It needs to be pointed out that some sections of society had had ambivalence about or actually have been opposed to the use of novel therapies for infertility. In the Catholic tradition, for example, the Vatican[8] has indicated that assisted reproductive technology is not licit and should not be used. While an example has been cited of the Roman Catholic tradition, there are other traditions that frown upon the use of certain technologies. For example, Islam does not allow in vitro fertilization if donor gametes, either of the male or female, are used. For that matter, Islam does not sanction the use of donor gametes, regardless of the method of fertilization.[9]

It needs to be noted that in many countries there are governmental regulatory agencies which control fertility practices. For example, in Great Britain the Human Fertilization and Embryology Authority (HEFA) issues licenses to programs wishing to practice assisted reproductive technology and specific licenses for various aspects of that, as for example, a special license is required if intracytoplasmic sperm injection (ICSI) is used. There have been numerous reports of studies by worldwide governmental and lay organizations about infertility and by 1987 at least 85 reports had been issued on this subject.[10] It is safe to say that no medical procedure has been subjected to such intense ethical and societal scrutiny as those with infertility, particularly those with assisted reproduction.

For many, indeed for most couples, infertility is a major life crisis. The emotional experience seems to pass through several phases, beginning with disbelief and denial, moving into anger and frustration, and only after a considerable period of time, to acceptance. These emotional problems are accompanied by a realization that monetary costs for treatment and support can be very high and this aspect of the problem is often greatly aggravated when it is found that insurance does not cover costs for this particular problem when the couple has had the expectation that their insurance would cover all health problems.

The care of the psychological and emotional aspects of infertility must be considered a responsibility of the treating physician. To be sure, help can be obtained in suitable cases by referral to those experienced in the psychological aspects of this problem. There is a large literature on the subject which has been well-summarized in a volume from a symposium on this subject held by the American Psychological Association.[11]

However, it needs to be emphasized that the physicians who see these couples—including the initial physician and any physician involved in consultative services—needs to communicate to the couple the fact that the physician is aware of their emotional crisis. This can be indicated by suitable questions and statements and help can be offered in meeting social situations that are embarrassing and stressful to the couple, such as inquiries about infertility from friends and particularly from relatives who do not understand, such as in-laws, siblings, parents, and the like. The physician may make available to the patient various books that have been produced for the general public or, as mentioned above, he may prefer to refer the couple to an experienced counselor for supplementary care.

Couples with infertility seem to be helped by two particular circumstances. One is the realization that there are other couples with the same problem. Thus, group therapy and ancillary groups, such as Resolve, can be useful in this regard. The second point that seems to be helpful is the provision of information to the couple. Again, there is an obligation for the physician to supply the fundamental and simple details to patients, but many books have been written for the infertile couple and many of these are kept up-to-date, are useful, and can be recommended by the physician. However, the complete physician should be able to understand and treat the emotional needs of most couples with infertility.

An overview

At mid-20th century, infertility was often a taboo subject. Infertility was commonly considered untreatable. The physician frequently had to convey the unwelcome news that no further treatment was available and that the only avenue to parenting was adoption, which was never easy and became more difficult as elective abortion became more widespread.

Times have changed. Extracorporeal mammalial fertilization, now known as in vitro fertilization, was first accomplished in 1958 by Chang in the rabbit[12] and 20 years later by Edwards et al in the human.[13] During the 1980s and 1990s, in vitro fertilization has revolutionized the treatment of infertility and has overcome all forms of infertility, except those associated with oocyte depletion and absence or severe deformity of the uterus. Even couples whose male partner has very serious sperm defects may be helped in certain cases. Regardless of all of this, provided that the couple without gametes is willing to accept donated gametes and the couple without a womb is willing to allow the use of a surrogate one, for the first time in history the physician is able to offer all couples some method of forming a family exclusive of adoption.

While much has been accomplished, it would be a mistake to say that nothing remains to be done, particularly with the goal of providing members of a nuclear family with the same genetic lineage. New information will be forthcoming in several areas. There is reason to believe that knowledge will be forthcoming on the physiology of the oocyte and an understanding of the factors which would allow their prolonged preservation. Very little is known about the causes of abnormal spermatogenesis; studies in this area would be useful. A strategy for coping with sexually transmitted disease in terms of both prevention and treatment would be a step forward. Furthermore, a wider acceptance of infertility by society in general as a legitimate health problem and the acceptance of the responsibility for infertility by the insurance industry are surely goals that must be accomplished in the near future. If all of this is done, the emotional health of the infertile will improve because of the possibility for the nuclear family to have an offspring of their own genetic lineage.

REFERENCES

1. US Congress, Office of Technology Assessment. *Infertility: Medical and Social Choices*, OTA-BA-358. Washington, DC: US Government Printing Office, May 1988.
2. Mosher WD. Reproductive impairments in the United States, 1965–1982. *Demography* 1988; **22**:415–430.
3. Statistical Abstract of the United States 116th edn. Washington, DC, 1996.
4. Greenhall E, Vessey M. The prevalence of subfertility: a review of the current confusion and a report of two new studies. *Fertil Steril* 1990; **54**:978–983.
5. Tietze C. Reproductive span and rate of reproduction among Hutterite women. *Fertil Steril* 1957; **8**:89.
6. Holst N, Maltau JM, Forsdahl F, Hansen LJ. Handling of tubal infertility after introduction of in vitro fertilization: changes and consequence. *Fertil Steril* 1991; **55**:140–143.
7. Van Voorhis BJ, Sparks AE, Allen BD *et al*. Cost-effectiveness of infertility treatments: a cohort study. *Fertil Steril* 1997; **67**: 830–831.
8. Instruction on respect for human life in its origin and on the dignity of procreation: replies to certain questions of the day. Congregation for the Doctrine of the Faith: Rome, 1987.
9. Serour GI. Traditional sexual practices in the Islamic world and their evolution. Benagiano G, Di Renzo GC, Cosmi EV, eds. *The Evolution of the Meaning of Sexual Intercourse in the Human*. Cortona: Editrice Grafica L'Etruria, 1996.
10. Walters L. Ethics and new reproductive technologies: an international review of committee statements. *Biomedical Ethics: A Multinational View*. Hastings Center Report, Special Supplement, June 1987.
11. Stanton AL, Dukel-Schetter C. *Infertility: Perspectives from Stress and Coping Research*. New York: Plenum Press, 1991.
12. Chang MC. The maturation of rabbit oocytes in the culture and their maturation, activation, fertilization, and subsequent development in the fallopian tube. *J Exp Zool* 1955; **128**:379–405.
13. Edwards RG, Steptoe PC, Purdy JM. Establishing full term human pregnancies using cleaving embryos grown in vitro. *Br J Obstet Gynaecol* 1980; **87**:737.

2 The many faces of the pelvis: normal physiology as seen with ultrasound

Steven R Goldstein

The introduction of the vaginal probe afforded a degree of structural detail of pelvic organs that has opened new doors in the application of ultrasound to the practice of gynecology and is specifically relevant for the infertile patient. The vaginal probe affords a degree of image magnification that is actually a form of 'sonomicroscopy'.

Before embarking on the use of ultrasound in infertile women a thorough understanding of the normal pelvis is essential. Vaginal ultrasound can provide more than just anatomic findings such as the size and location of pelvic structures. Correlation of ovarian cyclical changes and their expression on endometrial epithelium is the basis from which to start using ultrasound in such patients. This introduction will go through the normal phases of the menstrual cycle both in terms of ovarian anatomy and structure, uterine epithelial cyclical changes, endocervical mucous and cul-de-sac fluid, as well as some of the more common pathological entities that one encounters.

Hoeckelore et al.[1] first used ultrasound to detect the development of a follicle in the normal menstrual cycle. Many clinicians think that ultrasound in infertility is just for follicle measurements or perhaps as an adjunct for oocyte retrieval for in vitro fertilization (IVF). However, ultrasound is a window to normal physiologic changes seen cyclically in the female pelvis. The pelvis is a dynamic place. It undergoes a cyclical journey each month, sometimes culminating in a menses and sometimes culminating in a pregnancy. There should be synchrony between ovarian findings and their expression in the endometrium. With menses comes a sloughing of the endometrium down to a low basal superficial epithelium. Sonographically this appears as a thin, linear echogenicity (*Fig. 2.1*). The ovary has numerous small

sonolucencies which represent the recruitment of multiple follicles (*Fig. 2.2*). Under the influence of estrogen further proliferation of the endometrial epithelium takes place. Sonographically this is seen as a multilayered trilaminar appearance with a central linear echogenicity surrounded on each side by a sonolucent 'halo' culminating in an echogenic interface to the compact inner myometrium (*Fig. 2.3*). This is accompanied by the development of a dominant follicle some time after day 8–9. A single sonolucency will grow exponentially and culminate in rupture, i.e. ovulation, at around 20–25 mm at approximately day 14 in an idealized cycle (*Fig. 2.4*). Under the influence of progesterone that is secreted after ovulating, the endometrium converts to secretory type. In the first 24–48 hours this may produce a 'peppered' effect. Later in the luteal phase the endometrium becomes thick and echogenic (*Fig. 2.5*). At this stage in the cycle it should be possible to identify the corpus luteum within one of the ovaries (*Fig. 2.6*). It

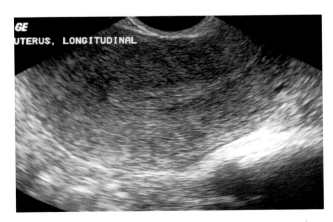

Figure 2.1 Long axis transvaginal ultrasonogram reveals a thin linear homogenous endometrial echo typical of the early proliferative phase of the cycle.

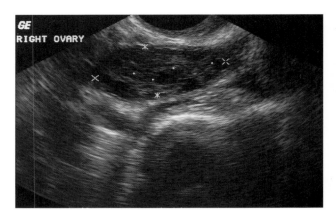

Figure 2.2 Transvaginal depiction of the right ovary of the patient whose endometrium is displayed in Fig. 2.1. Overall the ovary measures 2.5 × 3.3 cm. The small sonolucencies contained within it are follicles being recruited in the early proliferative phase.

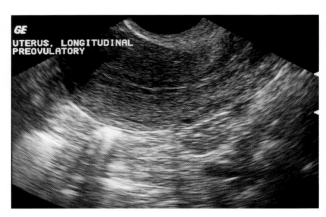

Figure 2.3 Transvaginal ultrasound of the uterus in long axis reveals a typical periovulatory multilayered endometrium. Notice the two sonolucent linear stripes on either side of the central midline echogenicity. These are then bounded by an echogenic outer layer, the vasalis layer.

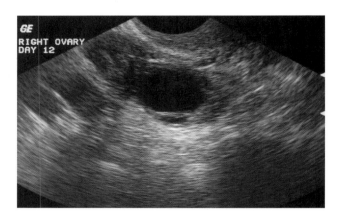

Figure 2.4 This is the right ovary on day 12 of the cycle, taken from the patient depicted in Fig. 2.3. Notice the central sonolucency corresponding to a dominant follicle. Of the numerous follicles recruited in the early proliferative phase only one becomes dominant, attaining a size of 20–25 mm prior to rupture (ovulation).

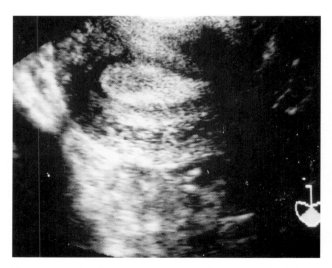

Figure 2.5 This long axis transvaginal ultrasound of the uterus depicts a typical thickened fiercely echogenic endometrial echo in the luteal (secretory) phase. Note the intact hypoechoic zone surrounding the endometrial echo corresponding to a normal junctional zone leading into the myometrium itself.

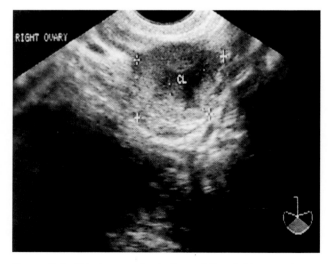

Figure 2.6 This transvaginal view of the right ovary is taken from the patient depicted in Fig. 2.5. The irregular, crenated, collapsed structure centrally located and labeled CL corresponds to the fresh corpus luteum.

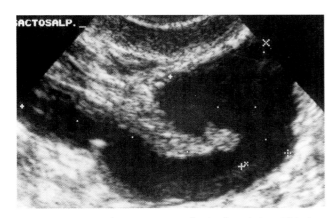

Figure 2.7 Typical appearance of a hydrosalpinx. This is a patient in whom previous pelvic infection has caused agglutination of the fimbriated end and collection of fluid. This should not be mistaken for a septum in an ovarian cyst. Notice that the echogenic solid portion does not reach the contralateral wall of the fallopian tube.

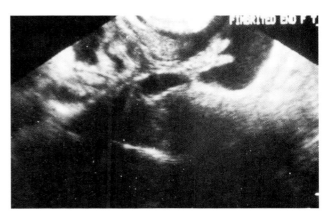

Figure 2.8 This transvaginal ultrasound depicts a normal appearing fallopian tube with the fimbriated end clearly identified and labeled. This is not normally seen in transvaginal scanning. The sonolucent backdrop here is the result of a ruptured follicle cyst the fluid background of which allows delineation of the fallopian tube floating.

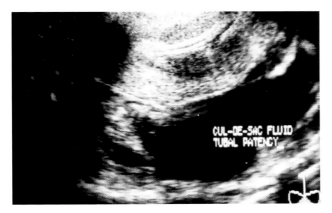

Figure 2.9 The sonolucent area posterior to the uterus represents cul-de-sac fluid present after the performance of a saline infusion sonohysterography. This proves tubal patency on at least one side.

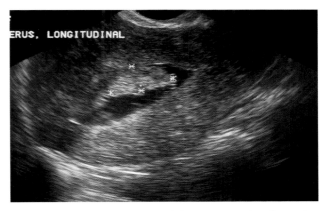

Figure 2.10 Long axis view of the uterus at the time of saline infusion sonohysterography. The structure outlined by the calipers represents an anterior wall mid-uterine segment polyp measuring 2.0 × 1.0 cm.

appears as a thick-walled, often crenated, irregular structure, sometimes containing internal echoes, corresponding to blood and debris.

In contrast to the pelvic findings in normal premenopausal women, other clinical entities may appear markedly different. For instance, the postmenopausal patient without estrogenic stimulation would be expected to have a very fine, thin, linear echogenicity with an intact hypoechoic zone surrounding it. Ovarian findings in such a patient should be devoid of any follicular development. Likewise, a patient on oral contraceptive pills has a fairly thin, low basilar inactive endometrium and may have multiple small follicles (< 10 mm) which are not undergoing development as a result of suppression by the contraceptive pill.

Ultrasound provides a way to see grossly abnormal fallopian tubes (*Fig. 2.7*) or sometimes normal fallopian tubes (*Fig. 2.8*) or even sometimes to diagnose tubal patency (*Fig. 2.9*).

Ultrasound provides a way to diagnose endometrial pathologies such as polyps (*Fig. 2.10*), as distinct from dysfunctional anovulatory changes (*Fig. 2.11*) or from submucous myomas (*Fig. 2.12*).

Ultrasound is an excellent method for differentiating endometriomas from hemorrhagic corpus lutea. Endometriomas have a diffuse uniform internal echo pattern when seen with the vaginal probe (*Fig. 2.13*). This is very different from their variable appearance on transabdominal ultrasound where they may appear sonolucent (*Fig. 2.14*). These should not be

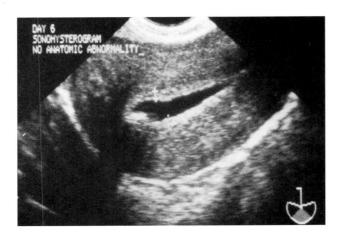

Figure 2.11 Long axis view of a patient with several months of irregular abnormal menstrual bleeding. Saline infusion sonohysterography done on day 6 of the current bleeding cycle reveals a normal appearing endometrial cavity displaying no anatomic abnormality. The sonolucent fluid has distended the anterior and posterior walls, which measure 1.9 × 2.0 cm, respectively. This ultrasound picture is compatible with dysfunctional uterine bleeding and no further diagnostic work-up is indicated.

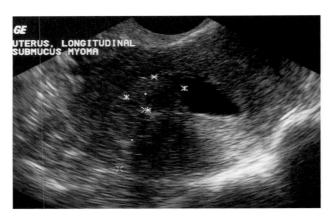

Figure 2.12 Saline infusion sonohysterography reveals this submucous myoma protruding into the endometrial cavity. Overall it measures 1.5 × 1.0 cm.

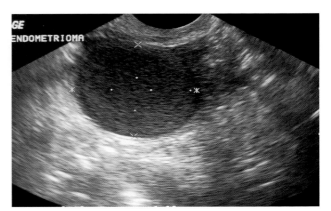

Figure 2.13 This 'solid appearing' cyst with very fine homogenous internal echoes is typical of the transvaginal ultrasound appearance of an endometrioma. This measures 3.2 × 2.8 cm.

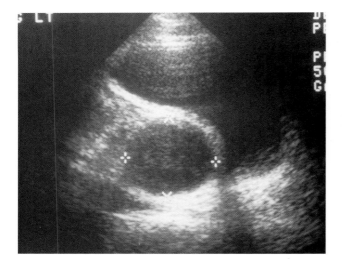

Figure 2.14 Transabdominal ultrasound view of a cystic mass measuring 4.5 × 5.0 cm. With transabdominal ultrasound, endometriomas often appear to be sonolucent and the fine 'ground glass' internal echoes as depicted in Fig. 2.13 are not appreciated.

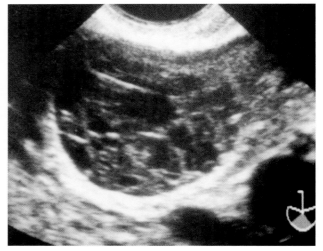

Figure 2.15 Transvaginal ultrasound depicts a typical appearance of a hemorrhagic corpus luteum. This cystic structure (as evidenced by increased through transmission to the posterior wall) has internal echoes. This cobweb-like appearance represents coagulation of blood; this should not be mistaken for the fine reticular pattern typical of an endometrioma seen in Fig. 2.13.

confused with a solid mass, for they will demonstrate posterior wall acoustic enhancement. Hemorrhagic corpus lutea are functional cysts, which represent bleeding into the site of ovulation. As the blood organizes, the sonographic appearance depends on when along the maturation process it is viewed. It begins as diffusely echogenic (although less uniform than endometriomas) (*Fig. 2.15*). Through a process of clot retraction it will develop a reticular cobweb-like pattern that can sometimes even mimic papillary projections.

In infertility, ultrasound is able to diagnose the success—an early intrauterine gestation (*Fig. 2.16*)— and then follow its normal progress until it is time to return that patient to the obstetrician (*Figs 2.17* and *2.18*), although sadly that is sometimes not the outcome (*Fig. 2.19*). Ultrasound is an excellent way to diagnose twins (*Fig. 2.20*), triplets (*Fig. 2.21*), and higher-order multiple gestations (*Fig. 2.22*).

In summary, the pelvis is a dynamic place undergoing constant cyclical change. The morphologic appearance of these physiologic changes serves as the basis for the recognition of normal as distinct from pathologic states. A thorough understanding of this area serves as the fundamental basis for the successful incorporation of ultrasound imaging in the diagnosis, management and, ultimately, successful treatment of the infertile couple.

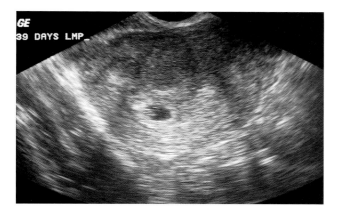

Figure 2.16 Transvaginal view of a patient at 39 days last menstrual period (LMP). This 4 mm gestational sac shows a typical echogenic rind (choriodecidual reaction) around a sonolucent center.

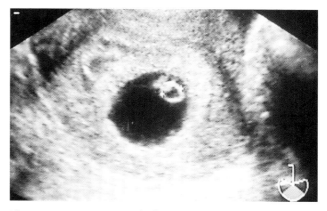

Figure 2.17 Transvaginal ultrasound of a patient with a gestational sac. A normal appearing yolk sac (calipers) measures 4.2 mm. The beginning of an embryonic pole can be seen as a thickening at the upper left-hand corner of the yolk sac.

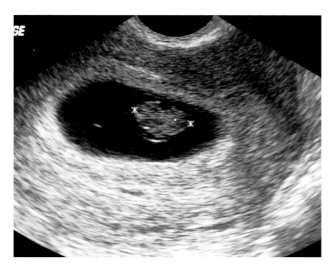

Figure 2.18 A 14 mm embryonic structure (calipers) in a typical C-shape seen in this transvaginal ultrasound of a patient with a pregnancy whose LMP was 56 days (8 weeks) prior.

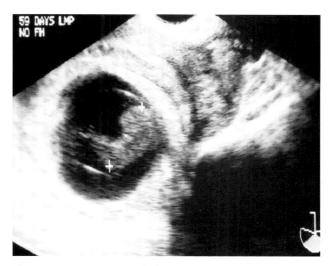

Figure 2.19 Transvaginal ultrasound of a failed intrauterine gestation. Patient was 59 days LMP and a 20 mm embryonic structure (calipers) is shown. No embryonic cardiac activity was discernible.

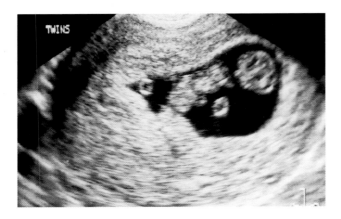

Figure 2.20 Transvaginal ultrasound view of a twin gestation. Twin A is clearly seen in the upper right-hand portion of the gestational sac. The yolk sac of twin A is seen slightly inferior and to the right of the embryo. A small portion of the second-twin gestational sac showing its yolk sac is seen in the left-hand portion of the uterine cavity. This depiction of both yolk sacs in the same scanning plane is typical of a twin gestation.

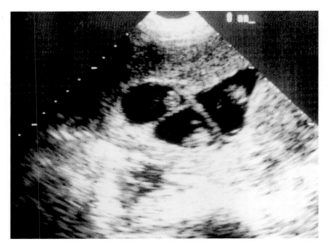

Figure 2.21 Transvaginal ultrasound of a triplet gestation in which three distinct gestational sacs in the same scanning plane are clearly visible.

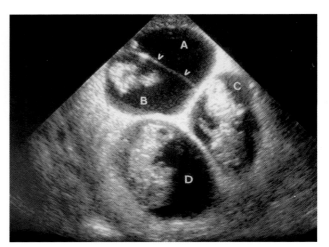

Figure 2.22 Transvaginal ultrasound of a quadruplet pregnancy. Each gestational sac is lettered A–D.

REFERENCE

1. Hoeckelore B, Fleming R, Robinson H *et al*. Correlation of ultrasonic and endocrinologic assessment of human follicular development. *Am J Obstet Gynecol* 1979; **135**:1.

FURTHER READING

Dimitry ES, Subak-Sharpe R, Mills M *et al*. Nine cases of heterotopic pregnancies in 4 years of in vitro fertilization. *Fertil Steril* 1990; **53**:107–110.

Fleischer AC, Pennell RG, McKee MS *et al*. Ectopic pregnancy: features at transvaginal sonography. *Radiology* 1990; **174**:375–378.

Goldstein SR. Incorporating endovaginal ultrasonography into the overall gynecologic examination. *Am J Obstet Gynecol* 1990; **162**:625–633.

Goldstein SR. *Endovaginal Ultrasound* 2nd edn. New York: Wiley Liss, 1991.

Goldstein SR, Timor-Tritsch IE. *Ultrasound in Gynecology*. New York: Churchill Livingstone, 1995.

Goldstein SR, Nachtigall M, Snyder JR *et al*. Endometrial assessment by vaginal ultrasonography before endometrial sampling in patients with postmenopausal bleeding. *Am J Obstet Gynecol* 1990; **163**:119–123.

Sassone A, Timor-Tritsch I, Artner A. Transvaginal sonographic characterization of ovarian disease: evaluation of new scoring system to predict ovarian malignancy. *Obstet Gynecol* 1991; **78**:70–76.

Stiller RJ, de Regt RH, Blair E. Transvaginal ultrasonography in patients at risk for ectopic pregnancy. *Am J Obstet Gynecol* 1989; **161**:930–933.

Timor-Tritsch IE. Is office use of vaginal sonography feasible? *Am J Obstet Gynecol* 1990; **162**:983–985.

3 Endometriosis

James M Shwayder

The incidence of endometriosis in the general population is unknown. In selected populations the range is 0.7–77%.[1–3] Patients undergoing laparoscopy for sterilization were found to have endometriosis in 1.6–45.3% of cases.[4] In an infertile population laparoscopy revealed endometriosis in 21–49%.[4–7] Recent analyses indicate improved pregnancy rates in patients treated surgically rather than medically for endometriosis, not only with moderate to severe disease, but even with minimal to mild disease.[8,9]

The appropriate care of the infertile patient depends on precise diagnosis and treatment of underlying conditions. With more couples seeking care for infertility, often at an older age, it is particularly important to identify those patients who may warrant early surgical intervention or alternative treatments such as in vitro fertilization (IVF). The goal of this chapter is to highlight the value of ultrasound in identifying those patients with endometriosis and in diagnosing endometriosis at various sites, and to compare ultrasound to other available imaging modalities. In addition, the application of ultrasound in the triage of patients to appropriate medical and/or surgical treatment will be addressed.

Sites of endometriosis

Jenkins et al reported on the location of endometriosis found at the time of laparoscopy in a group of infertile patients (Table 3.1).[10] The ovary was the most common site of involvement, with 54.9% of patients having either unilateral or bilateral involvement. In decreasing frequency, endometriosis was found in the posterior broad ligament, anterior cul-de-sac, posterior cul-de-sac, and the uterosacral ligament. Ultrasound has been shown to be effective in the diagnosis of endometriosis at these and other sites.

Pelvic locations

Ovary

The most easily recognized sonographic feature associated with endometriosis is an endometrioma. The presence of homogeneous low-level echoes in a cystic pelvic mass is a common finding in endometriomas, present in 82–93% of those confirmed by laparoscopy (Figs 3.1 and 3.2).[11,12] Using this finding alone, transvaginal sonography (TVS) has a sensitivity of 79–86%, with a specificity of 89–97.7% (Table 3.2).[12,13] This feature can be found dispersed throughout a lesion or may involve one or more sites in a multiloculated mass. Less frequently, septations (29% of patients) and fluid levels (5% of patients) are identified in endometriomas (Fig. 3.3).[14] The above sonographic characteristics are not pathognomonic for endometriomas;

Table 3.1 **Location of endometriosis in infertile patients at laparoscopy.**[10]

Location	% of patients
Ovary	54.9
Posterior broad ligament	35.2
Anterior cul-de-sac	34.6
Posterior cul-de-sac	34.0
Uterosacral ligament	28.0

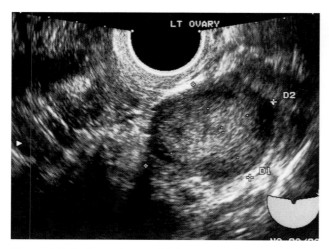

Figure 3.1 Endometrioma of left ovary with minimal cystic degeneration.

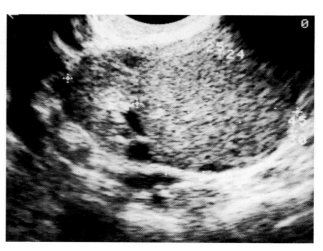

Figure 3.2 Endometrioma of right ovary with classic diffuse homogenous appearance.

Table 3.2 **Morphologic evaluation of endometriomas with transvaginal sonography.**

Year	Reference	Number of patients	Sensitivity (%)	Specificity (%)	PPV (%)	NPV (%)
1993	13	236	75.0	99.0	78.0	98.0
1995	12	50	82.4	97.7	94.0	92.3
1995	60	251	83.0	89.0	77.0	92.0
1995	15	943	86.5	99.1	91.5	98.1
Average			81.73	96.20	85.11	95.11

PPV, positive predictive value; NPV, negative predictive value.

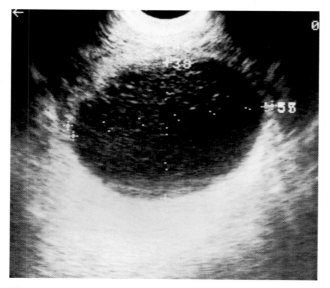

Figure 3.3 Endometrioma with fluid level and slight 'debris' within an endometrial cyst.

Table 3.3 **Differential diagnosis for endometriomas.**

- Hemorrhagic corpus luteum
- Tuberculous ovarian abscess
- Mature benign cystic teratoma (dermoid)
- Mucinous cystadenoma
- Granulosa cell carcinoma

differential diagnosis includes ovarian masses such as hemorrhagic corpus lutea (*Table 3.3*).[15,16] A hemorrhagic corpus luteum often has a complex, rather 'moth-eaten' appearance, as a result of hemorrhage within the cyst. In these cysts, clot formation is followed by retraction and dissolution, forming a characteristic cystic and solid component of clot and liquefied blood (*Fig. 3.4*). If a hemorrhagic mass is followed for 6–8 weeks, it will typically resolve, confirming the presence of a functional structure. Persistence of the mass suggests an endometrioma, which may warrant additional investigation.

In most studies, endometriomas are diagnosed by ultrasound when they are relatively large, with the average size at diagnosis being 53.4 mm (*Table 3.4*). The improved sensitivity of vaginal sonography allows earlier diagnosis, often at times when pelvic examination and laparoscopy are 'normal' (*Fig. 3.5a* and *b*). Preoperative evaluation with ultrasound allows diagnosis of smaller lesions and directs appropriate surgical management. Of note, in these studies the average age of diagnosis was over 30, an age when fertility potential begins to decline. This again highlights the importance of early diagnosis and treatment.

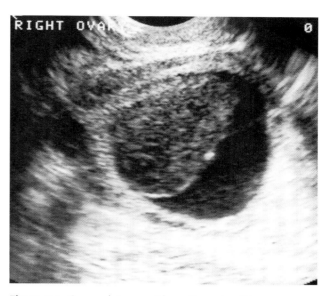

Figure 3.4 Corpus luteum with cystic and solid component, representing retraction and liquefaction of clot.

Table 3.4 **Characteristics at time of sonographic diagnosis of endometriomas.**

| Year | Reference | Size (mm) | | Patient's age (years) | | Bilateral |
		Range	Average	Range	Average	(%)
1993	16	10–100	61.0	15–45	31.3	7.8
1992	14	18–144	52.0			23.3
1995	12	15–130	5.5	18–55	31.0	13.5
1993	13	17–65	38.0			
1995	15	29–93	61.0	26–36	29.1	9.8

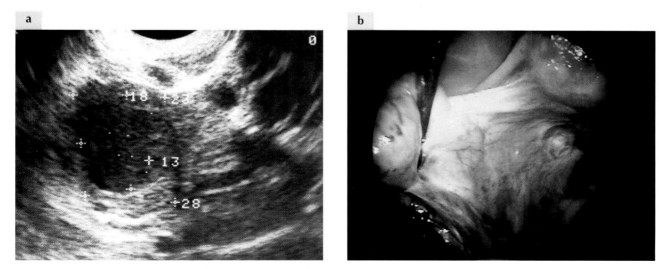

Figure 3.5 (a) Homogenous mass of left ovary detected in transvaginal sonography in infertility patient with normal pelvic examination. (b) Laparoscopy revealing a relatively normal appearance of the ovary. Subsequent excision confirmed the diagnosis of an endometrioma.

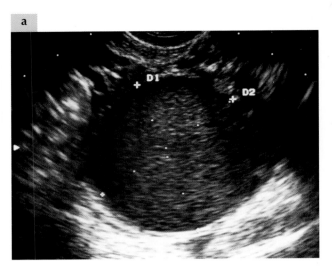

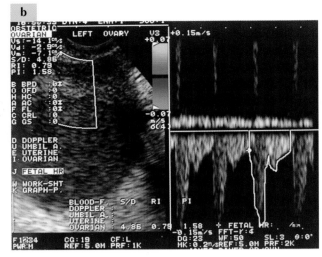

Figure 3.6 (a) Homogenous mass of left ovary consistent with diagnosis of an endometrioma. (b) Color Doppler analysis of hilar vessel. Spectral parameters consistent with a benign lesion with resistance index (RI) > 0.4 and pulsatility index (PI) >1.00.

Further assessment of possible endometriomas using color and pulsed Doppler sonography has been evaluated by several authors.[17,18] Kurjak and Kupesic[17] identified vessels supplying endometriomas in 88.3% of patients, the most prominent vascular area being at the level of the ovarian hilus (*Fig. 3.6a* and *b*). Vascular quality was assessed in terms of resistance index (RI = peak systolic − end-diastolic Doppler shift/peak systolic Doppler shift). The RI values of endometriomas were usually high, > 0.45, with only 5.83% found to have an RI < 0.40.

Low RIs (< 0.40) are associated with low resistance flow and neovascularization, which often accompanies malignant transformation. These authors developed a scoring system for the prediction of ovarian endometriosis based on morphologic assessment, Doppler findings, and CA-125 levels (*Table 3.5*). Based on this scoring system endometriomas were correctly identified in 102 patients undergoing surgical intervention for endometriomas, with two false positives being a cystic teratoma and a hemorrhagic cyst. Sensitivity, specificity, and negative and

Table 3.5 Evaluation of endometriomas by morphology, color Doppler, and CA-125.

Year	Reference	Number of patients	Criteria	Sensitivity (%)	Specificity (%)	PPV (%)	NPV (%)
1994	17	544	Morphology	83.9	97.1		
			CFD+CA-125	99.0	99.6	98.1	99.8
			CA-125 > 35	63.1	83.3	36.9	93.6
1997	18	78	Morphology	88.9	91.0	84.2	94.5
			CFD	76.2	88.9	82.4	82.4
			CA-125 > 35	79.3	84.6	79.3	84.6
Average			TVS	86.4	94.1	42.1	47.3
			CFD	87.6	94.3	90.3	91.1
			CA-125	71.2	83.9	58.1	89.1

TVS, transvaginal sonography; CFD, color flow Doppler.

positive predictive values of the combined scoring system were all high, above 98%.[17] In contrast, Alcazar et al, using similar parameters, found that color velocity imaging and pulsed Doppler did not improve on the accuracy of transvaginal sonography alone.[18] However, color velocity imaging and pulsed Doppler assessment are helpful in predicting those masses which are probably benign (RI > 0.40 or pulsatility index > 1.0) and may thus be observed over time for possible resolution. In addition, patients with benign Doppler parameters may be triaged to initial laparoscopic evaluation and treatment rather than immediate laparotomy.

Broad ligament

Diagnosis of endometriosis of the broad ligament is particularly challenging. Papadimitriou et al reported on the use of power Doppler as an alternative in diagnosis.[19] These authors used a 5 MHz transvaginal probe at a pulse repetition frequency of 800 Hz. All patients underwent laparoscopy after 10 days. Soft-tissue hyperemia, described as a diffuse 'blush' of virtually the entire symptomatic site, was seen on power Doppler in 22 symptomatic patients. Specificity was 52.4% and sensitivity 47.1% with a positive predictive value of 53.2%. This technique relies on the presence of implants with vascular activity (*Fig. 3.7*). Unfortunately, a large percentage of implants represent scarified areas, thus having no significant vascular activity;[20] power Doppler may be of less value in these patients. However, with over 40% of cases of endometriosis having penetration of >4 mm, it is postulated that transvaginal sonography may be useful in diagnosing these deeply infiltrating lesions[21] (*Figs 3.8* and *3.9*). In addition, the demon-

stration of 'point tenderness' with movement of the transducer has been noted with broad ligament implants.[22] The inability to demonstrate the 'sliding organ sign' is suggestive of adhesions, associated with more advanced endometriosis.[23]

Posterior cul-de-sac

Endometriosis infiltrating the rectovaginal septum and uterosacral ligaments typically elicits severe symptoms of dysmenorrhea, dyspareunia, or lateralizing pelvic pain.[24,25] Findings on pelvic examination consistent with endometriosis include nodularity on the uterosacral ligaments or in the rectovaginal septum, a retroflexed uterus, or an adnexal mass.

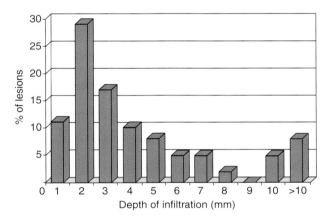

Figure 3.8 Depth of infiltration of endometriosis.[61]

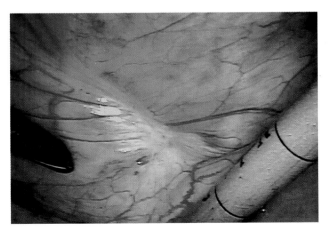

Figure 3.7 Peritoneal implant of endometriosis with vascular activity (red lesion) adjacent to scarified area. This lesion was not identified with standard vaginal sonography.

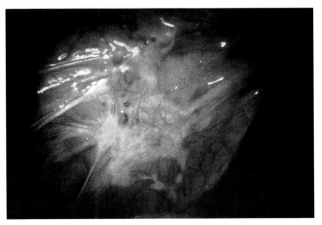

Figure 3.9 Peritoneal implant of endometriosis with red, brown and white (scarified) lesions. Patient had marked tenderness upon movement of the transducer against the left pelvic side wall.

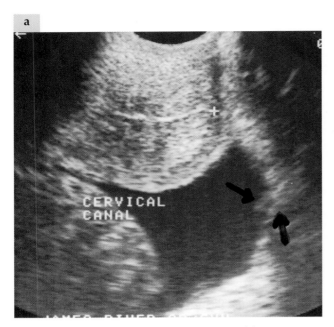
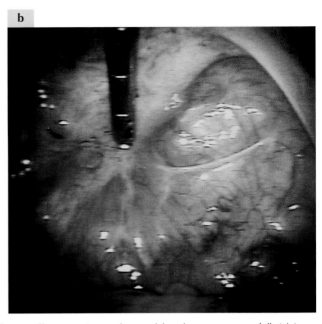

Figure 3.10 (a) Small nodule on uterosacral ligament. Note the small protrusion enhanced by the presence of fluid in the cul-de-sac. (b) Laparoscopy confirming a nodule of endometriosis. Excision revealed a nodule penetrating 3 mm into the uterosacral ligament.

Ohba et al reported on the use of transrectal sonography to diagnose endometriosis of the uterosacral ligaments.[26] Normal ligaments were characterized by low echoic homogeneous areas on both sides of the cervix. Those with nodules of endometriosis showed thick and irregularly shaped ligaments, some with small cystic lesions (*Fig. 3.10*). Their results suggest that the thickness of uterosacral ligaments was associated with the degree of involvement of endometriosis, with an average thickness of 11.2 ± 2.1 mm in non-affected patients, 12.8 ± 4.7 mm with superficial endometriosis, and 14.5 ± 3.5 mm with deep infiltrative endometriosis. In patients with ligaments > 14 mm thick, 94.1% were found to have tenderness on palpation of the uterosacral ligament on rectal examination. It is recognized that a normal fluctuation of peritoneal fluid occurs throughout the cycle.[27] The description of discriminatory volumes of fluid within the pelvis in patients with endometriosis has not been possible.[28,29] However, demonstrating free fluid in the pouch of Douglas may be helpful in determining those patients without significant involvement of the cul-de-sac with endometriosis or adhesions[30] (*Fig. 11a* and *b*).

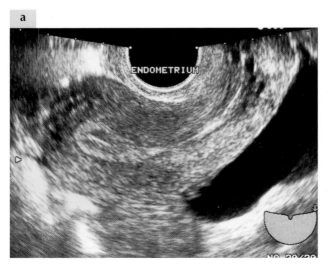
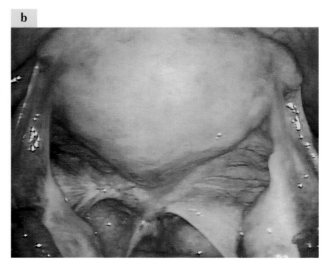

Figure 3.11 (a) Preoperative ultrasound in patient with infertility and pain. Fluid in posterior cul-de-sac. (b) Laparoscopy identifies implants of endometriosis on the uterosacral ligaments and peritoneum. Note the lack of significant adhesions or obliteration of the posterior cul-de-sac.

Mobility of the uterus, demonstrated by gentle advancing of the probe, also helps to rule out a retroflexed, fixed uterus.

Bianchi et al reported on the use of biplane ultrasonography in the assessment of 22 patients with pathologically confirmed rectovaginal endometriosis.[31] Identifying a homogenous mass, occasionally with cystic areas, correctly identified vaginal infiltration in 100% (22 of 22) of patients with vaginal infiltration of endometriosis. Infiltration into the rectal wall was found in 12 patients, and was correctly predicted by ultrasound in 83% of cases. The two cases (17%) that were not identified by ultrasound were found to have infiltration of < 5 mm. A case report by Hauge et al[32] describes a patient with cyclic perineal swelling, with confirmed endometriosis in the anal sphincter by transrectal sonography. Endosonography revealed a hypoechoic tumor within the external sphincter. Differentiation between the tumor and the hypoechoic internal sphincter was not possible. Initial suppressive medical therapy followed by surgical excision confirmed the finding of endometriosis. Thus, in several reports ultrasound has been useful in diagnosing endometriosis of the rectovaginal area, correctly predicting endometriosis in > 80% of patients. The performance of transrectal sonography may be quite useful in patients with significant pelvic and rectal pain.

Cervix

Cervicovaginal endometriosis may develop from spontaneous or iatrogenic endometrial dissemination, or local tissue metaplasia.[10] The reported involvement of the cervix ranges from 0.5% to 2.4% of women with endometriosis.[33] Nguyen et al reported on a patient with cervicovaginal endometriosis, presenting with menorrhagia, tenesmus, and dysuria.[34] Examination revealed a bulky cauliflower-like mass at the cervix, extending into the left vaginal apex. Transabdominal and transvaginal ultrasound demonstrated a complex multicystic mass at the cervix, measuring 4 cm in diameter. Magnetic resonance imaging showed multiple areas of high signal intensity of both T1- and T2-weighted images within an enlarged cervix. Definitive diagnosis was made with colposcopically directed biopsies.

Uterus–adenomyosis

Adenomyosis is considered a variant of endometriosis, with 'invasion' of the uterine wall by endometrial glands. Symptomatic patients complain of severe dysmenorrhea, dyspareunia, and menorrhagia. Physical findings include an enlarged uterus,

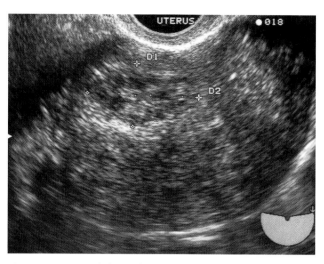

Figure 3.12 'Nodular' adenomyosis (adenomyoma) confirmed at the time of hysterectomy for abnormal uterine bleeding.

particularly during menses.[35,36] Descriptions of 'diffuse' and 'nodular' adenomyosis are found. The latter, often called adenomyomas, may be difficult to discern from intramural leiomyomas by ultrasound[37] (*Fig. 3.12*). Diffuse adenomyosis is characterized on transvaginal sonography by thickening and asymmetry of the anterior and posterior myometrial walls, heterogenous echogenicity of the myometrium, occasionally with indistinctly marginated areas (in the case of adenomyomas), and myometrial cysts.[38,39] Using these criteria, transvaginal sonography has a sensitivity of 80–86%, specificity of 74–96%, positive predictive value of 68–73%, and negative predictive value of 81–98%.[11,36,37,39] Hirai et al evaluated the use of transvaginal pulsed and color Doppler sonography in the evaluation of adenomyosis.[40] At a power of 210 mW/cm^2, spatial peak temporal average at 100% output, the wall filter set at 50–100 Hz, and a cut-off of RI = 0.43, the accuracy in diagnosis was 96%, with a sensitivity of 100% and a specificity of 83%.

Several authors have reported on the successful use of magnetic resonance imaging (MRI) in the diagnosis of adenomyosis.[36,38] The criteria for diagnosis with MRI include: (a) a myometrial mass with indistinct margins of primarily low signal intensity in all sequences (consistent with 'nodular' adenomyosis); and (b) diffuse or focal widening, > 0.5 cm, of the junctional zone on T2-weighted images and contrast-material-enhanced T1-weighted images. Ascher et al found MRI significantly ($P < 0.02$) better than transvaginal sonography.[38] Although the number of patients was small (17 with adenomyosis) MRI was accurate in 88% of patients (15 of 17) while TVS identified only 53% correctly (9/17).

Extrapelvic locations

Urinary tract

Endometriosis affects the urinary tract in 1–4% of patients with pelvic endometriosis.[41] The bladder is the most common site, accounting for 80–90% of cases of urinary tract involvement, while ureteral and renal lesions are quite rare.[42] Symptoms found in up to 80% of patients with bladder involvement include dysuria, urinary frequency, suprapubic pressure, and back pain. Ureteral lesions, occurring in 11–15% of patients with urinary tract disease, are found most commonly in the distal third of the ureter, below the pelvic brim, and more commonly on the left ureter than the right.[43] Symptoms associated with ureteral involvement include flank pain, dysuria, and urgency.

Whitman and McGovern reported the first case of vesical endometriosis detected by ultrasonography, which had eluded detection by urography and cystoscopy.[44] Sonography identified a 1.9 cm triangular plaque-like lesion of the posteroinferior bladder wall, which was confirmed on exploratory laparotomy to correspond to endometriosis. Filling the bladder enhanced the transabdominal visualization of this lesion, which was also seen on TVS.

Brough and O'Flynn reported on a patient who had previously undergone a total abdominal hysterectomy and bilateral salpingo-oophorectomy who developed recurrent pelvic endometriosis leading to bilateral ureteric obstruction, presumably secondary to estrogen replacement therapy.[45] An intravenous urogram and renogram demonstrated a completely obstructed right kidney and a partially obstructed left kidney. The initial lesion, detected by pelvic ultrasound and computed tomography, was a 9 cm homogenous mass anterior to the rectum, which proved to be endometriosis on cystoscopically directed biopsy. The patient was treated by withdrawal of her estrogen therapy and the introduction of a gonadotropin-releasing hormone agonist. Decrease in the size of the mass was documented with computed tomography, with subsequent return of renal function.

Gastrointestinal endometriosis

Intestinal involvement is found in 5–15% of patients with endometriosis-related pelvic pain or infertility.[46] Gastrointestinal (GI) endometriosis is usually asymptomatic, thus making detection difficult. Involvement of the appendix has been documented in 5–20% of patients with chronic pelvic pain.[47] Imaging studies have been somewhat disappointing in their ability to diagnose endometriosis of the gastrointestinal tract. Barium enema may demonstrate extrinsic bowel compression, an abdominal mass, or stenosis of the bowel. Ultrasound has not been useful in the diagnosis of GI endometriosis, with a reported sensitivity of < 11%.[48] Computed tomography has similar limitations. Magnetic resonance imaging has been proposed as the superior imaging technique for diagnosis.[49] However, data regarding its effectiveness in diagnosing and monitoring gastrointestinal endometriosis are still lacking.

Symptoms

Patients with endometriosis may present with a variety of symptoms or may be asymptomatic[4] (*Table 3.6*). In the symptomatic patient the prevalence of each symptom varies with the stage of the disease[24] (*Table 3.7*). Although ultrasound is quite useful in the evaluation of patients with pelvic masses, a significant challenge is encountered in diagnosing endometriosis without significant uterine or adnexal disease.

Table 3.6 **Endometriosis staging in asymptomatic women.**						
Reference	Number	% of patients				
		I	II	III	IV	
1	85	32.5	9.3	1.1	2.3	
4	115	91.3	4.8	4.0	0.0	

Patients undergoing laparoscopy for chronic pelvic pain were found to have endometriosis in 12–47% of cases.[4] Melis et al found endometriosis in 43% of patients presenting with pain, characterized by dysmenorrhea, dyspareunia, or lateralizing pelvic pain.[24] This author's experience is similar, with endometriosis in 47% of symptomatic patients[7] (*Table 3.8*).

Infertility

The mechanism of infertility in patients with endometriosis is the development of significant adhesional or tubal disease. Several associated factors are implicated when less severe disease is

Table 3.7 Symptoms related to stage of endometriosis.[24]

Symptom	n	Stage I	II	III	IV
Infertility	18	55.6%	11.1%	22.2%	11.1%
Pelvic pain	18	50.0%	16.7%	16.7%	16.7%
Benign ovarian cysts	28	17.9%	0.0%	46.4%	35.7%
Uterine fibroids	12	33.3%	25.0%	33.3%	8.4%

Table 3.8 Laparoscopic findings in 188 patients presenting with pelvic pain.[7]

Findings	n	% with finding
Endometriosis	88	46.8
Adhesions	87	46.3
Fibroids	2	13.3
Ovarian cyst	1	7.9
Ectopic pregnancy	8	4.3
Uterine septum	7	3.7
Hydrosalpinx	6	3.2
Endo Polyp/Fibroid	5	2.6
Polycystic ovaries	2	1.1
Corpus luteum	2	1.1
Synechiae	1	0.5
Salpingitis/Tubo-ovarian abscess	1	0.5
Dermoid	1	0.5
Ovarian cancer	1	0.5

Table 3.9 Possible causes of endometriosis-related infertility.[50]

- Adhesional disease
- Hormonal factors
- Immunologic factors
- Ovulatory dysfunction
- Luteal phase defects
- Impaired tubal transport
- Disturbed implantation
- Spontaneous abortion

Table 3.10 Criteria to establish diagnosis of luteinized unruptured follicle.[51,52]

1. Rise in basal body temperature
2. Sonographic findings after administration of human chorionic gonadotropin (hCG)
   - Persistent and enlarged follicles
   - Lack of collapse of large follicle
   - Lack of free fluid in pouch of Douglas
   - A degenerated oocyte mass in the context of persistent follicles
3. Serum progesterone > 5 ng/ml in the midluteal phase

present[50] (*Table 3.9*). These include luteinized unruptured follicle syndrome (LUFS), luteal phase defect (LPD), and increased prostanoid concentrations in peritoneal fluid. Ultrasound is useful in the diagnosis of ovulatory dysfunction and LUFS. Mio evaluated 70 patients with unexplained infertility, of whom 47 (67%) were found to have endometriosis at laparoscopy, 85% with mild to moderate disease.[51] The diagnosis of luteinized unruptured follicle was established by a constellation of specific findings (*Table 3.10*). He found that the incidence of luteinized unruptured follicle was higher ($P < 0.05$) in patients with endometriosis (35% per patient, 25% per cycle) than in those who did not have endometriosis (11% per patient, 7% per cycle). Brosens et al described LUFS in 79% of patients with endometriosis, versus only 6% of control patients.[52] Although the existence of this syndrome has been challenged and its association with endometriosis is unclear, a finding of LUFS may lead to earlier performance of laparoscopy for diagnosis and treatment of possible endometriosis.

Luteal phase defect (LPD) is a relatively uncommon cause of primary infertility, being found in < 5% of infertile patients. There appears to be a higher incidence of LPD in patients with endometriosis than in those without it.[53] Ultrasound is useful in diagnosing LPD by demonstrating a discrepancy between endometrial thickness and ovarian morphology in the luteal phase. The endometrial thickness is influenced by the inadequate progesterone levels found in patients with LPD rather than a lack of preovulatory endometrial response in patients with endometriosis.[54]

Increased prostanoid concentrations in cul-de-sac fluid, in concert with an increased volume of fluid, has been postulated as a cause for endometriosis-mediated infertility. However, as noted earlier, discriminatory amounts of fluid in patients with endometriosis have not been identified. The primary benefit of identifying fluid in the pouch of Douglas is to exclude an obliterated cul-de-sac.

Familial inheritance

A familial incidence of endometriosis has been demonstrated, which appears to be polygenic/multi-factorial in inheritance. A female patient who has an affected first-degree relative has an approximately 10-fold increased risk of developing the disease.[55] Another possible congenital mechanism includes patients with Mullerian anomalies.[3] When outflow obstruction is present the incidence of endometriosis increases from 37% to 77%.[4] These abnormalities can be visualized easily by transvaginal sonography.[56]

Sonographic findings correlated with pelvic examination

Nezhat et al compared transvaginal sonography and bimanual examination in patients with endometriosis and pain. Laparoscopic evaluation revealed ovarian endometriosis in 48% of patients, pelvic endometrial implants with adhesions in 41% of patients, and involvement of both ovaries and uterus in 11% of patients. In all, 53% of women had abnormal pelvic examinations, based on the findings of pain, nodularity, enlarged adnexa, abnormal uterine configuration, fixation of the uterus, or a mass in the rectal vaginal septum. Ultrasound findings were unremarkable in 41% of patients. However, with involvement of the ovaries and uterus, 89% had abnormal ultrasonographic evaluation compared with 11% with peritoneal implants only.[57] The concordance between examination and ultrasound was 65%. The advantage of pelvic examination is that it offers an enhanced subjective assessment of a patient's discomfort. However, vaginal sonography, being a dynamic study, is quite useful in detecting pelvic adhesions, a common component of more advanced endometriosis, i.e. Stages III and IV. Adhesions are suspected with decreased mobility of the ovary, the lack of the so-called 'sliding organ sign,' particularly when associated with the production of pain[23,58] (*Fig. 3.13a* and *b*). In the author's experience this finding was confirmed at laparoscopy in 74% of patients[7] (*Table 3.11*).

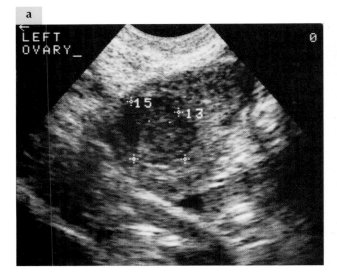
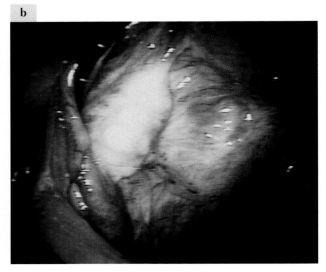

Figure 3.13 (a) Infertility patient, with complaints of dyspareunia, with the finding of a small endometrioma of the left ovary. With movement of the transducer the ovary had decreased mobility associated with reproduction of pain experienced with coitus. (b) Laparoscopy confirmed the presence of adhesions of the left ovary to the left posterior broad ligament. Excision of the mass confirmed the presence of an endometrioma.

Table 3.11	**Transvaginal sonography (TVS) versus pelvic examination in the diagnosis of endometriosis and pelvic adhesions.**[7]

Finding	Number of patients	% confirmed at laparoscopy	
		TVS	Exam
Endometriosis	140	43	23
Adhesions	125	74	22

Conclusion

The age of patients seeking treatment of infertility continues to rise. As a result, this patient population has a relatively high incidence of endometriosis. Early diagnosis of endometriosis in these patients is paramount to the success of treatment. The use of transvaginal sonography, augmented with abdominal ultrasound examination when necessary, is particularly valuable in their initial triage. Utilizing preoperative sonography allows the surgeon to anticipate the intraoperative findings, thus allowing appropriate patient counseling, planning of surgery, and realistic expectations regarding the outcome of surgical intervention.

REFERENCES

1. Rawson JMR. Prevalence of endometriosis in asymptomatic women. *J Reprod Med* 1991;**36**:513–515.
2. Wheeler JM. Epidemiology of endometriosis-associated infertility. *J Reprod Med* 1989;**34**:41–46.
3. Olive DL, Henderson DY. Endometriosis and Mullerian anomalies. *Obstet Gynecol* 1987;**69**:412–415.
4. Sangi-Haghpeykar H, Poindexter AN. Epidemiology of endometriosis among parous women. *Obstet Gynecol* 1995;**85**:983–992.
5. Damario MA, Rock JA. Exploring causes of infertility associated with endometriosis. *Contemp Obstet Gynecol* 1993;**38** Fertility Supplement:38–48.
6. el-Yahia AW. Laparoscopic evaluation of apparently normal infertile women. *Aust N Z J Obstet Gynaecol* 1994;**34**:440–442.
7. Shwayder JM, Burcher D. Use of transvaginal sonography prior to operative endoscopy. *J Am Assoc Gynecol Laparosc* 1994;**1**:S31.
8. Adamson GD, Pasta DJ. Surgical treatment of endometriosis-associated infertility: meta-analysis compared with survival analysis. *Am J Obstet Gynecol* 1994;**171**:1488–1505.
9. Marcoux S, Maheux R, Berube S. Laparoscopic surgery in infertile women with minimal or mild endometriosis. Canadian Collaborative Group on Endometriosis. *N Engl J Med* 1997;**337**:217–222.
10. Jenkins S, Olive DL, Haney AF. Endometriosis: pathogenic implication of the anatomic distribution. *Obstet Gynecol* 1986;**37**:335–338.
11. Atzori E, Tronci C, Sionis L. Transvaginal ultrasound in the diagnosis of diffuse adenomyosis. *Gynecol Obstet Invest* 1996;**42**:39–41.
12. Volpi E, DeGrandis T, Zuccaro G, LaVista A, Sismondi P. Role of transvaginal sonography in the detection of endometriomata. *J Clin Ultrasound* 1995;**23**:163–167.
13. Mais V, Guerriero S, Ajossa S, Angiolucci M, Paoletti AM, Melis GB. The efficiency of transvaginal ultrasonography in the diagnosis of endometrioma. *Fertil Steril* 1993;**60**:776–780.
14. Kupfer MC, Schwimer SR, Lebovic J. Transvaginal sonographic appearance of endometriomata: spectrum of findings. *J Ultrasound Med* 1992;**11**:129–133.
15. Dogan MM, Ugur M, Soysal SK, Soysal ME, Ekici E, Gokmen O. Transvaginal sonographic diagnosis of ovarian endometrioma. *Int J Gynecol Obstet* 1996;**52**:145–149.
16. Fried AM, Rhodes RA, Morehouse IR. Endometrioma: analysis and sonographic classification of 51 documented cases. *Southern Med J* 1993;**86**:297–301.
17. Kurjak A, Kupesic S. Scoring system for prediction of ovarian endometriosis based on transvaginal color and pulsed Doppler sonography. *Fertil Steril* 1994;**62**:81–87.
18. Alcazar JL, Laparte C, Jurado M, Lopez-Garcia G. The role of transvaginal ultrasonography combined with color velocity imaging and pulsed Doppler in the diagnosis of endometrioma. *Fertil Steril* 1997;**67**:487–491.
19. Papadimitriou A, Kalogirou D, Antoniou G, Petridis N, Kalogirou O, Kalovidouris A. Power Doppler ultrasound: a potentially useful alternative in diagnosing pelvic pathologic conditions. *Clin Exp Obstet Gynecol* 1996;**23**:229–232.
20. Martin DC, Hubert GD, VanderZwaag R, El-Zeky FA. Laparoscopic appearances of peritoneal endometriosis. *Fertil Steril* 1989;**51**:63–67.
21. Koninckx PR, Oosterlynck D, D'Hooghe T, Meuleman C. Deeply infiltrating endometriosis is a disease whereas mild endometriosis could be considered a non-disease. *Ann NY Acad Sci* 1994;**734**:333–341.
22. Parsons A. Personal communication, 1996.
23. Timor-Tritsch IE, Bar-Yam Y, Elgali S, Rottem S. The technique of transvaginal sonography with the use of a 6.5 MHz probe. *Am J Obstet Gynecol* 1988;**158**:1019–1024.
24. Melis GB, Ajossa S, Guerriero S et al. Epidemiology and diagnosis of endometriosis. *Annal NY Acad Sciences* 1993;**734**:352–357.
25. Ramzy I. Endometriosis: contemporary concepts in clinical management. In: Schenken RS, ed. *Endometriosis, Contemporary Concepts in Clinical Management.* Philadelphia: J.B. Lippincott Co., 1985.

26. Ohba T, Mizatani H, Maeda T, Matsuura K, Okamura H. Evaluation of endometriosis in uterosacral ligaments by transrectal ultrasonography. *Human Reprod* 1996;**11**:2014–2017.

27. Schellpfeffer MA. Sonographic detection of free pelvic peritoneal fluid. *J Ultrasound Med* 1995;**14**:205–209.

28. Rock JA, Dubin NH, Ghodgaonkar RB, Berquist CA, Erozan YS, Jr. AWK. Cul-de-sac fluid in women with endometriosis: fluid volume, protein and prostanoid concentration during the proliferative phase - days 8 to 12. *Fertil Steril* 1982;**37**:747–750.

29. Rezai N, Ghodgaonkar RB, Zacur HA, Rock JA, Dubin NH. Cul-de-sac fluid in women with endometriosis: fluid volume, protein and prostanoid concentration during the periovulatory period - days 13 to 18. *Fertil Steril* 1987;**48**:29–32.

30. Yano K, Suginami H, Matsuura S. Ultrasonographic diagnosis of cul-de-sac endometriosis. *Nippon Sanka Fujinka Gakkai Zasshi* 1987;**39**:2011–2016.

31. Bianchi S, Fedele L, Portuese A, Borruto F, Dorta M. Transrectal ultrasonography in the assessment of rectovaginal endometriosis. ASRM annual meeting. San Antonio, TX, 1996.

32. Hauge C, Nielsen MB, Rasmussen OO, Christieansen J. Clinical findings and endosonographic appearance of endometriosis in the anal sphincter. *J Clin Ultrasound* 1993;**21**:48–51.

33. Veiga-Ferreira MM, Leiman G, Dunber F et al. Cervical endometriosis: Facilitated diagnosis by fine needle aspiration cytologic testing. *Am J Obstet Gynecol* 1987;**157**:849–856.

34. Nguyen BD, Georges NP, Hamper UM, Zerhouni EA. Primary cervicovaginal endometriosis: sonographic findings with MR imaging correlation. *J Ultrasound Med* 1994;**13**:809–811.

35. Fedele L, Bianchi S, Dorta M, Arcaini L, Zanotti F, Carinelli S. Transvaginal ultrasonography in the diagnosis of diffuse adenomyosis. *Fertil Steril* 1992;**58**:94–97.

36. Reinhold C, McCarthy S, Bret P et al. Diffuse adenomyosis: comparison of endovaginal US and MR imaging with histopathologic correlation. *Radiology* 1996;**199**:151–158.

37. Fedele L, Bianchi S, Dorta M, Zanotti F, Brioschi D, Carinelli S. Transvaginal ultrasonography in the differential diagnosis of adenomyoma versus leiomyoma. *Am J Obstet Gynecol* 1992;**167**:603–606.

38. Ascher S, Arnold L, Patt R et al. Adenomyosis: prospective comparison of MR imaging and transvaginal sonography. *Radiology* 1994;**190**:803–806.

39. Reinhold C, Atri M, Mehio A, Zakarian R, Aldis A, Bret P. Diffuse uterine adenomyosis: morphologic criteria and diagnostic accuracy of endovaginal sonography. *Radiology* 1995;**197**:609–614.

40. Hirai M, Shibata K, Sagai H, Sekiya S, Goldberg BB. Transvaginal pulsed and color Doppler sonography for the evaluation of adenomyosis. *J Ultrasound Med* 1995;**14**:529–532.

41. Jubanyik KJ, Comite F. Endometriosis: extrapelvic endometriosis. *Obstetrics and Gynecology Clinics* 1997;**24**:411–440.

42. Abeshouse BS, Abeshouse G. Endometriosis of the urinary tract: a review of the literature and a report of four cases of vesicle endometriosis. *J Int Coll Surg* 1960;**37**:43.

43. Markham SM, Carpenter SE, Rock JA. Extrapelvic endometriosis. *Obstet Gynecol Clin North Am* 1989;**16**:193–219.

44. Whitman GJ, McGovern FJ. Endometriosis of the bladder detected by pelvic ultrasonography. *J Ultrasound Med* 1994;**13**:155–157.

45. Brough R, O'Flynn K. Recurrent pelvic endometriosis and bilateral ureteric obstruction associated with hormone replacement therapy. *Br Med J* 1996;**312**:1221–1222.

46. Weed JC, Ray JE. Endometriosis of the bowel. *Obstet Gynecol* 1987;**69**:727–730.

47. Howard F. Laparoscopic evaluation and treatment of women with chronic pelvic pain. *J Am Assoc Gynecol Laparosc* 1994;**1**:325–323.

48. Friedman H, Vogelzang RL, Mednelsohn EB et al. Endometriosis detection by ultrasound with laparoscopic correlation. *Radiology* 1985;**157**:217–220.

49. Olive DL, Schwartz LB. Endometriosis. *New Eng J Med* 1993;**328**:1759–1769.

50. Olive DL, Haney AF. Endometriosis-associated infertility. Critical review of therapeutic approaches. *Obstet Gynecol Survey* 1986;**41**:538–555.

51. Mio Y, Toda T, Harada T, Terakawa N. Luteinized unruptured follicle in the early stages of endometriosis as a cause of unexplained infertility. *Am J Obstet Gynecol* 1992;**167**:271–273.

52. Brosens IA, Koninckx PR, Corveleyn PA. A study of plasma progesterone, oestradiol-17, prolactin, and LH levels, and of the luteal-phase appearance of the ovaries in patients with endometriosis and infertility. *Br J Obstet Gynaecol* 1978;**85**:246–250.

53. Pittaway D, Maxson W, Daniell J, Herbert C, Wentz A. Luteal phase defects in infertility patients with endometriosis. *Fertil Steril* 1983;**39**:712–713.

54. Check JH, Dietterich C, Lurie D, Adelson HG, O'Shaughnessy A. Relationship of endometrial thickness and sonographic echo pattern to endometriosis in non-in vitro fertilization cycles. *Gynecol Obstet Invest* 1995;**40**:113–116.

55. Cramer DW. Epidemiology of endometriosis. In: Wilson EA, ed. *Endometriosis* vol 5. New York: Alan R. Liss, Inc, 1987.

56. Timor-Tritsch IE, Rottem S, Boldes R. Scanning the uterus. In: Timor-Tritsch IE, Rottem S, eds. *Transvaginal sonography*. New York: Elsevier, 1988.

57. Nezhat C, Santolaya J, Nezhat FR, Nezhat C. Comparison of transvaginal sonography and bimanual pelvic examination in patients with laparoscopically confirmed endometriosis. *J Amer Assoc Gynecol Laparosc* 1994;**1**:127–130.

58. Timor-Tritsch I, Rottem S. *Transvaginal Sonography*. New York: Elsevier, 1991.

59. Timor-Tritsch IE. Transvaginal sonography in gynecologic office practice. *Curr Opin Obstet Gynecol* 1992;**4**:914–920.

60. Guerriero S, Mais V, Ajossa S et al. The role of endovaginal ultrasound in differentiating endometriomas from other ovarian cysts. *Clin Exp Obstet Gynecol* 1995;**22**:20–22.

61. Martin DC, Hubert GD, Levy BS. Depth of infiltration of endometriosis. *J Gynecol Surg* 1989;**5**:55–60.

4 Inflammatory diseases of the female pelvis

Ilan E Timor-Tritsch and Ana Monteagudo

Introduction

Inflammatory diseases of the female pelvis, more specifically those of the fallopian tubes and/or the ovaries, are common. According to Westrom,[1] in the late 1970s the annual incidence of inflammatory tubal disease was 1% of women of reproductive age. McCormac[2] reported that about one million American women develop inflammatory disease of the pelvis each year. About 25–35% of females with tubal damage following acute salpingitis were thought to become infertile[2,3] and it was estimated that about 13% of women might become infertile after only one attack of acute salpingitis.[4]

It has also been estimated that about 10–15% of all women in the reproductive years suffer at least one bout of inflammatory tubal disease. Furthermore, about 50% of ectopic pregnancies can be attributed to a previous episode of such a pelvic inflammatory process.[5,6]

Even more importantly—as will be alluded to later on in this chapter—a rather significant number of women with infertility suspected to be caused by one of the major agents never had clinical symptoms.[2] This explains the fact that at times sonography detects markers of chronic tubal disease without any clear recall by the patient of suffering from what would be attributed to a previous inflammatory disease. One report stated that patients treated by microsurgery for tubal occlusion had overt salpingitis with flattened mucosal folds and the tubes were devoid of epithelial cilia regardless of whether the patient had overt clinical signs and symptoms of salpingitis or whether they had a silent history.[7]

The need for a thorough sonographic investigation of the adnexa, but more specifically of an affected fallopian tube, became quite evident after the widespread use of assisted reproductive technolo-gies. It seems that an existing hydrosalpinx interacts negatively with the pregnancy and implantation rate after in vitro fertilization (IVF) with embryo transfer (ET).[8–10] Other articles claim that the aspiration of hydrosalpinges increases the success rate of pregnancies in those patients.[11] At times, the induction of ovulation, which in a parallel fashion may increase the secretions in the tube, leads to the formation of hydrosalpinx.[12] The need for a proper evaluation of the adnexa was stressed in reports claiming that in a small number of patients, after oocyte retrieval, the development of severe inflammatory reaction of the tube and the ovary (tubo-ovarian abscess) occurs.[13–17]

Finally, ultrasound was found to provide an effective method of draining abscesses as well as loculated inclusion cysts created postoperatively or following pelvic inflammatory disease.[16,18–26] Targeted aspiration of chronic hydrosalpinges has also been reported.[11,27–32]

The value of transabdominal sonography (TAS) was described during the 1970s and 1980s. There is no practical value at this time in reviewing articles dealing with the use of this imaging modality to detect tubal disease, since its use became almost obsolete after the introduction of transvaginal sonography (TVS).

After the introduction of TVS and after its value in gynecologic ultrasound was established,[33–35] a series of comparative reports were published. These reports analysed the comparative clinical utility of TAS and TVS[7,36–39] or compared TVS with laparoscopy.[40]

Soon the scanning technique of TVS to image the female pelvis prevailed as the most useful and clinically meaningful, as well as simple and relatively inexpensive, imaging modality.

Most reports agree upon the reliability of TVS in diagnosing inflammatory changes of the tubes and ovaries. The first transvaginal sonographic images of normal and abnormal fallopian tubes were presented as a light poster presentation at the Annual Meeting of the American Institute of Ultrasound in Medicine in 1982. Following this, a series of peer-reviewed articles appeared.[34,35,41–45]

The clinical use of TVS in examination of the tube was described in 1988, stressing its clinical value.[33,34] No specific distinction between acute and chronic sonographic features was made at that time. Tessler et al[35] recognized the usefulness of TVS in diagnosing hydrosalpinx by identifying a tubular structure with a well-defined echogenic wall as well as a folded configuration and linear echoes. They also distinguish dilated (motionless) tubes from bowel loops and from pelvic vessels and concluded that these findings were sufficiently characteristic to allow the diagnosis to be made with transvaginal sonography.

Not all reports are enthusiastic about the capabilities of TVS for use in the diagnosis of upper genital tract infections. A study by Boardman et al[46] reported that the specificity for detection of hydrosalpinx on ultrasound was 97%; however, the sensitivity was only 32% and the detection of tubo-ovarian abscess was 42%. However, if the reader scrutinizes the article carefully, it is possible to see the reasons for the low sensitivities obtained in the study. First, the ultrasound equipment used was less than adequate for a good pelvic examination; second, the physicians themselves did not routinely scan the patients; and third, a radiologist rather than an obstetrician/gynecologist performed the scans. In most cases radiologists are better at the technical aspects of imaging as compared with the imaging skills of obstetricians/gynecologists. However, they probably scanned the patients without the benefit of clinical information, leading them to produce an unnecessarily broad list of differential diagnoses, which is clinically counter-productive. These were (most probably) the reasons behind the fact that this particular study yielded results that lead to the wrong conclusions regarding the utility of TVS in diagnosing inflammatory diseases of the adnexa.

Taipale et al[41] studied 86 patients with pelvic inflammatory disease using TVS, within 1–3 days, 14 days, and 90 days after their hospitalization. The diagnosis was confirmed in 37% of their patients by surgical means. In the patients with acute disease (31%), an echogenic tube with thick walls (> 5 mm in diameter) raised the suspicion of pyosalpinx. Those patients developing chronic hydrosalpinx after 3 months had a sonolucent, fluid-filled struc-

ture with a wall thickness that measured < 5 mm. Of the total of 86 patients, only 6% showed a hydrosalpinx after 3 months. Therefore, these authors found TVS to be useful in the diagnosis of inflammatory diseases of the pelvis and particularly of the fallopian tube, and recommended a rescan after 3 months following the acute phase, to detect any sequel of the disease.

Although hydrosalpinx is usually the result of an earlier acute salpingitis, it was also described in patients who had had a hysterectomy or tubal ligation/cauterization by Krivak et al.[47] Their observations in this regard match our experience. Several of our patients showed clear presence of hydrosalpinges after total abdominal hysterectomy, without salpingectomy, or after bilateral tubal ligation or cauterization.

Natural history of pelvic inflammatory disease

In order to understand the rationale behind the description of the sonographic attributes of inflammatory tubal disease, it is first necessary to discuss the natural history and progression of the infection resulting in the acute and chronic changes in the fallopian tube and the ovaries.

The disease is usually the result of an infection by *Neisseria gonorrhoeae* or by chlamydia. This is an ascending infection from the lower to the upper genital tract and usually occurs immediately after the menstrual period. The pathogens move from the vagina, through the cervical os, into the uterus, and then the fallopian tubes. The inner lining of the tube contains an abundance of folds, which are thin, slender and lined with ciliated endothelia. *Figure 4.1* shows a drawing of a normal tube cross-sectioned at the ampullar region. First, during the acute phase, if the normal tubal mucosa is involved in the inflammatory process its wall becomes thick and extremely edematous, and some, but not a large amount, of purulent exudate fills the lumen. Some of the exudate may also spill into the cul-de-sac through the still open fimbrial end of the tube. The adnexa are usually extremely tender and the distended thick-walled tube may kink and form a convoluted structure which resembles the glass retorts employed in laboratories. These are known as 'retort-shaped tubes.'

If the process of tubal occlusion continues at both ends and the process heals owing to intervention or to its self-limiting nature, the picture transforms into that of the chronic hydrosalpinx. The tube is now overly distended by fluid, which may or may not

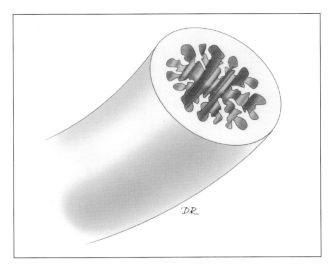

Figure 4.1 Artist's impression of the cross-section of a normal tube at the ampullary level. The branching of the thin longitudinal endosalpingeal folds is shown.

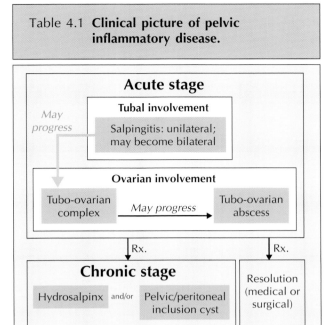

Table 4.1 **Clinical picture of pelvic inflammatory disease.**

contain particulate matter, its walls become thin, and the previously rich and tortuous endosalpingeal folds flatten, fibrose and are barely visible. At times they may be detected only in the pathology laboratory through the microscope, as tags or longitudinal flat folds extruding from the inner lining of the tubal wall. The chronic hydrosalpinx is pear- or oval-shaped and often has a 'beak' as it approaches the cornual area of the uterus, and most of the time, owing to its size, it kinks or folds within the pelvis.

If the tube does not occlude, some of the pus spills into the pelvis and—at the time of ovulation (in the reproductive years of the patient)—the bacteria take advantage of the small defect on the ovary itself caused by the ovulation and invade that one ovary. This is the first phase of ovarian involvement, which in a certain number of cases can result in more extensive pelvic inflammatory processes. At first, the anatomy involved is not broken down, and if laparotomy or laparoscopy is performed an inflammatory conglomerate with ovary and tube still recognizable as separate entities can be observed. Only at a later stage and after several days does the process spread to the other side, involving the contralateral adnexa. This is the reason why, quite frequently, the two adnexa have an out-of-phase appearance. First, the tube in which the process started advances to a tubo-ovarian abscess stage and then the other side, which still lags behind, shows all the signs of a still recognizable tubo-ovarian entity or complex, in which the anatomy has not yet broken down.

If conventional antibiotic treatment fails or is not applied, the acute inflammatory process progresses, resulting in the full-blown tubo-ovarian abscess. This process is illustrated in *Table 4.1*. Of course, if the process is recognized in its earliest stages, complete healing may take place as a result of successful medical treatment. Once again, the anatomy may be completely restored or the process in the tube may progress into the chronic phase already described.

Most commonly in the acute phase, small amounts of fluid may be seen persisting for a variable length of time in the cul-de-sac or different parts of the pelvis. Later on, adhesions between various organs in the pelvis may appear. These adhesions persist for months or even years. Fluid may be trapped between the adhesions and the pelvic organs and this becomes evident as pelvic peritoneal inclusion fluid or a pelvic peritoneal inclusion cyst.

Tubo-ovarian complex/tubo-ovarian abscess

Unfortunately, in the literature the terms 'tubo-ovarian complex' and 'tubo-ovarian abscess' are used interchangeably and in a rather undefined fashion.[35,39–41,43–45,48] These two entities are clinically distinct and are usually treated by different therapeutic approaches. In addition to this, even sonographically, they present with different pictures. The only thing that these two entities have in common is that they only occur in the acute phase of the tubal disease and, if not diagnosed and treated in time, the first evolves into the second entity.

Tubo-ovarian complex is a first step in the inflammatory process that may or may not lead to subsequent abscess formation. Tubo-ovarian complex should therefore be diagnosed on the basis of the sonographic picture when there are clear sonographic attributes of this process, such as thick walls and an irregular sonolucent core and when the tube and the ovary can still be recognized on the image. The sonographic signs of tubo-ovarian complex are discussed in a subsequent section of this chapter.

In contrast to the tubo-ovarian complex, the term or the diagnosis of *tubo-ovarian abscess* should be reserved for a much later phase in the inflammatory process when the adnexal structure, such as the ovary and the tube, on one or both sides, are totally broken down as anatomic entities. If such an abscess develops, the ultrasound will show the presence of loculated, speckled fluid in the cul-de-sac, which will be consistent with a multi-loculated debris (pus)-filled space above the cross, or the longitudinal section of the rectum.

The various individual researchers and the clinical practitioners interested in imaging have described (quite competently) the sonographic picture of the diseased salpinx and that of the tubo-ovarian inflammatory process as well as the cul-de-sac. However, it was necessary to 'merge' the natural history or the clinical evolution of this pelvic inflammatory process with the different transvaginal sonographic attributes of this process. A recent report described a study of 77 patients scanned by transvaginal sonography and divided into two groups according to their clinical picture. One group had an acute inflammatory process and the second had a history of chronic PID or had no history at all but a serendipitously found pelvic adnexa mass which turned out to represent chronic inflammatory processes of the pelvis. Looking at the different sonographic markers, which are described below, it was possible to construct a 'sonographic history' of the evolution of the pelvic inflammatory disease involving the tube and the ovary.[49]

Sonographic markers of pelvic inflammatory disease

Using transvaginal sonography (the gold standard of sonographic evaluation of the female pelvis), the basic building blocks or sonographic attributes of the different pictures involving the tube and the

Table 4.2 Sonographic attributes of pelvic inflammatory disease.

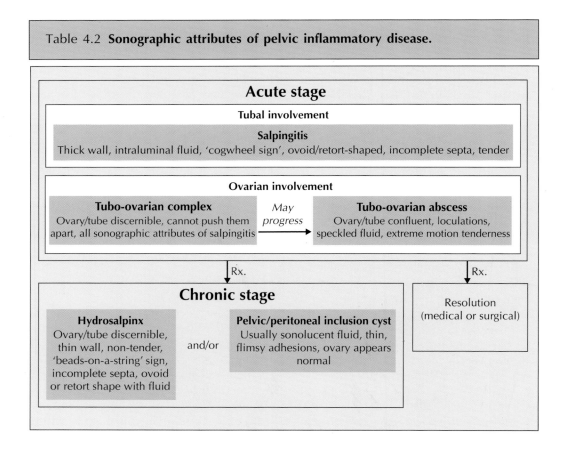

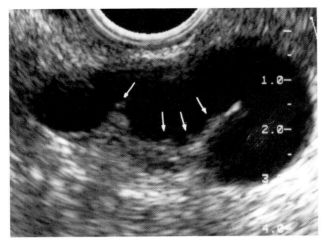

Figure 4.2 This fluid-filled fallopian tube assumes the shape of a pear with a beak or tapered shape towards the left side of the picture. The arrows mark incomplete septae.

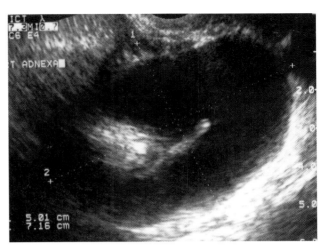

Figure 4.3 The longitudinal section of a right-sided, chronic hydrosalpinx in a patient status post bilateral tubal ligation. Note the retort shape and the incomplete septum resulting from the kinking of the distended tube, as well as the thin wall and the sonolucent fluid within the lumen.

ovary as well as the cul-de-sac are presented in *Table 4.2*. In this table the most commonly recognized ultrasound features of inflammatory disease of the female pelvic organs are added into the flowchart shown in *Table 4.1*. The basic data from a report published earlier[49] have been used to show the main 'building blocks' of the sonographic pictures seen in the clinically acute and chronic phases of infectious pelvic disease in the female patient.

Shape. On the longitudinal section, the fluid-filled tube, regardless of the clinical picture (i.e. acute or chronic), is a pear-shaped, ovoid, or retort-shaped structure containing sonolucent or sometimes various degrees of low-level echoes (*Figs 4.2* and *4.3*).

The wall structure demonstrates the following distinguishing features on the longitudinal or coronal section. (a) Incomplete septa, which are defined as hyperchoic septa that originate as a triangular protrusion from one of the walls but do not reach (in the overwhelming majority of cases) the opposite wall. Applying pressure with the tip of the transvaginal probe as well as the abdominally placed second hand of the operator, an attempt can be made to force the fluid from one compartment to flow into another one, confirming the nature of the incomplete septa (*Figs 4.2* and *4.3*). (b) The 'cogwheel sign,' which was first suggested by Timor-Tritsch et al[50] and consists of a sonolucent cogwheel-shaped structure seen on the cross-section of the tube with thick walls (*Fig. 4.4*). The 'cogwheel

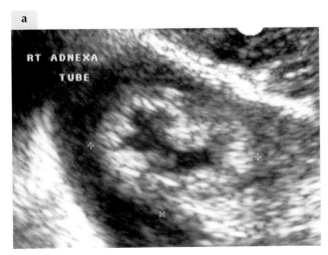
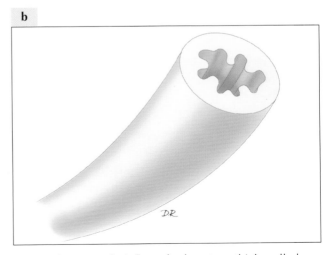

Figure 4.4 The 'cogwheel sign' in acute salpingitis. (a) Cross-section of an acutely inflamed edematous thick-walled fallopian tube. There is a scant amount of fluid in the lumen. The shape of the sonolucent fluid gives it the appearance of a cogwheel. (b) Artist's impression of the 'cogwheel sign.'

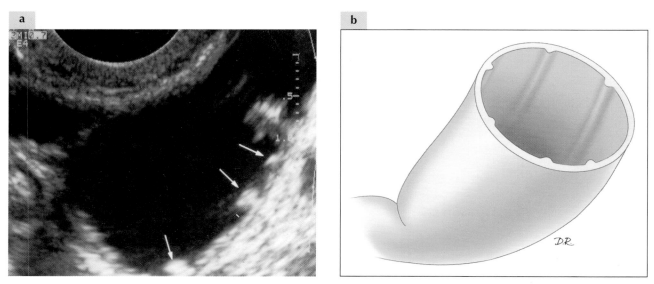

Figure 4.5 The 'beads-on-a-string sign' is of chronic salpingitis. (a) Cross-section of a chronic, thin-walled hydrosalpinx. The arrows mark the fibrosed protrusions of the flattened endosalpingeal folds. (b) Artist's impression of the 'beads-on-a-string sign.'

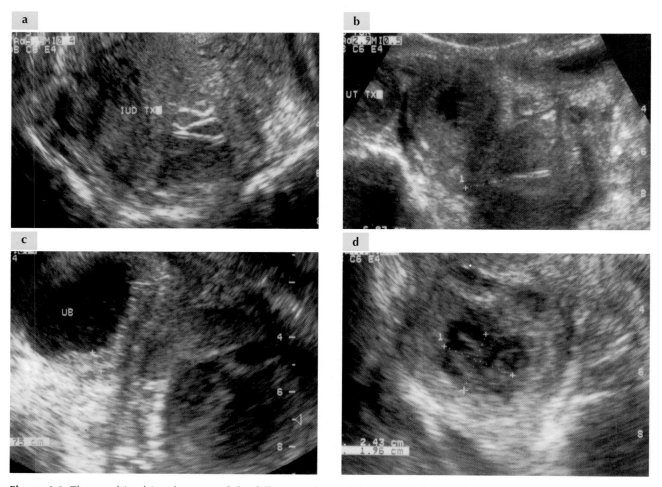

Figure 4.6 The combined involvement of the fallopian tube and the ovary: tubo-ovarian complex. In a patient with a Lippes loop (a), a pelvic inflammatory process develops. The dilated, thick-walled and inflamed right tube is shown in front and on the right of the uterus (b). The left ovary (c) is still seen close to the tube. The right tube is seen on the cross-section filled with a small amount of fluid (d).

sign' is the result of the acutely inflamed edematous thick tube and the interdigitated fashion of the thick endosalpingeal folds and the shape of the sonolucent fluid, which is trapped within the tube. Once again it should be said clearly that in the acute phase there is only a small amount of intraluminal fluid. The shape of this sonolucent fluid in the lumen resembles a cogwheel. (c) The 'beads-on-a-string' sign, which is defined as hyperechoic mural nodules of about 2–3 mm seen on the cross-section of the fluid-filled distended tube. These echogenic mural papillarities are the remnants of the fibrosed and flattened endosalpingeal folds (*Fig. 4.5*). The thin wall with the bright echoes described above appears as beads-on-a-string or a rosary.

The wall thickness is determined as being thick if it is ≥ 5 mm and thin if it is < 5 mm (*Figs 4.3–4.5*).

The ovarian involvement is defined as follows. (a) 'None' if the ovary appears normal and can be distinguished clearly on the sonographic image. (b) Tubo-ovarian complex (*Fig. 4.6*), in which the ovaries and the tubes can be identified and recognized, but the ovaries cannot be separated by pushing the structure with the tip of the vaginal probe. In addition, the patient demonstrates all the clinical signs and symptoms of an acute pelvic inflammatory process. At times, there is a stage which is considered to be a transient stage between the tubo-ovarian complex and the overt abscess. This is when the ovary is involved in such a manner that it is 'consumed' by the inflammatory process and it is filled by pus but has not yet ruptured. The thick-walled, inflamed tube is also seen separately (*Fig. 4.7*). Since the ovary is filled with pus and by definition this may represent an 'ovarian abscess,' many would call this stage a tubo-ovarian abscess. However, the real tubo-ovarian abscess is present when these structures rupture into the pelvis and

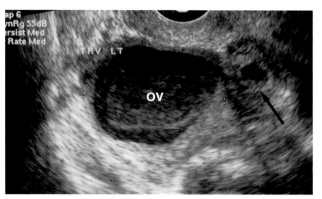

Figure 4.7 The 'intermediary' or transient' stage between tubo-ovarian complex and tubo-ovarian abscess. Note that the cross-section of the thick-walled tube (arrow) is distinctly separate from the low-level, echo-filled ovary (OV) within which no ovarian structure, as such, is seen. This ovary may indeed rupture at any time, creating the full-blown picture (sonographic and clinical) of a tubo-ovarian (pelvic) abscess.

the pelvis is filled with pus. (c) Tubo-ovarian abscess (*Fig. 4.8*) in which the patient is acutely ill with significant tenderness at the touch of the ultrasound probe or the abdominally placed hand of the operator. Of course, all the classical signs and symptoms of a pelvic abscess are present. In this case, a total or significant breakdown of the normal architecture of one or both adnexa, i.e. the tube and the ovaries, with formation of a conglomerate is seen. Neither the ovary nor the tubes can be recognized separately. The classical pelvic abscess appears as speckled fluid or as a web of thin and thick septa criss-crossing the area of interest, locking in fluid between these septa.

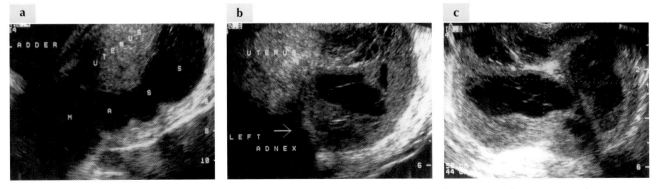

Figure 4.8 The combined involvement of the fallopian tube and the ovary: the tubo-ovarian abscess. Here the sonographic picture shows a totally 'broken down' image of the adnexa, free pelvic fluid behind the uterus. The patient demonstrated the clinical picture of severe pelvic infection. (a) The median section. (b) The left adnexa. (c) Transverse image of the cul-de-sac.

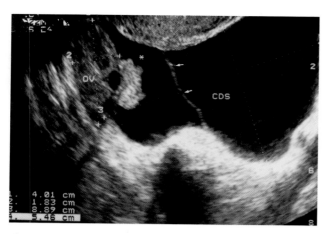

Figure 4.9 Late sequel of pelvic infection. The cross-section of the cul-de-sac (CDS) filled with sonolucent fluid. The typical thread-like adhesion (arrows) is diagnostic. The right ovary and a section of the right fallopian tube are also seen (OV and FT).

The presence of *free or loculated cul-de-sac fluid* is also considered to be a sonographic marker of a previous pelvic inflammatory process, after which adhesions lock in fluid between the pelvic wall and the pelvic organs and the bowel. At times thin adhesions fluctuating within sonolucent fluid stretched within the different organs in the pelvis are seen (*Fig. 4.9*). There is usually no tenderness upon touch with the vaginal probe and there are no clinical signs or symptoms of an acute illness.

A thick wall was present in 100% of the patients with acute disease and, conversely, a thin wall occurred much more often in patients with chronic disease (97%). In the acute group, none of the examinations revealed a thin tubal wall. This was significant at a P value of < 0.001.

Looking at the wall structure, 86% of the patients showed the cogwheel sign, i.e. the thickened tubal wall with edematous endosalpingeal folds, whereas only two of the patients with chronic disease demonstrated this marker (P < 0.001). The beads-on-a-string sign was present in 57% of the patients with chronic disease; however, none of the patients with acute tubal disease showed this sign (P < 0.001). Incomplete septa were present in 93% of the chronic cases and 86% of the acute cases. The presence of incomplete septa was not discriminatory between the chronic and the acute cases (P = 0.3); however, as this sonographic marker was present in a total of 92% of all cases within the study, this sign is considered a very good sonographic marker of tubo-inflammatory disease.

Tubo-ovarian complex was present in five of the patients with acute disease (36%) and only one of the 60 patients with chronic disease. However, it should be pointed out that this one patient was in the process of healing after extensive antibiotic treatment and showed no signs of acute tubal disease.

Cul-de-sac fluid was seen most commonly in the acute cases: 50% of these patients showed some fluid in the cul-de-sac. In the chronic group only 10% of patients had a small amount of fluid present.

Palpable pelvic findings were common both in the acute and in the chronic group. It is also understandable that 100% of the acute cases had palpatory findings of tenderness and an adnexal mass, but only 72% of the chronic cases demonstrated palpatory findings. This, of course, was non-discriminatory (P = 0.03).

The medical and surgical histories of these patients were quite revealing and were more common in women who had acute disease (57%). In the chronic group only 25% of the patients had the recollection of a significant inflammatory history (P = 0.003). However, the previous surgical history was non-discriminatory: 21% of patients with acute disease and 30% of patients with chronic disease reported prior surgical procedures. However, it is interesting that 20 of the 74 patients studied had had previous surgical procedures, such as an operation for an ectopic pregnancy, bilateral tubal ligation, or total abdominal hysterectomy.

The drawback of this study was that only a small percentage of the patients had surgical confirmation of the sonographic diagnosis. However, it is to be expected that patients in whom a hydrosalpinx was found during a routine ultrasound examination and did not have acute symptoms, or did not have any other reason for surgical exploration, were not candidates for laparoscopy or surgical confirmation of their findings. Nevertheless it is important to state that the sonographic findings in the acute and in the chronic group cannot be explained by any disease other than those of the tubes and the ovaries caused by inflammatory processes.

False positive cases were also encountered in this study and these included an ovarian cystadenoma in which the sonographic finding was re-read within a matter of weeks and the diagnosis changed. Another case was that of an appendiceal mucocele mimicking a pyosalpinx.

The sonographic pictures reported in the above study[49] reflect the pathological changes occurring in the process of the acute and chronic disease of the tube and those involving the ovary and the cul-de-sac. In the acute phase when the tube becomes occluded at the fimbrial or at the cornual end and pus fills the tube, slightly distending it, this leads to the entity called pyosalpinx. The edematous endosalpingeal folds and the fluid within the lumen produce the cogwheel sign in this tube. If the same tube becomes convoluted and kinked, the retort-shaped tube with incomplete septa appears.

If the inflammatory process ends, either spontaneously or as a result of successful medical treatment, complete healing may take place. However, the process may enter another phase, namely the chronic phase which, as described earlier, is characterized by a completely blocked tube in which a larger amount of fluid accumulates, distending the wall, which in turn becomes extremely thin. On the internal wall within the lumen, the endosalpingeal folds almost disappear or become fibrosed or flattened. On the sonographic cross-section of the tube, these are

demonstrated as hyperechoic protrusions, which have been called beads-on-a-string. On a histological or pathological specimen, the microscopic sections demonstrate these remnants of the fibrosed endosalpingeal folds. This was a rather reliable marker of chronic tubal disease and it was present in 57% of the chronic cases, but in none of the acutely ill patients.

Both in the acute and in the chronic tubal diseases, the progressive filling and ballooning of the occluded tube leads to a kinking or doubling up of the hydrosalpinx or pyosalpinx, respectively. The sonographic equivalent of this process is the incomplete septum, which appears in acute, as well as chronic tubal disease. This was one of the most important findings in the study described,[49] since it was present both in the chronic and in the acute group (93% and 86%, respectively), rendering this sonographic marker an extremely reliable sign of tubal disease.

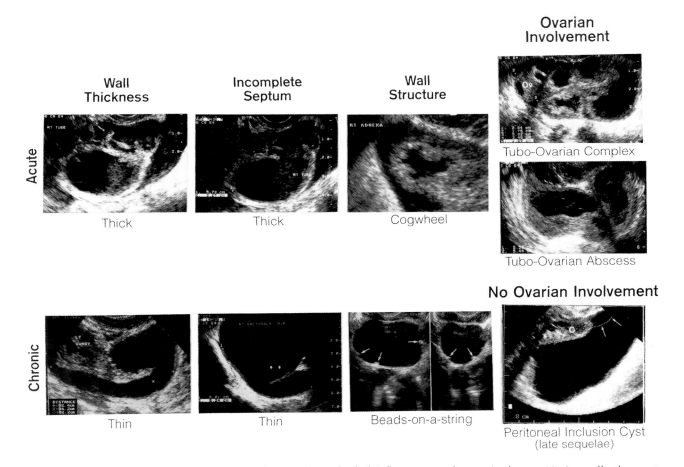

Figure 4.10 A pictorial table of the sonographic markers of tubal inflammatory disease is shown. Horizontally the acute and the chronic disease is shown as a function of the sonographic markers such as wall thickness, incomplete septa, wall structure and ovarian involvement. Using this guide, it is easy to evaluate ultrasound images for the acuteness of the process. (Reproduced with permission from Timor-Tritsch et al.[49])

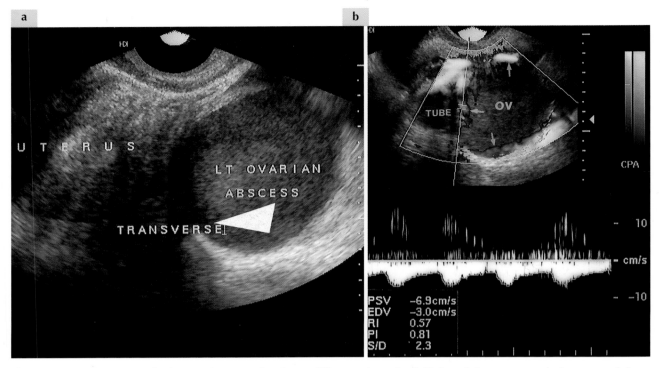

Figure 4.11 (a) Unruptured tubo-ovarian complex (on a different plane the follicles of the ovary, and also parts of the tube could be recognized) with a clear pus collection in the ovary. (b) Color flow (power amplitude) image shows the intensive blood flow (arrows) at the surface of the ovary. The resistance-to-flow indices are relatively low, but cannot be considered pathognomonic.

As for the presence of fluid in the pelvis in the acute or the chronic inflammatory processes, the presence of the fluid was seen more in the acute than in the chronic phases. However, since these patients were not followed longitudinally, it is not possible to comment on the length of time that the pelvic fluid persisted. The amount of the fluid was non-discriminatory and non-pathognomonic for acute or chronic disease in this study.

As a visual summary of the sonographic markers of inflammatory disease of the fallopian tube, a pictorial representation of these markers was constructed as a function of their clinical stage. This figure may help in recognizing the disease on the basis of its appearance on TVS (*Fig. 4.10*).

Doppler velocimetry of tubo-ovarian infections

If the peritoneal surface of an acutely inflamed tube or a tubo-ovarian complex is observed by laparoscopy or at laparotomy, it is striking that its surface appears red and an abundance of dilated vessels is present. It was therefore logical to search for the sonographic sign of this hyperemia. It seems that the inflamed adnexa are somewhat more sonolucent than the surrounding tissues. It is also evident that the surface of the ovary or a tubo-ovarian complex demonstrates a clear and obvious layer of blood vessels much like the 'color-ring' around the fresh corpus luteum (*Fig. 4.11*). This increased blood flow on the surface of the tube and the ovaries can be demonstrated with relative ease by color Doppler flow studies (*Fig. 4.11*). Starting in the early 1990s, several reports regarding the use of blood flow velocimetry were published. Tinkanen and Kujansuu[51] studied 10 women with tubo-ovarian abscesses and found that the resistance index (RI) and the pulsatility index (PI) measured at the margin of the infection complex were < 0.5 in six patients. Fleischer et al[52] found two patients with tubo-ovarian abscesses among 47 patients with adnexal masses studied for their Doppler flow characteristics. Both patients had a low PI. In a subsequent series Fleischer et al[53] found an additional tubo-ovarian abscess with a similarly low PI measurement.

Summary

It is clear that the first and most important step in the algorithm of correctly diagnosing a pelvic inflammatory process, acute or chronic, is to take a good history from the patient. Past history of intrauterine contraception device use, episodes of pelvic inflammatory disease, pelvic surgery, or infertility are helpful in finding the reason for a so-called 'incidental' or 'serendipitous' finding of a sonolucent, pear-shaped structure with an incomplete septum, i.e. a hydrosalpinx. Conversely, it is significant (and somewhat less complicated) to reveal the clinical signs and symptoms of an acute pelvic infection.

However, it is even more important to share these clinical impressions with the imaging specialist at the time of the scan or on the requisition form. Without the historical and clinical information, even the most experienced and accomplished sonographer and/or sonologist will issue a report including a practically useless and endless 'laundry list' of differential diagnoses for the clinician. Instead of being helped to establish the diagnosis, the clinician will have to 'choose' from the diagnostic suggestions of the imaging specialist. The clinician now has to go back to square one with little help from what should have been the number one laboratory test in deciding whether to start a timely treatment (i.e. for acute disease) or to end the testing (i.e. an 'old' hydrosalpinx).

Throughout this chapter, the transvaginal sonographic building blocks of inflammatory processes have been suggested. They have been placed in the clinical prospective and supported by histopathologic evidence. Much of this—if not all—was known before. This chapter has sought to organize the sonographic data into a clinically useful algorithm. It represents the sonographic snapshots of the natural development of inflammatory tubal disease: the acutely ill fallopian tube is edematous, its walls are thick, and if one or both ends obliterate it may kink. All this can be recognized by ultrasound. It is also clear that a chronically affected hydrosalpinx is thin-walled, its endosalpingeal folds practically disappear, and similar to the acute pyosalpinx it kinks, giving rise to incomplete septa—which are considered by these authors to be the most important markers of tubal disease, regardless of its stage of the disease. The attentive ultrasound practitioner can also recognize all these features.

It is also hoped that attention has been drawn to the distinction between the tubo-ovarian complex and the tubo-ovarian abscess. These are two separate entities with some overlapping as one progresses into the other. It is our belief that the two can be recognized and that by using the information the appropriate and emergent medical or surgical treatment can be applied.

At this point in time, attempts to apply color Doppler velocimetry to aid in the diagnostic process have been only partially successful at best. More information regarding the detection of hyperemia within the wall or on the surface of the inflamed organ is needed. In the future this obvious and objective sign of increased blood vessel dilation in acute disease and its lack in chronic disease will surely be detectable sonographically by the use of more advanced and more sensitive flow detection.

Conclusions

Transvaginal sonography is the best tool for the study of inflammatory processes of the pelvis. Coupling the patient's history with the sonographic picture enables the operator (sonologist and sonographer) to come closer to an accurate diagnosis and significantly shorten the list of possible differential diagnostic entities.

REFERENCES

1. Westrom L. Incidence, prevalence and trends of acute pelvic inflammatory disease and its consequences in industrialized countries. *Am J Obstet Gynecol* 1980; **138**:880–892.

2. McCormac W. Pelvic inflammatory disease. *N Engl J Med* 1994; **330**:115–119.

3. Grimes ER *et al*. Management of the infertile couple. In: Speroff L, Simpson JL eds. *Gynecology and Obstetrics*. Philadelphia: Harper & Row, 1987.

4. Westrom L. Effect of acute pelvic inflammatory disease on fertility. *Am J Obstet Gynecol* 1975; **125**:707–713.

5. Expert committee on pelvic inflammatory disease. Research direction for the 1990s. *Sex Transm Dis* 1991; **18**:46–64.

6. Gales W, Wasserheit J. Genital chlamydial infections: epidemiology and reproductive sequelae. *Am J Obstet Gynecol* 1991; **164**:1771–1781.

7. Patton D, More D, Spadoni I, Soules M, Halbert S, Wang S. A comparison of the Fallopian tube's response to overt and silent salpingitis. *Obstet Gynecol* 1989; **73**:622–630.

8. Bloechle M, Schreiner T, Lisse K. Recurrence of hydrosalpinges after transvaginal aspiration of tubal fluid in an IVF cycle with development of a serometra. *Human Reprod* 1997; **12**:703–705.

9. Akman MA, Garcia JE, Damewood MD, Watts LD, Katz E. Hydrosalpinx affects the implantation of previously cryopreserved embryos. *Human Reprod* 1996; **11**:1013–1014.

10. Abd-el-Maeboud KH, al-Dein M, Khalifa E, el-Hussein ES. An increased number of replaced embryos counteracts the adverse effect of hydrosalpinges on IVF/ET outcome. *J Assist Reprod Genet* 1998; **15**:22–26.

11. Van Voorhis BJ, Sparks AE, Syrop CH, Stovall DW. Ultrasound-guided aspiration of hydrosalpinges is associated with improved pregnancy and implantation rates after in-vitro fertilization cycles. *Human Reprod* 1998; **13**:736–739.

12. Schiller VL, Tsuchiyama K. Development of hydrosalpinx during ovulation induction. *J Ultrasound Med* 1995; **14**:799–803.

13. Younis JS, Ezra Y, Laufer N, Ohel G. Late manifestation of pelvic abscess following oocyte retrieval, for in vitro fertilization, in patients with severe endometriosis and ovarian endometriomata. *J Assist Reprod Genet* 1997; **14**:343–346.

14. Sauer MV, Paulson RJ. Pelvic abscess complicating transcervical embryo transfer. *Am J Obstet Gynecol* 1992; **166**:148–149.

15. Marlowe SD, Lupetin AR. Tuboovarian abscess following transvaginal oocyte retrieval for in vitro fertilization: imaging appearance. *Clin Imaging* 1995; **19**:180–181.

16. Hsu YL, Yang JM, Wang KG. Transvaginal ultrasound-guided aspiration in the treatment and follow-up of tubo-ovarian abscess: a report of two cases. *Chung Hua I Hsueh Tsa Chih* 1995; **56**:211–214.

17. Curtis P, Amso N, Keith E, Bernard A, Shaw RW. Evaluation of the risk of pelvic infection following transvaginal oocyte recovery. *Human Reprod* 1991; **6**:1294–1297.

18. Worthen NJ, Gunning JE. Percutaneous drainage of pelvic abscesses: management of the tubo-ovarian abscess. *J Ultrasound Med* 1986; **5**:551–556.

19. Sperling DC, Needleman L, Eschelman DJ, Hovsepian DM, Lev-Toaff AS. Deep pelvic abscesses: transperineal US-guided drainage. *Radiology* 1998; **208**:111–115.

20. Shulman A, Maymon R, Shapiro A, Bahary C. Percutaneous catheter drainage of tubo-ovarian abscesses. *Obstet Gynecol* 1992; **80**:555–557.

21. Nelson AL, Sinow RM, Renslo R, Renslo J, Atamdede F. Endovaginal ultrasonographically guided transvaginal drainage for treatment of pelvic abscesses. *Am J Obstet Gynecol* 1995; **172**:1926–1932, 1932–1935.

22. McGahan JP, Brown B, Jones CD, Stein M. Pelvic abscesses: transvaginal US-guided drainage with the trocar method. *Radiology* 1996; **200**:579–581.

23. Feld R, Eschelman DJ, Sagerman JE, Segal S, Hovsepian DM, Sullivan KL. Treatment of pelvic abscesses and other fluid collections: efficacy of transvaginal sonographically guided aspiration and drainage. *Am J Roentgenol* 1994; **163**:1141–1145.

24. Caspi B, Zalel Y, Or Y, Bar Dayan Y, Appelman Z, Katz Z. Sonographically guided aspiration: an alternative therapy for tubo-ovarian abscess. *Ultrasound Obstet Gynecol* 1996; **7**:439–442.

25. Casola G, van Sonnenberg E, D'Agostino HB, Harker CP, Varney RR, Smith D. Percutaneous drainage of tubo-ovarian abscesses. *Radiology* 1992; **182**:399–402.

26. Aboulghar MA, Mansour RT, Serour GI. Ultrasonographically guided transvaginal aspiration of tuboovarian abscesses and pyosalpinges: an optional treatment for acute pelvic inflammatory disease. *Am J Obstet Gynecol* 1995; **172**:1501–1503.

27. Doust B, Quiroz F, Stewart J. Ultrasonic distinction of abscesses from other intra-abdominal fluid collections. *Radiology* 1977; **125**:213–218.

28. Uhrich P, Sanders RC. Ultrasonic characteristics of pelvic inflammatory masses. *J Clin Ultrasound* 1976; **4**:199.

29. Lawson T, Albarelli J. Diagnosis of gynecologic pelvic masses by gray scale ultrasonography: analysis of specificity and accuracy. *Am J Roentgenol* 1977; **128**:1003–1006.

30. Fleischer A, James AJ, Millis J, Julian C. Differential diagnosis of pelvic masses by gray scale sonography. *Am J Roentgenol* 1978; **131**:469–476.

31. Swayne L, Love M, Karasick S. Pelvic inflammatory disease: sonographic–pathologic correlation. *Radiology* 1984; **151**:751.

32. Spirtos N, Bernstine R, Crawford W *et al.* Sonography in acute pelvic inflammatory disease. *J Reprod Med* 1982; **27**:312.

33. Timor-Tritsch I, Bar Yam Y, Elgali S, Rottem S. The technique of transvaginal sonography with the use of a 6.5 MHz probe. *Am J Obstet Gynecol* 1988; **158**:1019–1024.

34. Timor-Tritsch I, Rottem S. Transvaginal ultrasonographic study of the Fallopian tube. *Obstet Gynecol* 1987; **70**:424–428.

35. Tessler FN, Perrella RR, Fleischer AC, Grant EG. Endovaginal sonographic diagnosis of dilated fallopian tubes. *Am J Roentgenol* 1989; **153**:523–525.

36. Mendelson E, Bohm-Velez M, Joseph N *et al.* Gynecologic imaging: comparison of transabdominal and transvaginal sonography. *Radiology* 1988; **166**:321.

37. Leibman A, Kruse B, McSweeney M. Transvaginal sonography: comparison with transabdominal sonography in the diagnosis of pelvic masses. *Am J Roentgenol* 1988; **151**:89.

38. Fleischer A, Gordon A, Entman S. Transabdominal and transvaginal sonography of pelvic masses. *Ultrasound Med Biol* 1989; **15**:529.

39. Bulas DI, Ahlstrom PA, Sivit CJ, Blask AR, O'Donnell RM. Pelvic inflammatory disease in the adolescent: comparison of transabdominal and transvaginal sonographic evaluation. *Radiology* 1992; **183**:435–439.

40. Patten RM, Vincent LM, Wolner-Hanssen P, Thorpe E. Pelvic inflammatory disease. Endovaginal sonography with laparoscopic correlation. *J Ultrasound Med* 1990; **9**:681–689.

41. Taipale P, Tarjanne H, Ylostalo P. Transvaginal sonography in suspected pelvic inflammatory disease. *Ultrasound Obstet Gynecol* 1995; **6**:430–434.

42. Slap GB, Forke CM, Cnaan A *et al*. Recognition of tubo-ovarian abscess in adolescents with pelvic inflammatory disease. *J Adolesc Health* 1996; **18**:397–403.

43. Cacciatore B, Leminen A, Ingman-Friberg S, Ylostalo P, Paavonen J. Transvaginal sonographic findings in ambulatory patients with suspected pelvic inflammatory disease. *Obstet Gynecol* 1992; **80**:912–916.

44. Atri M, Tran C, Bret P, Aldis A, Kintzen G. Accuracy of endovaginal sonography for the detection of Fallopian tubes. *Am J Roentgenol* 1989; **153**:523–525.

45. Bellah R, Rosenberg H. Transvaginal ultrasound in a children's hospital: is it worthwhile? *Pediatr Radiol* 1991; **21**:570–574.

46. Boardman LA, Peipert JF, Brody JM, Cooper AS, Sung J. Endovaginal sonography for the diagnosis of upper genital tract infection. *Obstet Gynecol* 1997; **90**:54–57.

47. Krivak T, Propst A, Horowitz G. Tubo-ovarian abscess: principles of contemporary management. *Female Patient* 1997; **22**:27–44.

48. Russin L. Imaging of hydrosalpinx with torsion following tubal sterilization. *Semin Ultrasound CT MR* 1988; **9**:175–182.

49. Timor-Tritsch I, Lerner J, Monteagudo A, Murphy K, Heller D. Transvaginal sonographic markers of tubal inflammatory disease. *Ultrasound Obstet Gynecol* 1998; **12**:56–66.

50. Timor-Tritsch I, Rottem S, Lewett N. The Fallopian tube. In: Timor-Tritsch I, Rottem S, eds. *Transvaginal Sonography*. New York: Chapman & Hall, 1991.

51. Tinkanen H, Kujansuu E. Doppler ultrasound findings in tubo-ovarian infectious complex. *J Clin Ultrasound* 1993; **21**:175–178.

52. Fleischer A, Cullinan J, Jones HR, Peery C, Bluth R, Kepple D. Serial assessment of adnexal masses with transvaginal color Doppler sonography. *Ultrasound Med Biol* 1995; **21**:435–441.

53. Fleischer A, Rodgers W, Kepple D, Williams L, Jones HR, Gross P. Color Doppler sonography of benign and malignant ovarian masses. *Radiographics* 1992; **12**:879–885.

5 Uterine factors in infertility

Donald N Di Salvo, Faye C Laing and Clare M C Tempany

Introduction

Infertility is estimated to affect 6.1 million women in the USA, or roughly 10% of women of reproductive age.[1] Although uterine pathology accounts for < 10% of cases, uterine imaging is important not only for establishing a specific diagnosis, but also for directing corrective therapy.[2,3] In addition, knowledge of uncorrected structural abnormalities can forewarn a clinician of potential pregnancy complications including spontaneous abortion, intrauterine growth retardation, preterm delivery, malpresentation, dystocia, and retained products of conception.[4]

Non-invasive diagnostic imaging modalities currently used to evaluate infertile women include hysterosalpingography, ultrasound, and magnetic resonance imaging. This chapter will review the use of these modalities to assess anatomic and physiologic uterine abnormalities.

Diagnostic imaging modalities

Hysterosalpingography

Hysterosalpingography (HSG) uses fluoroscopic control to introduce radiographic contrast material into the uterine cavity and fallopian tubes. While today it is used primarily to assess tubal patency, this technique also provides indirect evidence for uterine pathology through depiction of abnormal uterine cavity contours.

Technical considerations for evaluating uterine causes of infertility include (a) obtaining true coronal images of the uterus by using traction on the cervix or adjusting patient position, and (b) carefully observing the uterine cavity contour at the beginning of the examination before too much contrast has been introduced. This will optimize visualization of thin adhesions and small polyps or fibroids.

The advantages of HSG include long-standing historical acceptance of this technique, as well as excellent detection of diethylstilbestrol (DES)-related anomalies and intrauterine adhesions. The disadvantages include limited myometrial evaluation and inability to define the outer uterine contour. Additionally, it is a relatively invasive and uncomfortable procedure, and it requires ionizing radiation.

Sonography

Sonography is frequently used to evaluate uterine pathology because of its excellent diagnostic accuracy, minimal patient discomfort, low cost and widespread availability. With the addition of transvaginal sonography, color Doppler imaging, and sonohysterography, ultrasound has become a sensitive technique for detecting endometrial and myometrial pathology.

For infertility evaluation, careful coronal imaging of the uterine fundal and endometrial contours is critical. Although this may be accomplished transabdominally with partial bladder filling (since a full bladder will frequently displace the uterine fundus out of a true coronal plane), in most cases transvaginal scanning is required (*Fig. 5.1*). For some conditions (e.g. adhesions, endometrial polyps), it is important to perform the ultrasound scan at the appropriate time of the menstrual cycle, but for congenital anomaly evaluation, the timing of the ultrasound examination is not critical.[5]

The major drawback of this modality is its operator dependency. Additional limitations include factors that contribute to an unfavorable ultrasound image, such as a large body habitus and/or the presence of large fibroids. Recently, three-dimensional ultrasound has been developed and applied to gynecologic imaging.[6,7] This new approach may improve detection of uterine structural anomalies, although to date it has not consistently shown an

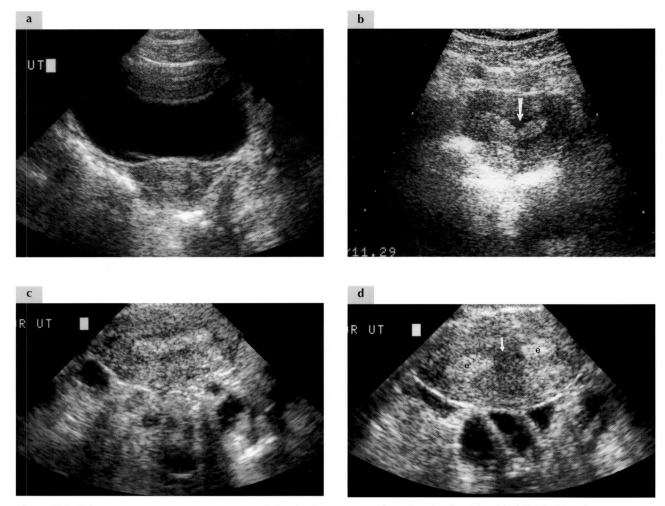

Figure 5.1 Subseptate uterus. Transverse transabdominal sonogram of uterine fundus (a) with full bladder shows no abnormality. Repeat imaging (b) following partial bladder void places uterus in a coronal plane and allows visualization of endometrial splitting by a small septum (arrow). The serosal uterine contour is smooth. Coronal transvaginal sonogram of fundus in the same patient is normal (c), but repeat image slightly more cephalad (d) shows splitting of endometrium (**e**) by small septum (arrow). This illustrates the importance of careful imaging through the entire uterine cavity.

advantage over sonohysterography or two-dimensional imaging.[8]

Magnetic resonance imaging

Magnetic resonance imaging (MRI), by virtue of its ability to demonstrate excellent inherent soft tissue contrast as well as its multiplanar capabilities, is well-suited for female pelvic imaging. Because it renders a global view of pelvic organs, it is superior to ultrasound for recognizing anatomic relationships, especially in clinical situations that limit ultrasound imaging (such as large uterine fibroids).

Recently introduced faster pulse sequences (e.g. single shot fast spin echo sequence), use of pelvic phased array coils, and chemical shift imaging have resulted in shortened examination times, improved resolution, and superior tissue characterization.[9,10]

Current standard imaging protocols for infertility evaluation include axial, sagittal, and coronal fast spin echo sequence images of the uterus, which can be supplemented by oblique views to obtain true coronal and axial images of the uterus. Large field of view images to look for associated renal anomalies should also be obtained. The major drawbacks of MRI are its high cost and limited availability.

Uterine cavity alterations

Müllerian duct anomalies (MDAs)

Definition and pathophysiology

Under normal circumstances, the Müllerian ducts give rise to the fallopian tubes, uterus, cervix, and upper two-thirds of the vagina. Müllerian duct anomalies, which represent a wide spectrum of malformations, result from failure of development, fusion and/or resorption of the paired embryologic Müllerian (paramesonephric) ducts (*Table 5.1*).[11] In the general population, reported prevalence rates range between 0.1% and 5%.[2,12] This wide range reflects these facts: (a) most women with MDAs are asymptomatic; and (b) detection rates vary depending on the population examined and the particular imaging modality used.[13,14] The most common MDAs are arcuate, septate, and bicornuate uteri, accounting for over half of all cases.[14–18]

Most studies suggest that the impact of MDAs on fertility is not in conception but in recurrent spontaneous abortion and/or obstetrical complications. In a study of 1035 women with reproductive dysfunction who were evaluated by HSG, congenital anomalies were detected in 26% of patients with prior miscarriage, compared with only 5% of patients with primary inability to conceive.[19] Septate uteri carry the highest risk for early miscarriage, presumably owing to placental implantation on the poorly vascularized septum.[20,21] Other obstetrical complications associated with congenital uterine anomalies include cervical incompetence (*Fig. 5.2*), preterm delivery, fetal malpresentation, uterine rupture, dystocia, and retained placenta.[4,22,23]

Table 5.1 American Fertility Society classification of Müllerian duct anomalies.[11]

I.   Hypoplasia/agenesis
A. Vaginal
B. Cervical
C. Uterine
D. Tubal
E. Combined
II. Unicornuate uterus
A. Rudimentary horn with communicating cavity
B. Rudimentary horn with noncommunicating cavity
C. Rudimentary horn without cavity
D. No rudimentary horn
III. Uterus didelphys
IV. Bicornuate uterus
A. Complete
B. Partial
V.   Septate uterus
A. Complete
B. Partial (subseptate)
VI. Arcuate uterus
VII. DES-related uterine anomalies

In addition to obstetrical complications, gynecologic and urologic problems may be seen in association with MDAs. Genital tract obstruction most often occurs in anomalies with a vaginal septum, but it may also occur at any level within a duplicated system (*Fig. 5.3a–c*). This obstruction leads to

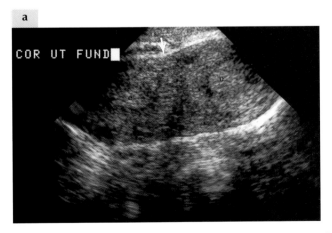
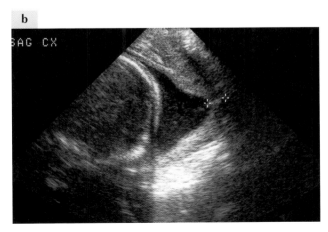

Figure 5.2 Bicornuate uterus with incompetent cervix. (a) Coronal transvaginal sonogram through fundus shows two endometrial cavities (**e**) separated by isoechoic myometrial tissue. Minimal fundal indentation is seen superiorly (arrow). (b) Sagittal midline translabial sonogram (same patient now 28 weeks pregnant) shows dilated internal os, cervical effacement, and residual cervical length of 1 cm (marked by calipers).

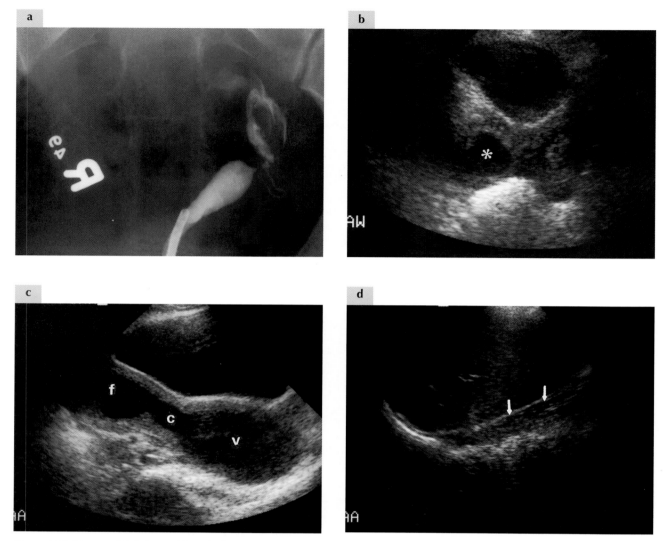

Figure 5.3 Uterus didelphys with right hematometrocolpos and right renal agenesis. (a) HSG shows opacification of left uterine horn only (note similarity with Fig. 5.7a, unicornuate uterus). (b) Transverse transabdominal sonogram through uterine fundus shows fluid-filled right horn (asterisk) and normal left horn (**e**). (c) Sagittal transabdominal sonogram through dilated fluid-filled right uterine fundus (**f**), cervix (**c**) and vagina (**v**). A right-sided obstructing transverse vaginal septum (not demonstrated) was found at surgery. (d) Sagittal transabdominal sonogram through right flank shows empty renal fossa (arrows) consistent with right renal agenesis.

dysmenorrhea, a palpable mass, or endometriosis via retrograde menstruation.[24,25] Renal abnormalities of number and/or position are found in 23% of women with MDAs, reflecting the linked embryologic development of the ureteric bud with the mesonephric (Wolffian) and paramesonephric ducts.[26] The most common renal anomaly is renal agenesis in association with either a unicornuate uterus or an obstructed uterine duplication[23] (*Fig. 5.3d*). Likewise, there is a 55–70% likelihood of genital malformation in a woman with unilateral renal agenesis.[24,27] Other less common clinical associations with MDAs include ovarian malposi-

tion, skeletal abnormalities (hemivertebra, fused vertebra), and connective tissue diseases.[23,28,29]

Imaging Müllerian duct anomalies

A summary of the key anatomic and clinical features of MDAs, including a diagrammatic representation of each class, is provided in *Table 5.2*.[30] The following sections describe in greater detail the clinical and imaging features for each anomaly.

Agenesis/hypoplasia (Class I). Agenesis or hypoplasia of any part of the genital tract (vagina, cervix,

Table 5.2 Summary of key anatomic/clinical features of MDAs.

Class	Diagram[30]	Key anatomic feature	Clinical features
I: Agenesis*		A. Vaginal agenesis B. Cervical agenesis C. Uterine (fundal) agenesis D. Tubal agenesis E. Combined agenesis	Primary amenorrhea rather than infertility is usual presentation; secondary hypoplasia may be due to ovarian failure, irradiation
IIA: Unicornuate uterus		Atretic horn with communicating cavity	Pregnancy in atretic horn may rupture
IIB: Unicornuate uterus		Atretic horn with non-communicating cavity	Fluid accumulation in atretic horn may cause palpable mass/cyclic pain
IIC: Unicornuate uterus		Atretic horn without cavity	Risk of preterm labor, intrauterine growth retardation
IID: Unicornuate uterus		No atretic horn	Risk of preterm labor, intrauterine growth retardation
III: Uterus didelphys		Complete fusion failure, complete cavity separation, vaginal septum in 75%	Least common duplication anomaly; minimal reproductive dysfunction; transverse vaginal septum may obstruct portion of system
IV: Bicornuate uterus		Partial fusion failure (upper uterus); deeply notched serosal fundal contour; cavities separated by myometrial tissue	Highest risk of cervical incompetence
V: Septate uterus		Fusion complete but medial wall persists (partial or complete); smooth or minimally indented fundal contour	Highest risk of recurrent spontaneous abortions
VI: Arcuate uterus		Mildest 'anomaly'; smooth or convex outer fundal contour; broad-based myometrial bulge on fundal endometrium	Questionable impact on reproductive function
VII: DES uterus		Global uterine hypoplasia; segmental cavity dilatations/constrictions	DES daughters exposed 1940s–1970s; vaginal/cervical abnormalities predictive of upper tract malformations

Diagrams reproduced with permission from Figs 21–26 in Karasick and Karasick.[30]
*Diagram shows Subtype I-C as an example of this class.

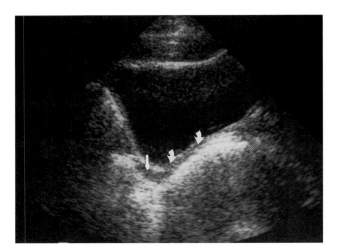

Figure 5.4 Uterine agenesis (Type I-C). Sagittal midline transabdominal sonogram shows normal vagina (curved arrows), small cervix (straight arrow), and absent uterus.

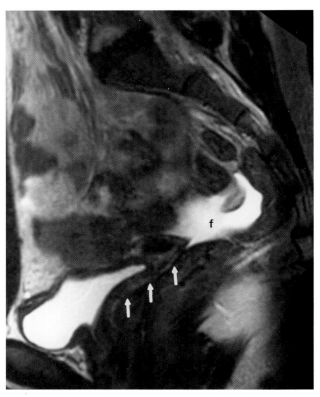

Figure 5.5 Uterine agenesis (Type I-C). Sagittal midline T2-weighted MRI shows normal vagina (arrows) with absent cervix and uterus. Free fluid (**f**) is seen posteriorly. Both ovaries and kidneys were present.

uterus, tube) may occur either in isolation or, more often, in combination. This relatively uncommon class of anomalies accounts for approximately 5% of MDAs and usually presents clinically with primary amenorrhea[31] (*Figs 5.4* and *5.5*). Vaginal agenesis is the most common subtype, and is often accompanied by uterine agenesis. On ultrasound or MRI, this anomaly is characterized by hematocolpos, rudimentary or absent uterus, and normal ovaries. Transperineal sonography may be used to define the distance between the caudal-most aspect of the vagina and the perineum for presurgical planning.[32,33] MRI has also been useful for delineating agenetic and/or obstructed segments.[34]

Women with acquired uterine hypoplasia due to drugs, pelvic irradiation, or ovarian failure may have a disproportionately small uterine corpus. In these patients, the ratio of the uterine body to the cervix is reduced to less than the normal 2:1, similar to a pre-menarchal uterus (*Fig. 5.6*).

Unicornuate uterus (Class II). This MDA consists of one normally developed Müllerian duct, with the contralateral duct either hypoplastic (Subtypes IIa, b, and c) or absent (Subtype IId). Types IIa–c comprise approximately 90% of cases.[17,35] Clinical complications include cyclic pain, intrauterine growth retardation, and preterm labor. A potentially lethal complication is uterine rupture, which can occur if a pregnancy implants in a rudimentary horn (Types II-B and II-C).[36]

Hysterosalpingography of this MDA reveals a banana-shaped cavity that is laterally flexed toward the devel-

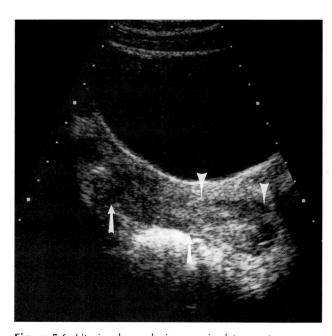

Figure 5.6 Uterine hypoplasia, acquired (premature ovarian failure). Sagittal transabdominal sonogram shows variant of hypoplasia, infantile uterus, wherein corpus and fundus are small (length marked by arrows) relative to the cervix (length marked by arrowheads). The transverse diameter of the fundus was < 4 cm.

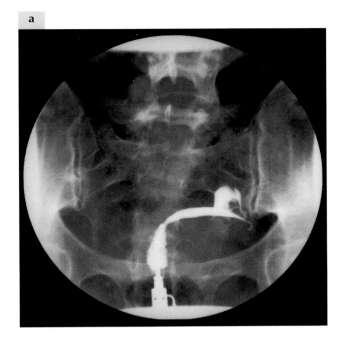

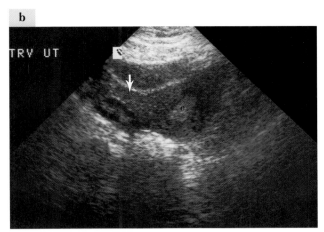

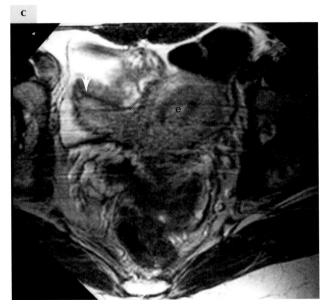

Figure 5.7 Left unicornuate uterus (Type II-C). (a) HSG shows uterine cavity deviated toward left side, with patent left fallopian tube (note similarity of uterine shape to Fig. 5.3a). (b) Transverse transabdominal sonogram shows single uterine cavity (**e**). Isoechoic tissue in the right cornual region (arrow) represents the rudimentary right horn, although this was mistaken for a fibroid. This patient also had right renal agenesis. (c) Axial T2-weighted MRI shows rudimentary right horn (arrow) without endometrium and normally formed left horn (**e**).

oped side (*Fig. 5.7a*). If the rudimentary horn is either non-communicating or lacks a cavity (Types IIb and c), it will not be detected by HSG. Sonographic findings, which are often subtle and easily overlooked, include a small uterine cavity, an asymmetric ellipsoid fundal shape, and lateral deviation of the uterus[20,37] (*Fig. 5.8*). If the rudimentary horn is present without a cavity, it may be mistaken for a fibroid or the broad ligament (see *Fig. 5.7b* and *c*). MRI findings are similar to those seen with ultrasound, but cavity detection in the rudimentary horn can be facilitated by using heavily T2-weighted imaging sequences to enhance endometrial conspicuity[9] (*Fig. 5.9*).

Uterus didelphys (Class III). This MDA results from complete failure of Müllerian duct fusion. It consists of two separate uterine and cervical cavities and, in 75% of cases, a longitudinal vaginal septum.[31] Uterus didelphys is the least common of uterine duplication anomalies and has the lowest incidence of reproductive dysfunction.[38,39]

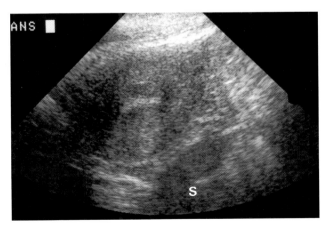

Figure 5.8 Right unicornuate uterus (Type II-C). Coronal transvaginal sonogram through uterine fundus. The uterine fundal contour has an ellipsoid shape and is displaced to the right of the spine (**s**). Although no rudimentary horn was seen by ultrasound, subsequent MRI (not shown) demonstrated a rudimentary left horn without endometrium.

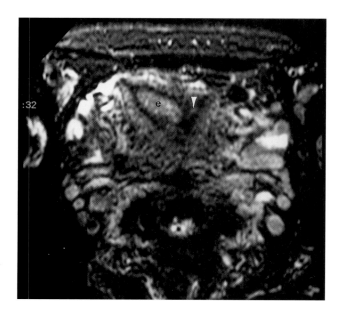

Figure 5.9 Right unicornuate uterus (Type II-A). Axial heavily T2-weighted MRI (TR:9000, TE:288) shows normal right uterine cavity (**e**) and very thin high signal left endometrial cavity (arrowhead). More caudal images showed a connection to the right side, indicating a communicating rudimentary left horn with endometrial tissue.

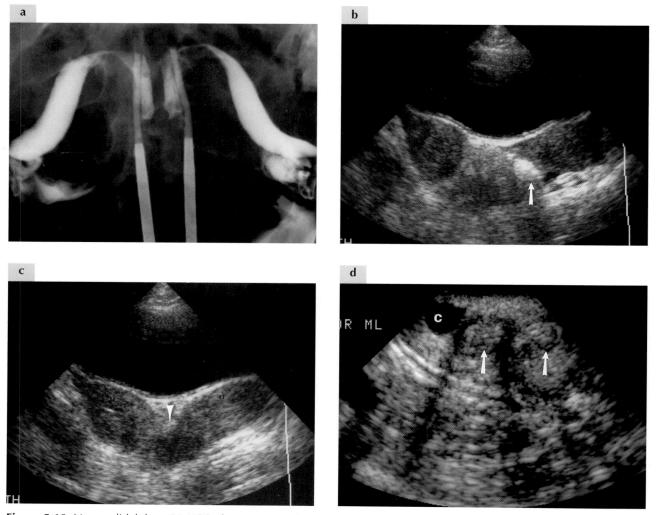

Figure 5.10 Uterus didelphys. (a) HSG shows separately cannulated cervices and widely spaced uterine cavities. (b) Transverse transabdominal sonogram shows widely separated uterine fundi with intervening bowel (arrow). (c) Transverse transabdominal sonogram caudal to (b) shows a deep cleft (arrowhead) between each hemi-uterus (**u**). (d) Coronal transvaginal sonogram at the level of the cervix shows two separate cervical stripes (arrows), indicating that this is a uterus didelphys. A nabothian cyst (**c**) is seen to the right.

With this MDA, HSG will clearly delineate the two separate uterine cavities if each cervix can be cannulated (*Fig. 5.10a*). In a small percentage of cases, however, the vaginal septum may prevent cannulation of one cervical canal, leading to the appearance of a unicornuate uterus (see *Fig. 5.3a*). Sonographic images reveal two widely spaced uterine fundi with myometrium and a deep cleft separating the two endometrial cavities (*Fig. 5.10b* and *c*). Two separate cervices may not be visible, since endocervical echoes are less prominent than endometrial echoes, but transvaginal imaging can demonstrate this finding better (*Fig. 5.10d*). Sonography is also useful for demonstrating hematocolpos, hematometra, and endometriosis in cases missed by HSG owing to an obstructing vaginal septum. Several series have noted a tendency for the right hemi-uterus to obstruct, in association with right renal agenesis[40] (see *Fig. 5.3a–d*). MRI is best performed with multiplanar scans. To improve visualization of the fundal contour, coronal images should be obtained in a plane parallel to the tubal ostia and internal os. MR findings are similar to those of sonography, with a deep separating cleft (> 3 cm) between the two uterine fundi.[41] The widely spaced uterine horns have an obtuse intercornual angle (usually > 110°), although occasional overlap with a bicornuate anomaly exists. Separate cervices and a vaginal septum (if present) can be demonstrated by caudal axial T2-weighted sections (*Fig. 5.11*).

Bicornuate uterus (Class IV). A bicornuate uterus results from partial failure of Müllerian duct fusion, leading to two separate uterine fundi joined either at the uterine corpus (bicornis unicollis subtype) or lower uterine segment (bicornis bicollis subtype).[23] In most cases there is a single cervix; however, since fusion failure may persist to the level of the cervix, there may be two cervical openings, creating an appearance similar to a patient with a septate uterus (Class V, see below). Of all classes of MDAs, it is the bicornuate uterus that has the strongest association with cervical incompetence.[39] It is crucial to differentiate between a bicornuate and septate uterus because (a) surgical correction of a bicornuate uterus is not generally warranted (since it is the cervical incompetence and not the cavity malformation that is the cause of the high spontaneous abortion rate with this anomaly), and (b) an abdominal metroplasty must be performed if surgical repair of a bicornuate uterus is undertaken, as opposed to hysteroscopic septoplasty (which is performed for a septate uterus).[42,43]

Hysterosalpingography of a bicornuate uterus will demonstrate separate uterine cavities with an intercornual angle that usually exceeds 105° (*Fig. 5.12*). With this imaging modality, however, the outer uterine contour cannot be evaluated, and overlap with the appearance of a septate uterus can occur (compare *Figs 5.12* and *5.15*). Not surprisingly, comparative studies of HSG and laparoscopy show

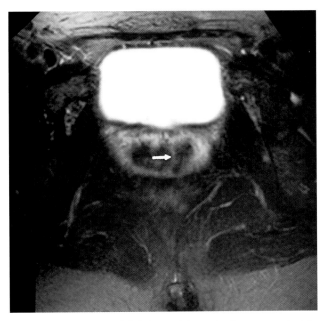

Figure 5.11 Uterus didelphys with vaginal septum. Axial T2-weighted MRI through level of upper vagina shows a thin longitudinal septum (arrow).

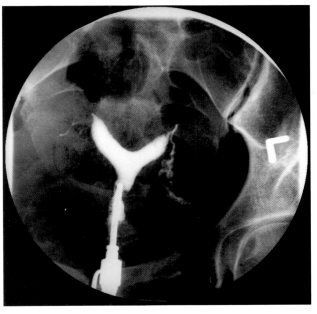

Figure 5.12 Bicornuate uterus. HSG shows widely splayed uterine horns (intercornual angle = 105°) consistent with bicornuate uterus.

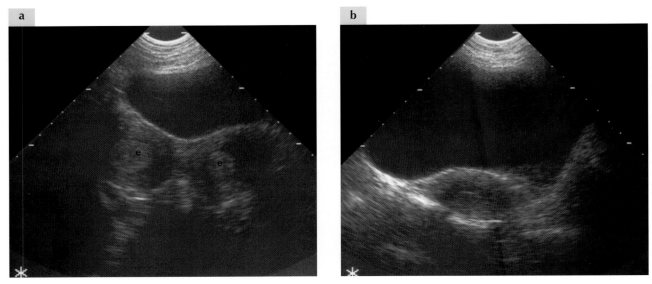

Figure 5.13 Bicornuate uterus. Transverse transabdominal sonogram (a) shows separation of uterine fundal endometria (**e**) with deep intercornual notch (note similarity to Fig. 5.10c). More caudal transverse image (b) through lower uterine segment shows a single cavity.

that the incidence of bicornuate uteri has been overestimated by HSG-based series due to inclusion of cases of septate uteri.[38,44] Sonographic diagnosis of a bicornuate uterus is made by analysis of both the outer fundal contour as well as visualization of a separate endometrial stripe in each horn. Sonographic criteria for making this diagnosis include fundal broadening (anteroposterior/transverse fundal ratio of ≤ 0.6), diverging endometrial cavities, and a fundal notch depth > 1 cm[20,45,46] (*Fig. 5.13a* and *b*). Despite these guidelines, sonographic differentiation of a bicornuate uterus from a septate uterus may be difficult. To optimize imaging of the fundal contour, transvaginal scans should be performed. An additional sonographic feature that is sometimes helpful for distinguishing between these anomalies is the echotexture of the tissue separating the two endometrial cavities. With a bicornuate uterus, the dividing tissue (muscular) is thick and isoechoic to the rest of the myometrium, whereas with a septate uterus the tissue (fibrous) is thin and hypoechoic[37] (compare *Fig. 5.2a* with *Fig. 5.16a* and *b*). Unfortunately, because septal tissue may contain both muscular and fibrous elements, reliance on this feature alone can be misleading.[47]

MRI diagnostic criteria are similar to those described for sonography. Imaging should be performed during the secretory phase to maximize contrast between the T2 signal of endometrium (bright), the junctional zone (dark), and the myometrium (medium intensity)[48] (*Fig. 5.14a–c*). On transaxial images, the intercornual distance exceeds 4 cm, and the tissue dividing the endometrial cavities is isointense with normal myometrium.[35,49] On coronal images of the

fundus, obtained in the plane of the tubal ostia, the serosal concavity exceeds 1 cm. Finally, careful attention should be given to the uterine–cervical junction to determine the most caudal extent of separation of the two uterine cavities.

Septate uterus (Class V). Septate uterus results from failure of resorption of the medial tissue following complete Müllerian duct fusion. In the majority of cases the midline septum is partial and extends for a variable distance from the fundus into the corpus or lower uterus segment (subseptate uterus) (see *Figs 5.1* and *5.18*). Less commonly, the septum extends to the level of the cervix, forming a complete septate uterus[45] (*Figs 5.15–5.17*). With a complete septate uterus, there may be two cervical openings, but this is owing to division of one canal, and not two separate cervices as occurs with a uterus didelphys (compare *Fig. 5.10d* with *Fig. 5.17*). Of all the MDAs, septate uterus has the highest association with recurrent spontaneous abortion.[50]

Hysterosalpingography of a septate uterus typically demonstrates two narrowly diverging cavities, yielding a V-shape configuration with relatively straight medial borders (*Fig. 5.15*). The angle formed by the medial borders of the two uterine hemi-cavities is usually $< 75°$, although some investigators have used 60° as a cut-off value.[44,45] Unfortunately, diagnosis of a septate uterus is often not possible by HSG because angle measurements may be difficult, the outer uterine contour cannot be imaged, and cannulation of one portion of the cavity may not be possible. To complicate matters even more, some septate uteri diverge by angles that exceed 75°.[15]

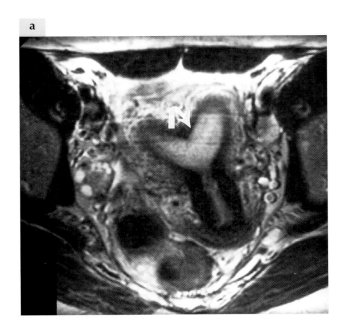

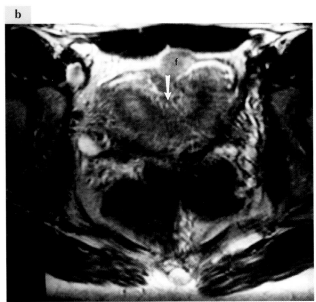

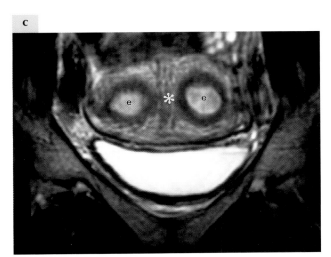

Figure 5.14 Bicornuate uterus. Coronal (a,b) and axial (c) T2-weighted MRI shows: (a) wide intercornual angle (curved arrow), (b) deep fundal cleft (arrow), and (c) medium intensity signal to the myometrial tissue (asterisk) dividing the two endometrial cavities (**e**), indicating a bicornuate uterus. Note in (b) the incidental subserosal fibroid (**f**) in the intercornual cleft.

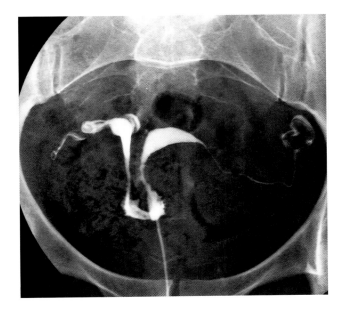

Figure 5.15 Complete septate uterus. HSG shows complete division of uterine cavity into two portions with a V-shaped configuration, narrow intercornual angle, and straightened medial borders. (Courtesy of IC Yoder MD, Massachusetts General Hospital, Boston, MA, USA.)

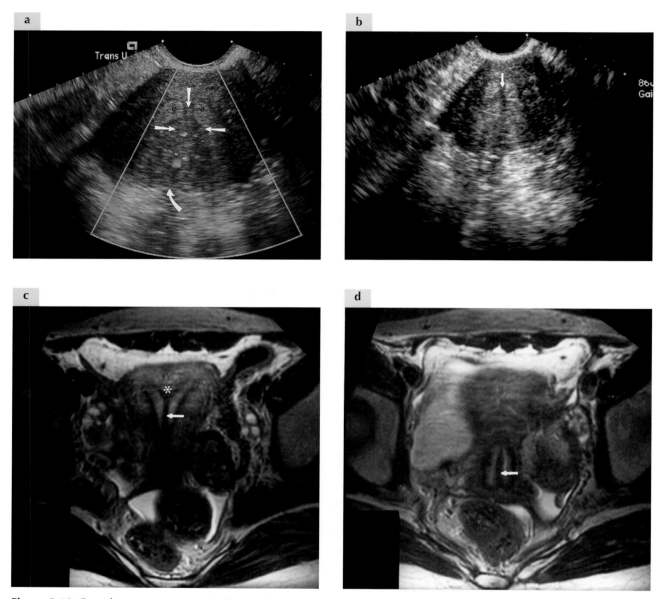

Figure 5.16 Complete septate uterus with mixed muscular/fibrous septum. (a) Coronal transvaginal color Doppler sonogram of retroverted uterine fundus shows fundal broadening, shallow fundal concavity (curved arrow), and splitting of endometrium (**e**) by septum. The upper portion of the septum (between straight arrows) is vascularized myometrial tissue (note color signals). (b) The lower portion of the septum (arrow) is hypoechoic avascular fibrous tissue. (c,d) Coronal T2-weighted MRI of uterine fundus in the same patient shows high signal myometrium (asterisk) forming upper muscular portion of septum in the fundus. The low signal portion of the septum in the corpus is fibrous (arrow) and continues (d) into the cervix (arrow).

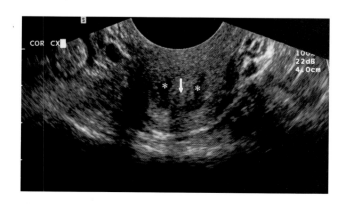

Figure 5.17 Complete septate uterus: cervix. Coronal transvaginal sonogram of cervical septum in a patient with a complete septate uterus. Small amounts of fluid in the split cervical canal (asterisks) outline the thick midline septum (arrow). Compare with Fig. 5.10d (double cervix of uterus didelphys).

a

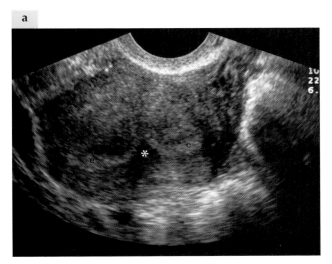

b

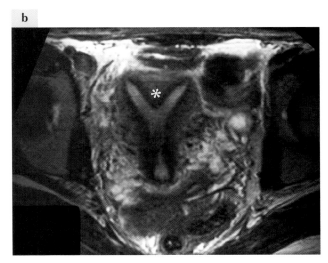

Figure 5.18 Subseptate uterus with muscular septum. (a) Coronal transvaginal sonogram of retroverted fundus shows fundal broadening, flat fundal contour and splaying of endometrial stripe (e) by hypoechoic septum (asterisk). The remainder of the cavity appeared normal. (b) Coronal MRI of uterus in same patient shows smooth outer contour and isointense muscular partial septum (asterisk). Uterine corpus and cervix are normal. In this case the sonographic appearance did not accurately predict the septal composition.

Sonography and MRI are each superior to HSG for diagnosing this MDA because these modalities permit evaluation of the outer uterine contour as well as the dividing septum. With a septate uterus the outer uterine contour is usually convex or flat (*Fig. 5.18a*). Occasionally there is a shallow fundal concavity whose depth is < 1 cm (see *Fig. 5.16a*). Transabdominal ultrasound can sometimes visualize and evaluate the fundal contour if the uterus is anteverted, but transvaginal scans are required if the uterus is retroverted. Coronal MRI allows the characteristic fundal changes of a septate uterus to be identified (e.g. flat or mildly concave serosal surface, intercornual distance < 4 cm)[35] (see *Figs 5.16c* and *5.18b*).

In addition to fundal contour, a second sonographic feature of a septate uterus is splitting of the endometrial echo by a hypoechoic band, most easily seen in the fundus (see *Figs 5.1d* and *5.16a* and *b*). Since it is often quite thin, this septum may easily be overlooked; however, since the presence of endometrial fluid facilitates visualization of subtle endometrial cavity changes (*Fig. 5.19*), sonohysterography will enhance septal detection.[51] In patients with a septate uterus, septal characterization should be attempted to assist surgical planning. Avascular fibrous septa can be safely resected hysteroscopically, whereas vascularized myometrial tissue within the septum requires a more invasive abdominal approach.[38,42] Based upon a single prospective sonographic report, a fibrous septum can be suggested when its echotexture is less than myometrial tissue, whereas muscular septal tissue is suggested when the

septum is isoechoic to myometrial echoes.[37] Unfortunately, refractive shadowing limits the ability of sonography to distinguish between fibrous and myometrial tissue (compare *Figs 5.18a* and *b*). On MRI with T2-weighting, fibrous tissue has a low signal equal to that obtained from the junctional zone, while muscular septal tissue has a medium intensity signal.[37,41,52] Since septal tissue is frequently both fibrous and muscular, MRI is the preferred modality for preoperative planning.

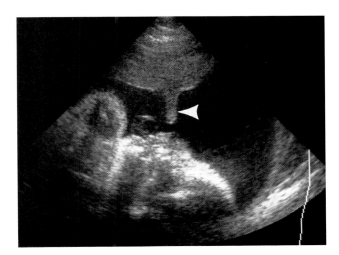

Figure 5.19 Subseptate uterus in pregnancy. Transverse transabdominal sonogram through fundus in patient with 28-week gestation shows partial septum (arrowhead) outlined by amniotic fluid. Fetal face and umbilical cord are just posterior to the septum.

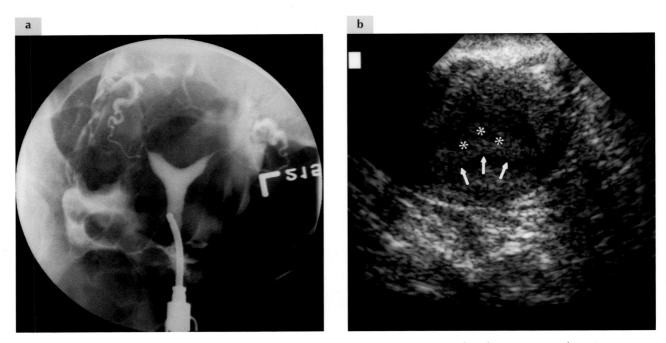

Figure 5.20 Arcuate uterus. (a) HSG shows saddle-shaped fundal cavity contour and wide separation of uterine cornua. Note the similarity of the uterine cavity outline to Fig. 5.12. (b) Coronal transvaginal sonogram through retroverted fundus in secretory phase of menstrual cycle shows smooth impression (arrows) on endometrial stripe (asterisks), with normal serosal contour, indicating arcuate uterus (contrast this appearance with the more angular indentation in a septate uterus, Figs 5.1b, 5.16a, and 5.18a).

Arcuate uterus (Class VI). Formerly, this MDA was classified as the mildest form of either a bicornuate or a septate uterus. In 1988, in an attempt to facilitate tracking patients with reproductive complications, the American Fertility Society issued a separate classification of 'arcuate' uterus.[11] Despite this effort, lack of precise diagnostic characterization has led to continued confusion. Some observers persist in considering complications of this mild anomaly to be similar to those associated with bicornuate and septate uterus; others, however, consider the arcuate uterus to be a normal variant without clinical consequences.[14,18,53,54]

Hysterographic examination of the arcuate uterus reveals a broad smooth indentation into the fundal cavity which causes a 'saddle-shaped' appearance (*Fig. 5.20a*). The indentation is approximately one-fifth the height of the uterus and results in > 100° separation of the cornua.[55] In contrast, septate or bicornuate uteri have a more V-shaped indentation and more acutely angled cornua (see *Fig. 5.15*).

Both MRI and sonography reveal a smooth outer fundal contour, associated with a subtle broad-based shallow indentation impressing the endometrial stripe (*Figs 5.20b* and *5.21*). Cephalad coronal trans-

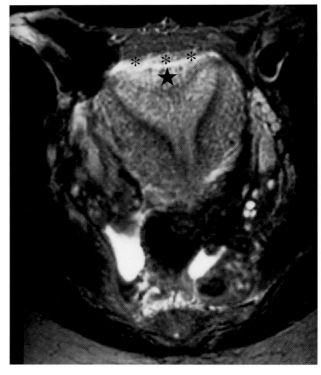

Figure 5.21 Arcuate uterus. Coronal T2-weighted MRI shows broad smooth indentation (star) on fundal endometrium and flat serosal contour (asterisks).

vaginal sonographic images may show lateral divergence of the endometrial stripe[4] (see *Fig. 5.20b*). Although the absence of serosal fundal contour depression may be appreciated by both sonography and MRI, distinguishing this entity from a normal uterus is often difficult.

DES-related uterine anomalies (Class VII)

Definition and pathophysiology

Between 1940 and 1970 diethylstilbestrol (DES), a synthetic estrogen, was administered to approximately 2 million pregnant women to prevent early spontaneous abortion. This drug caused characteristic genital tract abnormalities in the daughters of women who took it during their pregnancy. Most likely as a result of DES disrupting vaginal plate development and stromal differentiation, structural anomalies occurred in the fetal vagina, cervix, uterus, and tubes.[56]

The most common structural anomalies, encountered at physical examination, are vaginal adenosis and the presence of an anterior cervical ridge or hood. These physical findings should prompt the clinician to evaluate the patient for upper tract abnormalities.[57] Uterine cavity anomalies associated with DES exposure include hypoplasia, focal constrictions, bulbous dilatation of the lower uterine segment, and a T-shaped uterine configuration.[4,39] These uterine anomalies are associated with an increased incidence of spontaneous abortion, preterm labor, and ectopic pregnancy.[58]

Imaging

Hysterosalpingography is an excellent imaging modality for diagnosing DES-related uterine anomalies.[57] Typical cavity contour changes seen include scalloping and constriction bands, while uterine shape abnormalities are hypoplasia, T-configuration, and a bulbous lower uterine segment (*Fig. 5.22*).

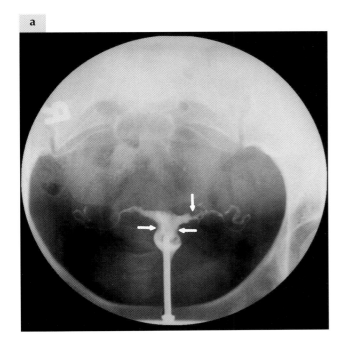

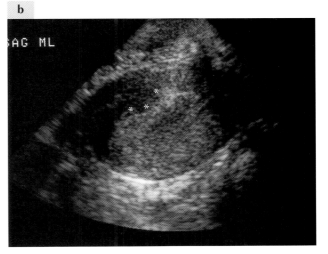

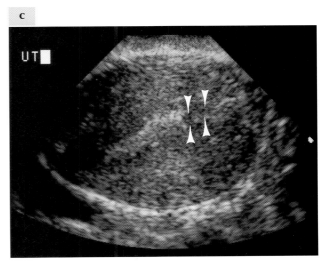

Figure 5.22 DES uterus (constrictions). (a) HSG shows left cornual and mid-cavity constrictions (arrows) in this infertility patient exposed to DES. Sagittal (b) and coronal (c) transvaginal sonograms on same patient as (a) show undulating endometrial stripe with relative narrowing in corpus (asterisks) and left cornual constriction (arrowheads).

To date, there has been a paucity of reported ultrasound or MRI studies to detect DES-related uterine changes. Most likely, this reflects relatively subtle findings on these examinations. One investigation, involving transabdominal ultrasound examinations on 18 DES-exposed women, noted a significant reduction in uterine volume in all patients and a lack of normal fundal expansion in three[5] (*Fig. 5.23*). Another study emphasized the importance of transvaginal imaging in the secretory phase to maximize detection of subtle cavity constrictions[60] (see *Fig 5.22b* and *c*). A comparative study of five DES-exposed women who were examined by MRI and HSG reported good imaging correlation for detecting cervical, uterine and cavity hypoplasia, uterine cavity constrictions, and T-shaped uterine morphology.[61] Mild contour abnormalities demonstrated on HSG were not visible on MRI imaging.

Although the number of women with DES-related anomalies will decline as the affected population ages, the fact that fewer diagnostic HSG examinations are currently performed may limit detection of uterine findings if only non-invasive imaging is done. This is particularly true with respect to sonography, as changes in uterine shape, endometrial thickness and configuration may be extremely subtle. Sonohysterography may potentially be useful to detect some of these findings. It is incumbent upon clinicians to be aware of current imaging limitations associated with ultrasound and possibly MRI, and to request an HSG if DES-related anomalies are suspected.

Asherman syndrome (intrauterine adhesions)

Definition and pathophysiology

This syndrome is defined by the combination of infertility, hypomenorrhea or amenorrhea, and a history of uterine curettage. It is estimated to occur in 68% of infertile women who have undergone two or more curettages and is seen in 1.5% of infertile women undergoing hysterosalpingography.[62] The pathophysiology consists of intrauterine adhesions (synechiae) that develop after traumatic endometrial injury, such as post-partum or post-abortion uterine curettage. Less commonly, it results from endometritis.[63] It is hypothesized that infertility occurs because uterine adhesions and scarring interfere with sperm migration and embryo implantation.

Imaging

Although hysteroscopy is considered the 'gold standard' for both diagnosis and treatment of intrauterine adhesions, imaging plays a role whenever cervical or lower uterine adhesions do not allow passage of a hysteroscope.

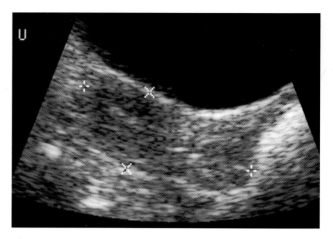

Figure 5.23 DES uterus (hypoplasia). Sagittal midline transabdominal sonogram shows mild diffuse uterine hypoplasia with loss of normal bulbous expansion of fundus. The uterine length was only 6 cm.

Typical HSG findings include multiple, irregular, angular, or serpiginous filling defects within the uterine cavity and reduced cavity volume[5,26] (*Fig. 5.24*). The filling defects are easily differentiated from the smoother and rounder filling defects seen with polyps or submucosal fibroids.

Ultrasound and MRI are not helpful in diagnosing a solitary uterine synechia in the nongravid uterus.

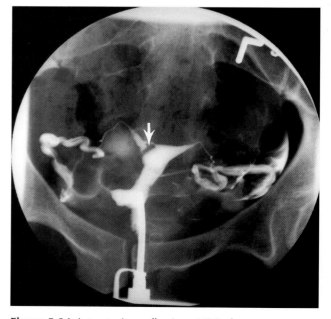

Figure 5.24 Intrauterine adhesion. HSG shows serpiginous filling defect in right cornual region (arrow), consistent with an adhesion. The cavity in the right lower uterine segment is a post-myomectomy scar. Neither abnormality was seen on transvaginal ultrasound.

During early pregnancy, however, sonography can detect an adhesion by demonstrating a linear indentation into the gestational sac.[64] Later in pregnancy, amniotic fluid facilitates detection of a synechia. It can be distinguished from the more serious amniotic bands by its rounded free edge and broad base at the uterine wall. Uterine synechiae are associated with malpresentation, leading to a higher rate of cesarean section, but other obstetric complications have not been found.[65]

In the nongravid patient, sonohysterography can demonstrate synechiae, and it may prove superior to HSG by its ability to detect fine filmy adhesions that dense radiographic contrast may obscure.[5] Conventional transvaginal ultrasound done during the secretory phase of the cycle can also diagnose intrauterine adhesions by noting subtle alterations in the endometrial thickness and homogeneity, and by detecting changes in the sharpness of the endometrial–myometrial interface (*Fig. 5.25a*). Using this approach to examine women with recurrent spontaneous abortion, one group of investigators correctly identified synechiae in 10 of 11 patients.[66] In that study, adhesions could be differentiated from polyps (which were hyperechoic and more distinctly demarcated from the underlying myometrium) and submucosal fibroids (which had variable echogenicity and were contiguous with the myometrium). MRI, using heavily T2-weighted sequences, can diagnose Asherman syndrome by revealing complete absence of the normal high signal endometrium in severe cases, or thin low signal bands traversing the endometrial or cervical canal in less severe cases[62] (*Fig. 5.25b*).

Myometrial abnormalities

Fibroids

Definition and pathophysiology

Uterine fibroids or leiomyomas are the most common neoplasm of the female genital tract, affecting 15–25% of women of reproductive age.[67] These tumors fluctuate in size depending on estrogen levels: they enlarge during early pregnancy and ovulation induction, and regress following delivery, in menopause, and during gonadotropin-releasing hormone analog therapy. Mechanisms proposed to explain the relationship of fibroids to reproductive dysfunction include mechanical blockage of the cervix or tubal ostia, interference with implantation, preterm labor, and increased risk of placental abruption.[68] Submucosal fibroids are thought to interfere with implantation, whereas subserosal or large intramural fibroids alter the relationship between fallopian tube and ovary, thus affecting egg transport into the tube following ovulation. Despite their prevalence, however, fibroids should not be assumed to be a primary cause of infertility; full investigation of other potential causal factors should be made. While several series have shown an improvement in fertility following myomectomy,[69–71] the risk of adhesion formation (especially after abdominal myomectomy) is high, indicating a need for caution before surgery is performed.[72,73]

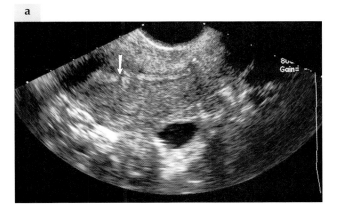

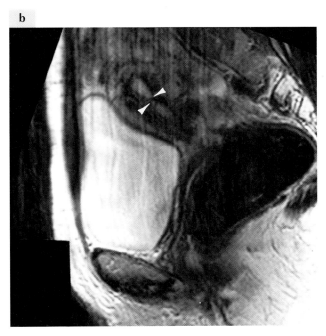

Figure 5.25 Intrauterine adhesion. (a) Sagittal transvaginal sonogram shows linear discontinuity in the endometrial stripe in the fundus (arrow). (b) Sagittal T2-weighted MRI scan shows linear interruption (arrowheads) of the normal high signal endometrium in the same location, consistent with an adhesion. (Although phase encoding artifacts are seen on this image, the focal endometrial discontinuity was present in the same location on all images.)

Imaging

HSG has limited usefulness in the evaluation of uterine fibroids. Sonography, on the other hand, has consistently demonstrated accuracy, speed, low cost, and better patient acceptance for evaluation of this condition. With ultrasound, fibroids can be localized as submucosal, intramural, or subserosal fibroids, whereas HSG is generally limited to detecting submucosal fibroids.

The most common sonographic appearance for a fibroid is a well-circumscribed, hypoechoic, sound-attenuating mass (*Figs 5.26* and *5.27*). Fibroids usually contain calcium or, rarely, fat. They may undergo degeneration and develop cystic or hemorrhagic areas.[74] Cystic degeneration usually begins centrally. It may occur during progestin or leuprolide therapy, or during pregnancy[67] (*Fig. 5.28*). Carneous degeneration, or acute hemorrhagic infarction, may follow a period of rapid growth, such as during early pregnancy (*Fig. 5.29*).

Small submucosal fibroids, which comprise 4–18% of all fibroids,[75] cause a focal hypoechoic indentation on the endometrial stripe and are best detected by transvaginal ultrasound during the periovulatory or secretory phase of the menstrual cycle (see *Fig. 5.27a* and *b*). Pedunculated fibroids may be confused with

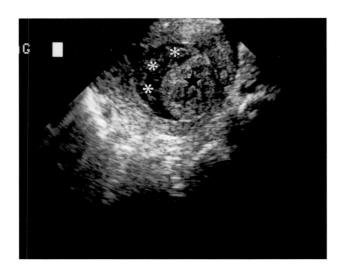

Figure 5.26 Intracavitary fibroid. Sagittal transvaginal sonogram shows an intracavitary heterogeneous mass (star) outlined by blood (asterisks). This somewhat atypical fibroid mimics a large endometrial polyp both in its location and echotexture.

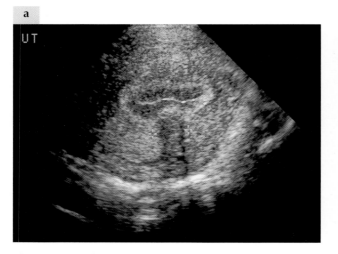 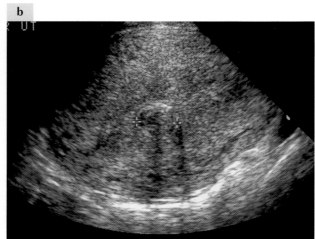

Figure 5.27 Submucosal fibroid in different phases of menstrual cycle. Coronal transvaginal sonogram of a small submucosal fibroid (calipers) was obtained in the same patient during different phases of the menstrual cycle. In (a) the patient was periovulatory, with a multi-layered endometrial stripe; in (b) she was perimenstrual, with a poorly defined stripe. The mass effect of the fibroid on the endometrium, and hence the conspicuity, is more apparent in (a). Note also the posterior acoustic shadowing and the contiguity of the mass with the myometrium, both features typical of a fibroid.

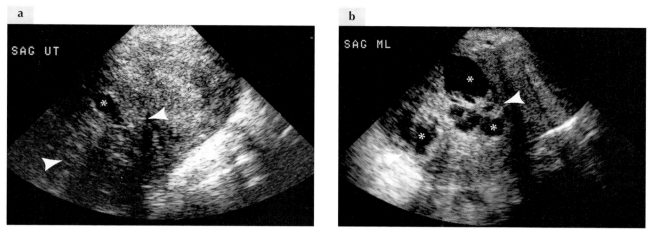

Figure 5.28 Cystic fibroid degeneration during ovulation induction therapy. Sagittal midline transvaginal sonogram of a retroverted uterus initially (a) shows a large subserosal fibroid (arrowheads) with a small fluid component (asterisk). The endometrium is marked by (**e**). The fibroid becomes progressively more cystic following one cycle of ovulation induction (b).

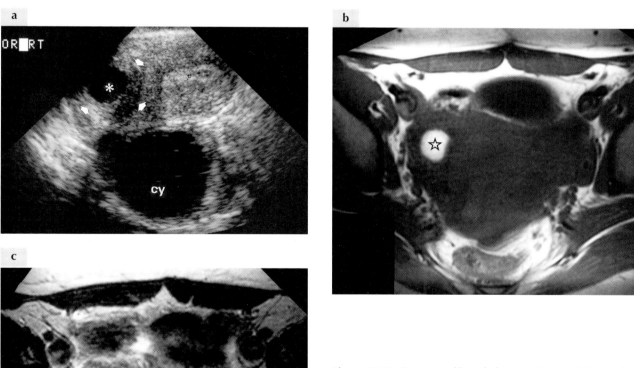

Figure 5.29 Carneous fibroid degeneration. (a) Coronal transvaginal sonogram shows a thick-walled right cornual mass (arrows) with a central complex fluid component (asterisk) that contained low level echoes. A right ovarian cyst (**cy**) is seen posterior to the fundus (**e**). (b,c) Axial T1-weighted MRI (b) shows hyperintense area (star) in center of right cornual mass which remains high signal on T2-weighted sequence (c). This area, which did not suppress with fat saturation sequences, corresponds to blood products in the center of a subserosal fibroid undergoing carneous degeneration. Normal high signal from fundal endometrium (**e**) is also seen.

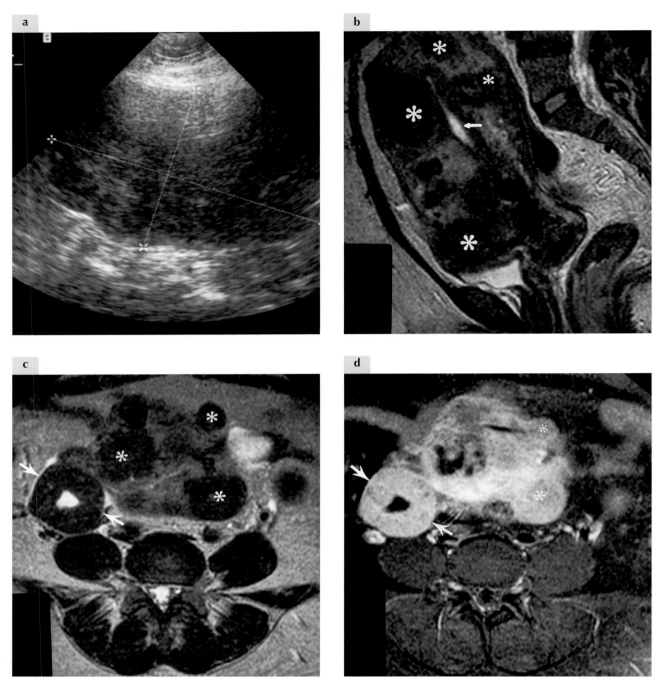

Figure 5.30 Multifibroid uterus. (a) Sagittal midline transabdominal sonogram shows enlarged heterogeneous uterus (outlined by measuring calipers) consistent with fibroids, but location and number of fibroids and the status of the endometrial cavity cannot be determined. (Transvaginal sonogram was equally unrevealing.) (b) Sagittal T2-weighted MRI shows multiple low signal intramural masses (asterisks) consistent with fibroids, as well as a normal high signal endometrial cavity (small arrow). (c,d) Axial T2-weighted image (c) through the fundus shows other low signal fibroids (asterisks) and a low intensity right subserosal mass (arrows) with a central high signal focus. Following intravenous gadolinium a T1 axial image through the same level (d) shows this mass (arrows) enhancing equally with the rest of the myometrium (asterisks), indicating that this is a subserosal fibroid. Note that the central portion is now low signal (i.e. fluid), consistent with cystic degeneration of this fibroid.

solid adnexal masses, but recognition of their typical sonographic texture coupled with identification of both ovaries as separate from the mass will usually help establish the correct diagnosis. In difficult cases, use of color Doppler to identify a feeding vessel that arises from the uterus may also be useful.[76]

MRI is also accurate for identifying and localizing fibroids.[77,78] Owing to the high cost of this modality, however, use of MRI is reserved for the following situations: (a) presurgical planning for selective myomectomy or for nonsurgical ablation (i.e. embolization, cryotherapy) when diffuse distribution limits sonographic visualization (*Fig. 5.30*); (b) differentiation of adenomyosis from fibroids (see next section); and (c) characterization of a sonographically atypical fibroid. MRI provides accurate three-dimensional information that can be used for pre-operative planning where volumetric information determines the therapeutic approach (laparoscopy, hysterotomy, or nonsurgical ablation).[79] On MR images, a typical fibroid has low signal on both T1- and T2-weighted images (*Fig. 5.30b*, and see *Fig. 5.33a* in next section); hyaline degeneration may cause interspersed areas of high signal on T2-weighted sequences.[80] As fluid content increases due to cystic degeneration, areas of confluent high signal become evident on T2 sequences (*Fig. 5.30c*); this is in contrast to areas of calcification, which show a signal void on all sequences. Carneous ('red') degeneration varies in its appearance because hemoglobin may have high signal on T1- and variable intensity on T2-weighting (see *Fig. 5.29b* and *c*).

Adenomyosis

Definition and pathophysiology

Adenomyosis is an elusive condition of unknown etiology, detected in 8–31% of hysterectomy specimens. It is defined by the presence of ectopic endometrial glands in the myometrium (at least 4 mm beneath the endomyometrial junction) which are surrounded by hypertrophied smooth muscle.[81,82] Adenomyosis typically affects the uterus in a diffuse manner; but when focal disease is present, adenomyomas result. Although this condition is not generally associated with infertility, it is important to distinguish adenomyosis from fibroids, because only the latter can be selectively resected.[83] In severe cases of generalized adenomyosis, hysterectomy may be indicated.

Imaging

In cases of extensive adenomyosis, HSG reveals glandular filling within myometrial tissue (*Fig. 5.31a*). This finding is present in only 25% of patients, however, since the ectopic glands often do not communicate with the uterine cavity. Subtle findings associated with localized disease may be overlooked or mistaken for venous intravasation.[82]

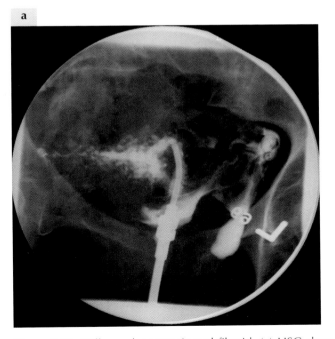
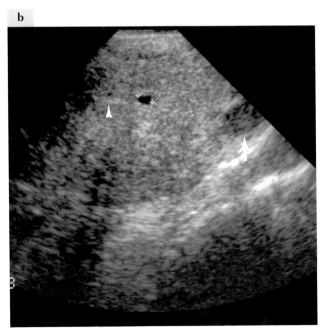

Figure 5.31 Diffuse adenomyosis and fibroid. (a) HSG shows diffuse irregular contrast outpouchings filling deeply imbedded endometrial glands in a retroverted uterus with extensive adenomyosis. (b) Sagittal transvaginal sonogram in the same patient shows a small subendometrial cyst (denoted by calipers), representing an ectopic endometrial gland filled with fluid. The endometrial stripe (arrowhead) is thin. The remainder of the myometrium is mildly heterogeneous. The focal hypoechoic mass in the fundus is a fibroid (arrow).

Transabdominal ultrasound findings include diffuse uterine enlargement without focal abnormality, diffuse posterior myometrial thickening, and myometrial sonolucencies[84] (*Fig. 5.32*). With transvaginal imaging of the myometrium, findings of adenomyosis include diffuse heterogeneity or poorly defined hypoechoic areas (owing to smooth muscle hypertrophy) and tiny myometrial cysts (owing to dilated ectopic glands)[85] (see *Fig. 5.31b*).

In pre-menopausal women, MRI is superior to ultrasound for diagnosing adenomyosis because of its improved definition of the junctional zone, which is located at the inner subendometrial portion of myometrium (also called the basal layer of myometrium).[86] To visualize and measure the junctional zone optimally, it is important to obtain short axis views of the endometrial cavity (perpendicular to the long uterine axis). On T2-weighted images, diffuse adenomyosis demonstrates diffuse junctional zone thickening (> 12 mm) that is due to hyperplastic smooth muscle surrounding the ectopic glands.[87] Specificity for diffuse adenomyosis is increased when punctate high signal foci, owing to the ectopic glands themselves, are seen within the thickened junctional zone (*Fig. 5.33*). Fibroids can often be distinguished from adenomyomas because the former are round and well-marginated, while the latter are oval and poorly defined.[80] Two recent series that compared transvaginal sonography with MRI for distinguishing adenomyosis from fibroids found higher sensitivity and specificity for MRI.[81,88].

Uterine motility

Definition and pathophysiology
Imaging of normal cervico-fundal uterine peristaltic contractions is accomplished by continuous videotaping of the uterus during transvaginal sonography. In the late proliferative phase of the menstrual cycle, contractions normally increase in frequency and intensity, and are preferentially directed toward the tubal ostium that contains the developing follicle.[89,90] In some infertile women and in those with mild endometriosis, there is hyperperistalsis in the early follicular and midluteal phases, while at mid-cycle the waves may appear disorganized and non-directional. This abnormal response may explain failure of sperm transport in these patients, and it may also be responsible for spreading peritoneal endometriosis.[91]

Imaging
In addition to documenting uterine peristalsis with continuous real-time vaginal sonography, radionuclide hysterosalpingography may be done as an alternative method, using sperm size macrospheres of labeled albumin placed within the

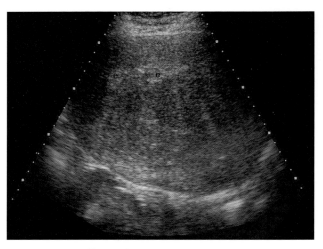

Figure 5.32 Diffuse adenomyosis. Transverse transabdominal sonogram through the fundus of the uterus shows severe global enlargement (uterine length was 20 cm) with diffuse thickening of the posterior myometrium without a discrete mass. Endometrial stripe (**e**) is normal.

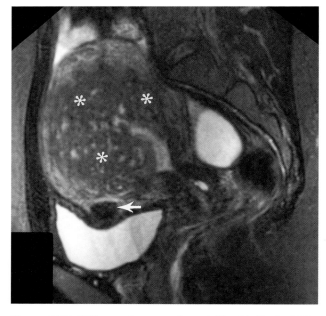

Figure 5.33 Diffuse adenomyosis and fibroid. Sagittal T2-weighted MRI with fat saturation shows diffuse junctional zone thickening (asterisks) with punctate high signal foci scattered throughout, indicating extensive adenomyosis. The focal well-demarcated low signal mass in the anterior corpus (arrow) is a fibroid. A left ovarian simple cyst is present in the cul-de-sac.

vagina. Using this method, it is possible to demonstrate changes in the speed with which these labeled particles reach the uterine cavity. This method can also trace the direction of movement in the fallopian tube.[90]

Conclusion

Uterine pathology is believed to be a contributing factor in up to 10% of cases of infertility; it is also associated with significant obstetric complications. With the exception of DES-related changes and Asherman syndrome, which should be evaluated by hysterosalpingography, most uterine abnormalities can be diagnosed by ultrasonography and/or magnetic resonance imaging.

While ultrasound is likely to remain the principal initial modality for investigating unexplained infertility, clinicians should understand the advantages and limitations of this form of imaging. They should also understand the particular circumstances when an MRI examination may be more appropriate.

With respect to Müllerian duct anomalies, ultrasound is reasonably sensitive in the detection of duplication anomalies such as bicornuate, septate, or didelphys uterus. In many of these cases, ultrasound can distinguish a septate from a bicornuate uterus, but it is limited in its ability to characterize the tissue that divides the two uterine cavities. For this reason, MRI should be used to evaluate these anomalies pre-operatively. MRI is the imaging modality of choice for differentiating the specific subtypes of unicornuate uterus and uterine/vaginal agenesis.

Acquired conditions that may result in infertility and/or pregnancy complications include endometrial polyps and submucosal fibroids. In most patients, transvaginal ultrasound, often in conjunction with sonohysterography, is both sensitive and specific for detection and diagnosis. In rare instances, where either body habitus or large fibroids impede sonographic imaging, MRI can be utilized. Adenomyosis, while not directly implicated in infertility, can be confused with fibroids, both clinically and during imaging. MRI is the best imaging modality for distinguishing between these two common conditions and is strongly recommended whenever there is doubt about the correct diagnosis, especially if surgical removal is being considered.

Prior to the development of these two powerful non-invasive imaging modalities, many women with uterine pathology and associated fertility problems were either not able to undergo satisfactory diagnostic evaluation or were misdiagnosed. Fortunately, as a result of increasingly sophisticated high resolution cross-sectional imaging, virtually all affected women can now be diagnosed correctly, and can often undergo appropriate corrective surgery.

REFERENCES

1. New York Times. February 22, 1998: 1,30.

2. Collins JI, Woodward PJ. Radiological evaluation of infertility. *Semin Ultrasound CT MR* 1995; **16**:304–316.

3. Lev-Toaff AS. Sonohysterography: evaluation of endometrial and myometrial abnormalities. *Semin Roentgenol* 1996; **31**:288–298.

4. Daya S. Ultrasonographic evaluation of uterine anomalies. In: Jaffe R, Pierson RA, Abramowicz JA, eds. *Imaging in Infertility and Reproductive Endocrinology.* Philadelphia: J B Lippincott, 1994:63–92.

5. Cullinan JA, Fleischer AC, Kepple DM, Arnold AL. Sonohysterography: a technique for endometrial evaluation. *Radiographics* 1995; **15**:501–514.

6. Raga F, Bonilla-Musoles F, Blanes J, Osborne NG. Congenital Müllerian anomalies: diagnostic accuracy of three-dimensional ultrasound. *Fertil Steril* 1996; **65**:523–528.

7. Wu MH, Hsu CC, Huang KE. Detection of congenital Müllerian duct anomalies using three-dimensional ultrasound. *J Clin Ultrasound* 1997; **25**:487–492.

8. Ayida G, Kennedy S, Barlow D, Chamberlain P. Contrast sonography for uterine cavity assessment: a comparison of conventional two-dimensional with three-dimensional transvaginal ultrasound; a pilot study. *Fertil Steril* 1996; **66**:848–850.

9. Tempany CM. MRI techniques and protocols. In: Tempany CM, ed. *MR and imaging of the female pelvis.* St Louis: Mosby Year Book, 1995: 55–74.

10. Woodward PJ, Wagner BJ, Farley TE. MR imaging in the evaluation of female infertility. *Radiographics* 1993; **13**:293–310.

11. American Fertility Society. The American Fertility Society classification of adnexal adhesions, distal tubal occlusion, tubal occlusion secondary to tubal ligation, tubal pregnancies, Müllerian anomalies and intrauterine adhesions. *Fertil Steril* 1988; **49**:944–955.

12. Jaffe R, Mesonero CE, Eggers PC. Ultrasonography of abnormal pelvic anatomy. In: Jaffe R, Pierson RA, Abramowicz JA, eds. *Imaging in Infertility and Reproductive Endocrinology.* Philadelphia: J B Lippincott, 1994:23–46.

13. Simon C, Martinez L, Pardo F. Tortajada M, Pellicer A. Müllerian defects in women with normal reproductive outcome. *Fertil Steril* 1991; **56**:1192–1193.

14. Makino T, Hara T, Oka C *et al.* Survey of 1120 Japanese women with a history of recurrent spontaneous abortions. *Eur J Obstet Reprod Biol* 1992; **44**:123–130.

15. Zanetti E, Ferrari LR, Rossi G. Classification and radiographic features of uterine malformations: hysterosalpingographic study. *Br J Radiol* 1978; **51**:161–170.

16. Buttram VC, Gibbons WE. Müllerian anomalies: a proposed classification (an analysis of 144 cases). *Fertil Steril* 1979; **32**:40–46.

17. Heinonen PK, Pystynen PP. Primary infertility and uterine anomalies. *Fertil Steril* 1983; **40**:311–316.

18. Acién P. Reproductive performance of women with uterine malformations. *Human Reprod* 1993; **8**:122–126.

19. Nicotra M, Stampone C, Piscitelli C, Coccia L, Orlandi A, Porfiri LM. Hysterosalpingographic abnormalities in infertile women: radiological and clinical interpretation. *Acta Eur Fertil* 1988; **19**:79–82.

20. Candiani GB, Ferazzi E, Fedele P, Vercellini P, Dorta M. Sonographic evaluation of uterine morphology: a new scanning technique. *Acta Eur Fertil* 1986; **17**:345–347.

21. Fedele L, Dorta M, Brioschi D, Guidici MN, Candiani GB. Pregnancies in septate uteri: outcome in relation to site of uterine implantation as determined by sonography. *Am J Roentgenol* 1989; **152**:781–784.

22. Daya S. The role of ultrasonography in the diagnosis and management of cervical incompetence. In: Jaffe R, Pierson RA, Abramowicz JA, eds. *Imaging in Infertility and Reproductive Endocrinology*. Philadelphia: J B Lippincott, 1994:93–115.

23. Golan A, Langer R, Bukovsky I, Caspi E. Congenital anomalies of the Müllerian system. *Fertil Steril* 1989; **51**:747–755.

24. Pinsonneault O, Goldstein DP. Obstructing malformations of the uterus and vagina. *Fertil Steril* 1985; **44**:241–247.

25. Sanfilippo JS, Wakim NG, Schikler KN, Yussman MA. Endometriosis in association with uterine anomaly. *Am J Obstet Gynecol* 1986; **154**:39–43.

26. Yoder IC, Hall DA. Hysterosalpingography in the 1990s. *Am J Roentgenol* 1991; **157**:675–683.

27. Li YW, Sheih CP, Chen WJ. Unilateral occlusion of duplicated uterus with ipsilateral renal anomaly in young girls: a study with MRI. *Pediatr Radiol* 1995; **25**:S54–S59.

28. Dabirashrafi H, Mohammed K, Moghadami-Tabrizi N. Ovarian malposition in women with uterine anomalies. *Obstet Gynecol* 1994; **83**: 293–294.

29. Rock JA, Parmley T, Murphy AA, Jones HW Jr. Malposition of the ovary associated with uterine anomalies. *Fertil Steril* 1986; **45**:561–563.

30. Karasick S, Karasick D. *Congenital Uterine Anomalies. Atlas of Hysterosalpingography*. Springfield, IL: Charles C Thomas, 1987:34–37.

31. Wagner BJ, Woodward PJ. Magnetic resonance evaluation of congenital uterine anomalies. *Semin Ultrasound CT MR* 1994; **15**:4–17.

32. Rosenberg HK, Sherman NH, Tarry WF, Duckett JW, Snyder HC. Mayer-Rokitansky-Küster-Hauser syndrome: US aid to diagnosis. *Radiology* 1986; **161**:815–819.

33. Scanlon KA, Pozniak MA, Fagerholm M, Shapiro S. Value of transperineal sonography in the assessment of vaginal atresia. *Am J Roentgenol* 1990; **154**:545–548.

34. Togashi K, Nishimura K, Itoh K *et al.* Vaginal agenesis: classification by MR imaging. *Radiology* 1987; **162**:675–677.

35. Carrington BM, Hricak H, Nuruddin RN, Secaf E, Laros RK Jr, Hill EC. Müllerian duct anomalies: MR imaging evaluation. *Radiology* 1990; **176**:715–720.

36. O'Leary JL, O'Leary JA. Rudimentary horn pregnancy. *Obstet Gynecol* 1963; **22**:371–375.

37. Pellerito JS, McCarthy SM, Doyle MB, Glickman MG, DeCherney AH. Diagnosis of uterine anomalies: relative accuracy of MR imaging, endovaginal sonography, and hysterosalpingography. *Radiology* 1992; **183**:795–800.

38. Buttram VC Jr. Müllerian anomalies and their management. *Fertil Steril* 1983; **40**:159–163.

39. Patton PE. Anatomic uterine defects. *Clin Obstet Gynecol* 1994; **37**:705–721.

40. Sardanelli F, Renzetti P, Oddone M, Toma P. Uterus didelphys with blind hemivagina and ipsilateral renal agenesis: MR findings before and after vaginal septum resection. *Eur J Radiol* 1995; **19**:164–170.

41. Fedele L, Dorta M, Brioschi D, Massari C, Candiani GB. Magnetic resonance evaluation of double uteri. *Obstet Gynecol* 1989; **74**:844–847.

42. Fielding JR. MR imaging of Müllerian anomalies: impact on therapy. *Am J Roentgenol* 1996; **167**:1491–1495.

43. March CM. Uterine surgical approaches to reduce prematurity. *Clin Perinatol* 1992; **19**:319–331.

44. Reuter KL, Daly DC, Cohen SM. Septate versus bicornuate uteri: errors in imaging diagnosis. *Radiology* 1989; **172**:749–752.

45. Fedele L, Ferrazzi E, Dorta M, Vercellini P, Candiani G. Ultrasonography in the differential diagnosis of 'double' uteri. *Fertil Steril* 1988; **50**:361–364.

46. Nicolini U, Bellotti M, Bonazzi B, Zamberletti D, Candiani GB. Can ultrasound be used to screen uterine malformations? *Fertil Steril* 1987; **47**:89–93.

47. Yoder IC. Diagnosis of uterine anomalies: relative accuracy of MR imaging, endovaginal sonography, and hysterosalpingography. *Radiology* 1992; **185**:343–344.

48. Zreik TG, Troiano R, McCarthy S, Arici A, Olive DL. Detection of myometrial tissue in uterine septa. *J Am Assoc Gynecol Laparosc* 1995; **2**:S62.

49. Ozsarlak O, De Schepper AMA, Valkenburg M, Delbeke L. Septate uterus: hysterosalpingography and magnetic resonance imaging findings. *Eur J Radiol* 1995; **21**:122–125.

50. Cooney MJ, Benson CB, Doubilet PM. Outcome of pregnancies in women with uterine duplication anomalies. *J Clin Ultrasound* 1998; **26**:3–6.

51. Salle B, Sergeant P, Gaudherand P, Guimant I, de Saint Hilaire P, Rudigoz RC. Transvaginal hysterosonographic evaluation of septate uteri: a preliminary report. *Human Reprod* 1996; **11**:1004–1007.

52. Mintz MC, Thickman DI, Gussman D, Kressel HY. MR evaluation of uterine anomalies. *Am J Roentgenol* 1987; **148**:287–290.

53. Raga F, Bauset C, Remohi J, Bonilla-Musoles F, Simon C, Pellier A. Reproductive impact of congenital Müllerian anomalies. *Human Reprod* 1997; **12**:2277–2281.

54. Tulandi T, Arronet GH, McInnes RA. Arcuate and bicornuate uterine anomalies and infertility. *Fertil Steril* 1980; **34**:362–364.

55. Whitehouse GH. Congenital abnormalities of the female genital tract. In: *Gynecologic Radiology*. Oxford: Blackwell Scientific Publications, 1981:56–72.

56. Parmley T. Embryology of the female genital tract. In: Kurman RJ, ed. *Blaustein's Pathology of the Female Genital Tract* 3rd edn. New York: Springer-Verlag, 1987:1–14.

57. Kaufman RH, Adam E, Binder GL, Berthoffer EA. Upper genital tract changes and pregnancy outcome in offspring exposed in utero to diethylstilbestrol. *Am J Obstet Gynecol* 1980; **137**:299.

58. Sedlis A, Robboy SJ. Diseases of the vagina. In: Kurman RJ, ed. *Blaustein's Pathology of the Female Genital Tract* 3rd edn. New York: Springer-Verlag, 1987:97–140.

59. Viscomi GN, Gonzalez R, Taylor KJ. Ultrasound detection of uterine anomalies after diethylstilbestrol (DES) exposure. *Radiology* 1980; **136**:733–735.

60. Lev-Toaff AS, Toaff ME, Friedman AC. Endovaginal sonographic appearance of a DES uterus. *J Ultrasound Med* 1990; **9**:661–664.

61. van Gils APG, Tham RTO, Folke THM, Peters AAW. Abnormalities of the uterus and cervix after diethylstilbestrol exposure: correlation of findings on MR and hysterosalpingography. *Am J Roentgenol* 1989; **153**:1235–1238.

62. Bacelar AC, Wilcock D, Powell M, Worthington BS. The value of MRI in the assessment of traumatic intrauterine adhesions (Asherman's syndrome). *Clin Radiol* 1995; **50**:80–83.

63. Kurman RJ, Mazur MT. Benign diseases of the endometrium. In: Kurman RJ, ed. *Blaustein's Pathology of the Female Genital Tract* 3rd edn. New York: Springer-Verlag, 1987:292–321.

64. Randel SB, Filly RA, Callen PW, Anderson RL, Golbus MS. Amniotic sheets. *Radiology* 1988; **166**:633–636.

65. Korbin CD, Benson CB, Doubilet PM. Placental implantation on the amniotic sheet: effect on pregnancy outcome. *Radiology* 1998; **206**:773–775.

66. Fedele L, Bianchi S, Dorta M, Vignali M. Intrauterine adhesions: detection with transvaginal ultrasound. *Radiology* 1996; **199**:757–759.

67. Stewart EA, Friedman AJ. Steroidal treatment of myomas: preoperative and long-term medical therapy. *Semin Reprod Endocrinol* 1992; **10**:344–357.

68. Krysiewicz S. Infertility in women: diagnostic evaluation with hysterosalpingography and other imaging techniques. *Am J Roentgenol* 1992; **159**:253–261.

69. Darai E, Dechaud H, Benifla JL, Renolleau C, Pavel P, Madelenat P. Fertility after laparoscopic myomectomy: preliminary results. *Human Reprod* 1997; **12**:1931–1934.

70. Duboisson JB, Chapron C, Chavet X, Gregorakis SS. Fertility after laparoscopic myomectomy of large intramural myomas: preliminary results. *Human Reprod* 1996; **11**:518–522.

71. Sudik R, Husch K, Steller J, Daume E. Fertility and pregnancy outcome after myomectomy in sterility patients. *Eur J Obstet Gynecol Reprod Biol* 1996; **65**:209–214.

72. Berkeley AS, De Cherney AH, Polan ML. Abdominal myomectomy and subsequent fertility. *Surg Gynecol Obstet* 1983; **156**:319–322.

73. Gehlbach DL, Sousa RC, Carpenter SE, Rock JA. Abdominal myomectomy in the treatment of infertility. *Intl J Gynaecol Obstet* 1993; **40**:45–50.

74. Cohen JR, Luxman D, Sagi J, Jossiphov J, David MP. Ultrasonic 'honeycomb' appearance of uterine submuccus fibroids undergoing cystic degeneration. *J Clin Ultrasound* 1995; **23**:293–296.

75. Fedele L, Bianchi S, Dorta M, Brioschi D, Zanotti F, Vercellini P. Transvaginal ultrasonography versus hysteroscopy in the diagnosis of uterine submucous myomas. *Obstet Gynecol* 1991; **77**:745–748.

76. Sladkevicius P, Valentin L, Marsal K. Transvaginal Doppler examination of uteri with myomas. *J Clin Ultrasound* 1996; **24**:135–140.

77. Dudiak CM, Turner DA, Patel SK, Archie JT, Silver B, Norusis M. Uterine leiomyomas in the infertile patient: preoperative localization with MR imaging versus ultrasound and hysterosalpingography. *Radiology* 1988; **167**:627–630.

78. Weinreb J, Barkoff N, Megibow A, Demopoulos R. The value of MR imaging in distiguishing leiomyomas from other solid pelvic masses when sonography is indeterminate. *Am J Roentgenol* 1990; **154**:295–299.

79. Tempany CM, Yousef N. Benign diseases of the uterus. In: Tempany CM, ed. *MR and Imaging of the Female Pelvis*. St Louis: Mosby Year Book, 1995:131–154.

80. Schnall MD. Magnetic resonance evaluation of acquired benign uterine disorders. *Semin Ultrasound CT MR* 1994; **15**:18–26.

81. Reinhold C, McCarthy S, Bret PM *et al*. Diffuse adenomyosis: comparison of endovaginal ultrasound and MR imaging with histopathologic correlation. *Radiology* 1996; **199**:151–158.

82. Yoder IC. Diseases of the uterus. In: *Hysterosalpingography and Pelvic Ultrasound: Imaging in Infertility and Gynecology*. Boston: Little, Brown, 1988:108–159.

83. de Souza NM, Brosens JJ, Schwieso JE, Paraschios T, Winston RML. The potential value of magnetic resonance imaging in infertility. *Clin Radiol* 1995; **50**:75–79.

84. Siedler D, Laing FC, Jeffrey RB, Wing VW. Uterine adenomyosis: a difficult sonographic diagnosis. *J Ultrasound Med* 1987; **6**:345–349.

85. Reinhold C, Atri M, Mehio A, Zakarian R, Aidis AE, Bret PM. Diffuse uterine adenomyosis: morphologic criteria and diagnostic accuracy of endovaginal sonography. *Radiology* 1995; **197**:609–614.

86. Maldjian C, Schnall MD. Magnetic resonance imaging of the uterine body, cervix, and adnexa. *Semin Roentgenol* 1996; **31**:257–266.

87. Outwater EK, Siegleman ES, Van Deerlin V. Adenomyosis: current concepts and imaging considerations. *Am J Roentgenol* 1998; **170**:437–441.

88. Ascher SM, Arnold LL, Patt RH *et al*. Adenomyosis: prospective comparison of MR imaging and transvaginal sonography. *Radiology* 1994; **190**:803–806.

89. Abramowicz JS, Archer DF. Uterine endometrial peristalsis – a transvaginal ultrasound study. *Fertil Steril* 1990; **54**:451–454.

90. Kunz G, Beil D, Deniger H, Einsanier A, Mall G, Leyendecker G. The uterine peristaltic pump: normal and impeded sperm transport within the female genital tract. *Adv Exp Med Biol* 1997; **424**:267–277.

91. Leyendecker G, Kunz G, Wilde L, Beil D, Deininger H. Uterine hyperperistalsis and dysperistalsis as dysfunctions of the mechanism of rapid sperm transport in patients with endometriosis and infertility. *Human Reprod* 1996; **11**:1542–1551.

6 The abnormal ovary

Douglas L Brown

Sonographic evaluation of the ovary in the infertile patient often reveals no abnormality. One may, however, identify abnormalities related to the infertility, such as endometriomas or evidence of polycystic ovarian disease. Benign masses, such as hemorrhagic cysts and teratomas, are not uncommon in premenopausal patients and may be encountered as incidental findings. The sonographic appearance of such lesions will be reviewed. We will focus on the ovary before hormonal stimulation, and consider the more common lesions one is likely to encounter.

Ovarian abnormalities possibly related to infertility

Endometriomas

While ultrasound is not reliable for the diagnosis of endometriosis, it is useful for identifying endometriomas that may occur in patients with endometriosis. Homogeneous low-to-medium-level echoes in a cystic ovarian mass without focal solid areas (*Fig. 6.1*) are very suggestive of an endometrioma.[1–5] Endometriomas may also be multilocular. The cyst wall can be thick or thin, and the thickness of the wall does not seem to be a useful criterion for diagnosing endometriomas.[5] Hyperechoic foci in the wall of the mass may be seen with endometriomas,[5] though it may be difficult to determine if such foci are within the wall or just in adjacent ovarian tissue. A small percentage of endometriomas will have focal solid areas[5] that may raise concern for neoplasm. Doppler sonography may be helpful in such cases,[6] as the absence of detectable flow would favor an endometrioma. However, some endometriomas have solid areas due to endometrial tissue and such areas may have detectable flow.

In summary, a cystic ovarian mass with homogeneous internal echoes, whether unilocular or multilocular, and without solid areas, is likely to be an endometrioma.

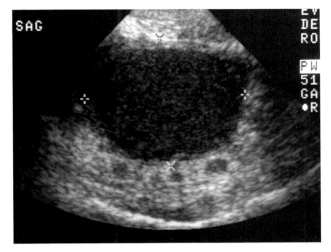

Figure 6.1 Endometrioma. Transvaginal scan demonstrates a cystic mass (outlined by cursors) with homogeneous internal echoes, and no solid component. This appearance is typical of an endometrioma.

If there are solid areas within the mass, then the diagnosis is problematic. Endometrioma is often still the likely diagnosis, as the focal, solid-appearing area may be due to clot or to endometrial tissue, but neoplasm becomes of more concern. Color Doppler may be helpful in such cases, but it may still be difficult to make an accurate diagnosis when there is a solid component to the mass.

Polycystic ovarian disease

The diagnosis of polycystic ovarian disease (PCOD) is generally made on clinical and biochemical grounds. Typical appearances of the ovaries in patients with PCOD have been described,[7–9] however, one cannot rely solely on ultrasound as the ovaries can appear normal in patients with PCOD. Ultrasound features that have been described for PCOD include: enlarged ovaries; multiple, small, peripherally located follicles; and increased

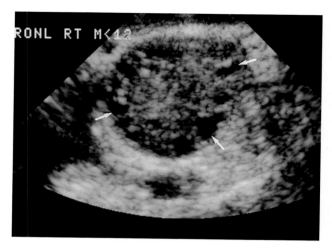

Figure 6.2 Polycystic ovarian disease. Transvaginal scan shows an ovary that was only slightly enlarged but has numerous small follicles (some indicated by arrows) that are located peripherally, which is a typical sonographic appearance of polycystic ovarian disease. The central stromal region of the ovary is subjectively increased in echogenicity.

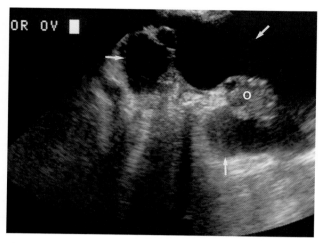

Figure 6.3 Peritoneal inclusion cyst. Transabdominal scan reveals a septated cystic mass (indicated by arrows) that surrounds a normal ovary (O).

echogenicity of the ovarian stroma (*Fig. 6.2*). Some patients with PCOD will have marked examples of these three features and present little problem in recognition. However, each of these features can be difficult to apply in less obvious cases. While volume can be measured, different upper limits of normal have been proposed. The number of follicles considered typical has also varied, from more than five to more than ten. The size of follicles has also been variably reported, though the follicles tend to be small, in the 5–8 mm range. Determination of increased stromal echogenicity is subjective and therefore may be difficult to assess.

In summary, for PCOD, enlarged ovaries with numerous small peripheral follicles and increased stromal echogenicity are a typical sonographic appearance and should suggest the diagnosis. However, some patients will have less obvious features and the sonographic diagnosis may be less certain. Additionally, the ovary can appear normal in patients with PCOD.

Extraovarian masses

While not strictly an ovarian abnormality, some adnexal masses arise outside the ovary and may be confused with ovarian masses. Hydrosalpinges, ectopic pregnancy, and peritoneal inclusion cysts are extraovarian masses that may be encountered in patients with infertility. Hydrosalpinges and ectopic pregnancy are discussed elsewhere in this text. Peritoneal inclusion cysts generally occur in patients with pelvic adhesions. Common predisposing factors are prior pelvic surgery, trauma, pelvic inflammatory disease, or endometriosis. Peritoneal inclusion cysts are often septated masses and, if one can recognize that such a mass surrounds a normal ovary (*Fig. 6.3*), particularly in a patient with a reason to have pelvic adhesions, the diagnosis can be strongly suggested.[10,11] If one is not aware of this entity and its typical ultrasound appearance, the cystic mass may be mistaken for an ovarian neoplasm.

Incidental ovarian abnormalities

Simple cysts

Simple cysts (i.e. anechoic, with thin walls, and distal acoustic enhancement) of the ovary are common. In premenopausal patients, we generally consider simple ovarian cysts less than 20 mm in greatest dimension to be normal follicles, though some individuals use a cut-off of 25 mm. Simple cysts greater than 20 mm may represent follicular or corpus luteal cysts.

Hemorrhagic cysts

A very fine network of thin linear-to-curvilinear echoes, sometimes called a 'fishnet' or 'reticular' pattern (*Fig. 6.4*), is strongly suggestive of a hemorrhagic cyst.[1,12–15] Such echoes are not true septations.

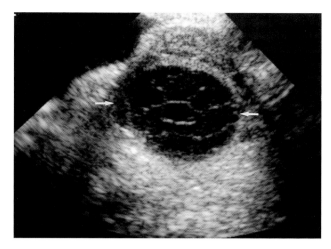

Figure 6.4 Hemorrhagic ovarian cyst. Transvaginal scan demonstrates a cystic mass (between arrows) that has low-level internal echoes and short, thin linear-to-curvilinear echoes within it, which have been referred to as a 'fishnet' pattern or a 'reticular' pattern. This appearance is very suggestive of a hemorrhagic ovarian cyst.

The appearance of hemorrhagic cysts and endometriomas may overlap, however, and not all hemorrhagic cysts or endometriomas have the typical appearance mentioned here. Hemorrhagic cysts or endometriomas may have a more solid nodular component due to clot that may be difficult to distinguish from the true solid tissue of a neoplasm.

One should also remember that internal echoes throughout a mass do not necessarily indicate it is solid. Sometimes, the clot within hemorrhagic cysts does not have the typical appearance discussed above, but instead suggests a solid mass. This possibility should be considered in premenopausal women, where hemorrhagic cysts are relatively common. In such cases, a follow-up sonogram should be performed. Color Doppler may also be helpful, as true solid masses would be more likely to have flow within them than would cysts filled with clot.

The corpus luteum may be seen during the latter portion of the menstrual cycle and has a variable appearance. A small corpus luteum may appear as a cystic mass with a thick wall and/or internal echoes due to hemorrhage. Larger corpus luteal cysts may appear as simple cysts or hemorrhagic cysts with the reticular pattern discussed above.

Mature cystic teratomas

A markedly hyperechoic nodule within a mass (*Fig. 6.5a*), particularly if it shadows, is generally a reliable sign of a teratoma.[16–24] Teratomas may also be uniformly hyperechoic, and such masses can be difficult to recognize and distinguish from bowel. Other sonographic features that are very suggestive of a teratoma include a fluid–fluid level (with the more echogenic fluid being non-dependent), and also what has been called the 'dermoid mesh', or 'hyperechoic lines and dots' (*Fig. 6.5b*).[24,25] Calcification may occur in teratomas, but calcification alone is not enough to make the diagnosis of a teratoma. The accuracy of sonography for teratomas improves when more than one typical sonographic

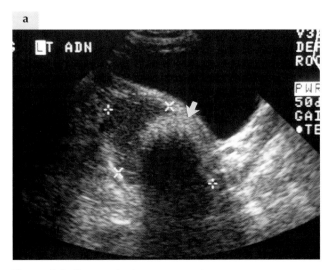

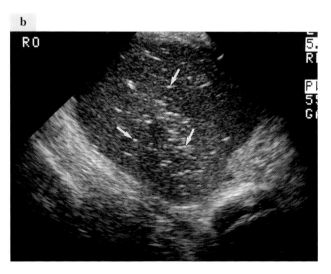

Figure 6.5 Two typical mature cystic teratomas.
(a) Transabdominal scan shows a cystic mass (outlined by cursors) which contains a hyperechoic nodule (arrow) that has distal shadowing. (b) Transvaginal scan shows a mass of overall medium echogenicity, within which there are 'hyperechoic lines and dots' (a few of which are indicated by arrows). This appearance has also been referred to as the 'dermoid mesh.'

feature is present.[24] The majority of teratomas have one or more typical ultrasound features; a small percentage will not have any suggestive sonographic features. MRI and CT are useful to demonstrate fat within the mass in the small percentage of teratomas that do not have a typical sonographic appearance.

Other masses

Ovarian malignancy is not generally of high concern in patients being evaluated for infertility. However, if an ovarian mass does not have any of the typical benign appearances discussed above, and the clinical situation does not help in suggesting the diagnosis (such as with pelvic inflammatory disease), benign or malignant neoplasm becomes of more concern. Sonographic characteristics that are generally associated with malignancy are septations (particularly when thick, which is generally defined as greater than 2 or 3 mm) and a solid component, which may be nodular in shape. A solid component, however, is the most significant gray-scale ultrasound feature.[26–28] Some benign neoplasms, particularly the epithelial neoplasms, will have solid areas and/or septations and can be difficult to distinguish from malignant neoplasms. A thick wall (generally defined as greater than 2 or 3 mm) is considered by some also to be a sign of malignancy, but many hemorrhagic cysts or endometriomas have a slightly thick wall. A thick wall, in and of itself, is not highly predictive of malignancy. In the past, size of the mass was considered useful, with larger masses more likely to be malignant. More recently, several studies have found no significant difference in size of malignant and benign ovarian masses.[28,29] This may be due to the more widespread use of sonography, leading to the detection of smaller masses, and also due to the improved characterization of masses based on sonographic features.

Incidental extraovarian masses may also be encountered in the infertile patient. Pedunculated fibroids are fairly common. They are generally heterogeneous, hypoechoic, solid masses but may present a confusing appearance, especially if there is cystic degeneration. The most helpful sonographic finding is to see a separate ipsilateral ovary. If one is not able to make this determination with ultrasound, MRI is generally useful. Paraovarian (or paratubal) cysts are generally simple cysts. Recognition that a simple cyst is separate from the ovary allows one to make a confident sonographic diagnosis.[30,31] Paraovarian cystadenomas are uncommon but typically appear as an extraovarian cyst with a small nodule and/or septations.[32]

Doppler evaluation of ovarian masses

Doppler evaluation of adnexal masses was initially proposed as a way to improve the accuracy of sonography for ovarian malignancy.[33] The neovascularization[34] that accompanies malignant tumors is associated with poor muscular support in the arterial walls, leading to less vascular resistance, which can potentially be detected by pulsed Doppler. Masses with a pulsatility index (PI) less than 1.0[33] or a resistive index (RI) less than 0.4[35] were initially considered to predict malignancy. Numerous studies have now been published evaluating the use of Doppler sonography for adnexal masses.[33,35–45] While most studies have shown a trend toward lower RI or PI with malignant masses, there is a broader overlap of the indices in benign and malignant masses than originally suspected.[42,44–47] Most investigators have found no reliable cut-off of PI or RI to distinguish benign from malignant ovarian masses.[42,44,45,47–50] Based on the literature as a whole, it appears that neither the PI nor the RI can be used alone to distinguish benign from malignant ovarian masses.

Other Doppler features such as the presence/absence of detectable flow, the presence/absence of a diastolic notch in the spectral waveform, and velocity criteria have also been evaluated for their ability to distinguish benign from malignant ovarian masses. As with the PI and RI, some general trends have been found, and variable conclusions have been reached. In this author's opinion, none of these other Doppler criteria alone is reliable.

Combined approaches, using gray-scale and Doppler ultrasound, have been investigated,[28,29,47,51,52] with variable performance reported, though generally better with a combined approach than either alone. We used stepwise logistic regression to analyze clinical, gray-scale, and Doppler features in 211 adnexal masses,[28] and found the solid component to be by far the most useful feature. Masses that had no solid component or a solid component that was markedly hyperechoic (i.e. typical of a teratoma) were always benign. For masses with a non-hyperechoic solid component, three other features were useful to predict malignancy: location of flow detected with color Doppler; amount of intraperitoneal fluid; and the presence and thickness of septations. The presence of flow centrally (in solid areas or septations) was more predictive of malignancy than no flow or only peripheral flow (*Fig. 6.6*). Not surprisingly, moderate or large amounts of intraperitoneal fluid were more predictive of malignancy than small amounts of free fluid. The absence of septations was more predictive of malignancy in our study, with thick

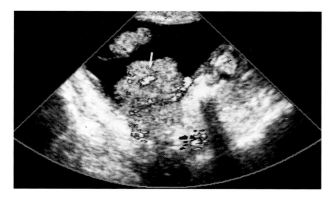

Figure 6.6 Malignant ovarian neoplasm. Transvaginal scan demonstrates a cystic mass containing irregular solid nodular areas. Flow is identified within one of the nodules (arrow) using color Doppler. This was an endometrioid adenocarcinoma of the ovary.

septations next most predictive, and thin septations the least predictive of malignancy. No other features improved the discrimination of benign from malignant ovarian masses. Using a scoring system based on the regression analysis and the cut-off score with the highest accuracy, the sensitivity for malignancy was 93% and specificity 93%. To achieve 100% sensitivity, the specificity dropped to 86%.

Conclusion

When imaging the ovary in the infertile patient, one should be aware both of abnormalities that can be related to infertility and of incidental abnormalities. One should try to determine whether a mass arises from the ovary or is extraovarian. For ovarian masses, one should determine if they have a typical ultrasound appearance for simple cyst, hemorrhagic cyst, endometrioma, or teratoma. If the mass does not have such a typical benign appearance, then the presence of a solid component that is not markedly hyperechoic is of concern for malignancy. However, clot may also appear as a solid component. Color Doppler may be useful for identifying flow in suspected solid areas, but it is still not fully reliable for distinguishing benign from malignant masses. If there is a non-hyperechoic solid component, then assessment of the location of detectable flow by color Doppler, presence and thickness of septations, and abnormal intraperitoneal fluid will help further distinguish benign from malignant masses.

REFERENCES

1. Filly RA. Ovarian masses ... what to look for ... what to do. In: Callen PW, ed. *Ultrasonography in Obstetrics and Gynecology*. Philadelphia: WB Saunders Company, 1994: 625–640.

2. Fried AM, Kenney CM, Stigers KB et al. Benign pelvic masses: sonographic spectrum. *RadioGraphics* 1996;**16**:321–334.

3. Kupfer MC, Schwimer SR, Lebovic J. Transvaginal sonographic appearance of endometriomata: spectrum and findings. *J Ultrasound Med* 1992;**11**:129–133.

4. Mais V, Guerriero S, Ajossa S et al. The efficiency of transvaginal ultrasonography in the diagnosis of endometrioma. *Fertil Steril* 1993;**60**:776–780.

5. Patel MD, Feldstein VA, Chen DC et al. Endometriomas: diagnostic performance of ultrasound. *Radiology* 1999;**210**:739–745.

6. Guerriero S, Ajossa S, Mais V et al. The diagnosis of endometriomas using colour Doppler energy imaging. *Human Reprod* 1998;**13**:1691–95.

7. Yeh H, Futterweit W, Thornton JC. Polycystic ovarian disease: US features in 104 patients. *Radiology* 1987;**163**:111–116.

8. Pache TD, Wladimiroff JW, Hop WCJ, Fauser BCJM. How to discriminate between normal and polylcystic ovaries: transvaginal US study. *Radiology* 1992;**183**:421–423.

9. Battaglia C, Artini PG, Salvatori M et al. Ultrasonographic patterns of polycystic ovaries: color Doppler and hormonal correlations. *Ultrasound Obstet Gynecol* 1998;**11**:332–336.

10. Hoffer FA, Kozakewich H, Colodny A, Goldstein DP. Peritoneal inclusion cysts: ovarian fluid in peritoneal adhesions. *Radiology* 1988;**169**:189–191.

11. Kim JS, Lee HJ, Woo SK, Lee TS. Peritoneal inclusion cysts and their relationship to the ovaries: evaluation with sonography. *Radiology* 1997;**204**:481–484.

12. Baltarowich OH, Kurtz AB, Pasto ME et al. The spectrum of sonographic findings in hemorrhagic ovarian cysts. *Am J Roentgenol* 1987;**148**:901–905.

13. Jain KA. Prospective evaluation of adnexal masses with endovaginal gray-scale and duplex and color doppler US: correlation with pathologic findings. *Radiology* 1994;**191**:63–67.

14. Okai T, Kobayashi K, Ryo E et al. Transvaginal sonographic appearance of hemorrhagic functional ovarian cysts and their spontaneous regression. *Int J Gynecol Obstet* 1994;**44**:47–52.

15. Stein SM, Laifer-Narin S, Johnson MB et al. Differentiation of benign and malignant adnexal masses: relative value of gray-scale, color Doppler, and spectral Doppler sonography. *Am J Roentgenol* 1995;**164**:381–386.

16. Atri M, Kintzen GM, Ye S et al. How accurate is endovaginal US in the diagnosis of ovarian dermoid? (Abstract). *Radiology* 1994;**193**(P):145.

17. Atri M, Reinhold C, Bret PM. Ovarian dermoid: correlation of endovaginal sonographic and MR imaging findings (Abstract). *Radiology* 1994;**193**(P):309.

18. Quinn SF, Erickson S, Black WC. Cystic ovarian teratomas: the sonographic appearance of the dermoid plug. *Radiology* 1985;**155**:477–478.

19. Mais V, Guerriero S et al. Transvaginal ultrasonography in the diagnosis of cystic teratoma. *Obstet Gynecol* 1995;**85**:48–52.

20. Cohen L, Sabbagha R. Echo patterns of benign cystic teratomas by transvaginal ultrasound. *Ultrasound Obstet Gynecol* 1993;**3**:120–123.

21. Laing FC, Van Dalsem VF, Marks WM et al. Dermoid cysts of the ovary: their ultrasonographic appearances. *Obstet Gynecol* 1981;**57**:99–104.

22. Sheth S, Fishman EK, Buck JL et al. The variable sonographic appearances of ovarian teratomas: correlation with CT. *Am J Roentgenol* 1988;**151**:331–334.

23. Caspi B, Appelman Z, Rabinerson D et al. Pathognomonic echo patterns of benign cystic teratomas of the ovary: classification, incidence and accuracy rate of sonographic diagnosis. *Ultrasound Obstet Gynecol* 1996;**7**:275–279.

24. Patel MD, Feldstein VA, Lipson SD et al. Cystic teratomas of the ovary: diagnostic value of sonography. *AJR* 1998;**171**:1061–1065.

25. George JC. Dermoid mesh: a sonographic sign of ovarian teratoma (Letter). *AJR* 1992;**159**:1349–1350.

26. Granberg S, Norstrom A, Wikland M. Tumors in the lower pelvis as imaged by vaginal sonography. *Gynecol Oncol* 1990;**37**:224–229.

27. Granberg S, Wikland M, Jansson I. Macroscopic characterization of ovarian tumors and the relation to the histological diagnosis: criteria to be used for ultrasound evaluation. *Gynecol Oncol* 1989;**35**:139–144.

28. Brown DL, Doubilet PM, Miller FH et al. Benign and malignant ovarian masses: selection of the most discriminating gray-scale and Doppler sonographic features. *Radiology* 1998;**208**:103–110.

29. Tailor A, Jurkovic D, Bourne TH et al. Sonographic prediction of malignancy in adnexal masses using multivariate logistic regression analysis. *Ultrasound Obstet Gynecol* 1997;**10**:41–1047.

30. Alpern MB, Sandler MA, Madrazo BL. Sonographic features of parovarian cysts and their complications. *Am J Roentgenol* 1984;**143**:157–160.

31. Athey PA, Cooper NB. Sonographic features of parovarian cysts. *Am J Roentgenol* 1985;**144**:83–86.

32. Korbin CD, Brown DL, Welch WR. Paraovarian cystadenomas and cystadenofibromas: sonographic characteristics in 14 cases. *Radiology* 1998;**208**:459–462.

33. Bourne T, Campbell S, Steer C et al. Transvaginal colour flow imaging: a possible new screening technique for ovarian cancer. *BMJ* 1989;**299**:1367–1370.

34. Folkman J, Watson K, Ingber D, Hanahan D. Induction of angiogenesis during the transition from hyperplasia to neoplasia. *Nature* 1989;**339**:58–61.

35. Kurjak A, Zalud I, Alfirevic Z. Evaluation of adnexal masses with transvaginal color ultrasound. *J Ultrasound Med* 1991;**10**:295–297.

36. Hata T, Hata K, Senoh D et al. Doppler ultrasound assessment of tumor vascularity in gynecologic disorders. *J Ultrasound Med* 1989;**8**:309–314.

37. Hata K, Hata T, Manabe A et al. A critical evaluation of transvaginal Doppler studies, transvaginal sonography, magnetic resonance imaging, and CA 125 in detecting ovarian cancer. *Obstet Gynecol* 1992;**80**:922–926.

38. Kurjak A, Zalud I, Jurkovic D et al. Transvaginal color Doppler for the assessment of pelvic circulation. *Acta Obstet Gynecol Scand* 1989;**68**:131–135.

39. Kurjak A, Schulman H, Sosic A et al. Transvaginal ultrasound, color flow, and Doppler waveform of the postmenopausal adnexal mass. *Obstet Gynecol* 1992;**80**:917–921.

40. Kawai M, Kano T, Kikkawa F et al. Transvaginal Doppler ultrasound with color flow imaging in the diagnosis of ovarian cancer. *Obstet Gynecol* 1992;**79**:163–167.

41. Fleischer AC, Rodgers WH, Rao BK et al. Assessment of ovarian tumor vascularity with transvaginal color Doppler sonography. *J Ultrasound Med* 1991;**10**:563–568.

42. Tekay A, Jouppila P. Validity of pulsatility and resistance indices in classification of adnexal tumors with transvaginal color Doppler ultrasound. *Ultrasound Obstet Gynecol* 1992;**2**:338–344.

43. Weiner Z, Thaler I, Beck D et al. Differentiating malignant from benign ovarian tumors with transvaginal color flow imaging. *Obstet Gynecol* 1992;**79**:159–162.

44. Brown DL, Frates MC, Laing FC et al. Ovarian masses: can benign and malignant lesions be differentiated by color and pulsed Doppler US? *Radiology* 1994;**190**:333–336.

45. Hamper UM, Sheth S, Abbas FM et al. Transvaginal color Doppler sonography of adnexal masses: differences in blood flow impedance in benign and malignant lesions. *Am J Roentgenol* 1993;**160**:1225–1228.

46. Bourne TH. Transvaginal color Doppler in gynecology. *Ultrasound Obstet Gynecol* 1991;**1**:359–373.

47. Timor-Tritsch IE, Lerner JP, Monteagudo A, Santos R. Transvaginal ultrasonographic characterization of ovarian masses by means of color flow-directed Doppler measurements and a morphologic scoring system. *Am J Obstet Gynecol* 1993;**168**:909–913.

48. Salem S, White LM, Lai J. Doppler sonography of adnexal masses: the predictive value of the pulsatility index in benign and malignant disease. *Am J Roentgenol* 1994;**163**:1147–1150.

49. Schneider VL, Schneider A, Reed KL, Hatch KD. Comparison of Doppler with two-dimensional sonogrpahy and CA 125 for prediction of malignancy of pelvic masses. *Obstet Gynecol* 1993;**81**:983–988.

50. Tekay A, Jouppila P. Controversies in assessment of ovarian tumors with transvaginal color Doppler ultrasound (Review). *Acta Obstet Gynecol Scand* 1996;**75**:316–329.

51. Kurjak A, Predanic M. New scoring system for prediction of ovarian malignancy based on transvaginal color doppler sonography. *J Ultrasound Med* 1992;**11**:631–638.

52. Pellerito JS, Taylor KJ, Quedens-Case C, Hammers LW. Endovaginal color flow scoring system: a sensitive indicator of pelvic malignancy (Abstract). *Radiology* 1994;**193**(P):276.

7 Sonohysterography in reproductive-aged women

Paulo Serafini and Jeffrey Nelson

Introduction

Despite the increased use of high-resolution transvaginal sonography (TVS) for the diagnosis of uterine pathology, its usefulness in evaluating the endometrial cavity has been less than optimal.[1-4] Small lesions, diffuse growths projecting into isoechoic surroundings, unusual distortions of the uterine anatomy, and phase of the menstrual cycle may pose significant diagnostic difficulties with conventional TVS.[1-3,5] Alternative diagnostic techniques such as hysterosalpingography (HSG) and office hysteroscopy, known as the 'gold standards', present important limitations such as expensive equipment, the necessity for dedicated suites and availability of radiographic fluoroscopy.[1-3,5,6]

Nannini et al[7] were the first to describe sonohysterography in 1981 and called the technique 'echohysteroscopy'. Sonohysterography is a term created by Parsons[8] to describe the infusion of saline into the uterus during sonography, and although it has some shortcomings, sonohysterography has major advantages owing to its simplicity, low cost, minimal invasiveness, and high level of diagnostic accuracy.[8-12] Sonohysterography is a relatively painless technique that provides information about the cervix, uterine cavity, and intraperitoneal adhesions, as well as indirect evidence of tubal patency.[8,9] In this chapter we will describe the sonohysterography technique, discuss indications for sonohysterography and interpretation of findings, advantages and limitations, and comment on the diagnostic potential of sonohysterography with naturally accumulated menstrual blood.

Technique and instrumentation

Various investigators have demonstrated that fluid enhances details in ultrasonographic imaging by virtue of distending the cavity, and outlining the endometrium with fluid.[1-3,5,6,13] Essentially, the saline infusion acts as a hysterosalpingogram for real-time sonographic evaluation. In addition, visualization of the pelvic organs can be extended for a longer period of time without fear of exposing the patient or the operator to ionizing radiation.

Sonohysterography is easy to learn and failure rates are low (< 1.8%). The examination can be carried out in the office on the first visit. It may be electively scheduled at a mutually convenient time in the early follicular phase, or performed under general anesthesia in patients scheduled to undergo either videohysteroscopy or laparoscopy/hysteroscopy procedures.[14]

The steps of sonohysterography are as follows:

(a) The physician should provide information about the examination, explaining benefits and potential complications. All questions should be answered before obtaining a written informed consent.

(b) Antibiotic prophylaxis (e.g. doxycycline, azithromycin) may be prescribed for patients with a previous history of pelvic inflammatory disease and those who require systemic bacterial endocarditis prophylaxis. Most investigators have not routinely used antibiotic prophylaxis.[1,2,8,13] Indeed, Chung and Parsons[2] have performed close to 1000 examinations, with 0.6% complicated by infection. Although this experience shows a low rate of infection, the stakes are too high for women with infertility; thus, routine prophylaxis is suggested in this patient population. Routine use of nonsteroidal analgesic 30 minutes before the procedure has been recommended to reduce discomfort.

(c) Pregnancy should be excluded before administering antibiotics and performing the examination. Sonohysterography should be performed in the first phase of the menstrual cycle (day 6–11

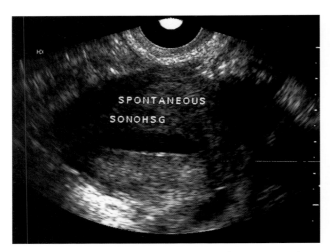

Figure 7.1 Spontaneous sonohysterography. Sonographic assessment of the endometrial cavity performed during the early phase of the menstrual cycle. The need for fluid infusion is avoided.

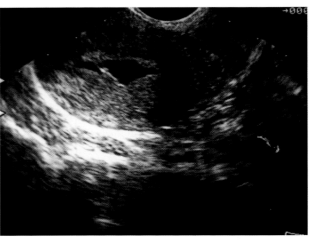

Figure 7.2 False appearances of 'polypoid' structure in the upper left portion of the uterine cavity and 'discontinuation' of the endometrial layer (lower central portion) caused by the infusion of saline during an examination conducted in the menstrual period.

of a 28-day cycle). This is also helpful because intracavitary lesions are more easily visualized on the background of a thin proliferative phase endometrium.

(d) Voiding before the sonohysterography is important.

(e) After positioning the patient in the dorsal lithotomy position, a comprehensive baseline ultrasound is performed to assess the size and position of the uterus, as well as to look for pathology. If pregnancy is detected, sonohysterography should be canceled. If the TVS exam is performed during menses, a uterine-filled cavity may be present, providing good endometrial–myometrial interface and negating the need for insertion of a catheter and injection of fluid. This is sometimes called 'spontaneous sonohysterography' (*Fig. 7.1*). Furthermore, the injection of fluid into the uterine cavity during menses may create artifacts from clots that may have similar characteristics to endometrial polyps (*Fig. 7.2*). If fluids such as dextran are infused during the menstrual period, care should be exercised because there is a greater tendency for the opening of venous sinuses in the uterus, increasing the chance of serious allergic reactions.

(f) After transvaginal sonography is performed (step (e)) the probe should be removed. A sterile, open-sided vaginal speculum is then inserted. The vagina and cervix are cleansed with antiseptic solution (povidone-iodine).

(g) The sonohysterography catheter is introduced into the uterine cavity just passing the internal cervical os. Gentle threading of the catheter is performed with either a sterile long uterine packing or ring forceps. When advancing the catheter, caution should be exercised to avoid striking the fundus of the uterus with the tip of the catheter, which can cause pain and sometimes produces a vasovagal response. The use of a cervical tenaculum is very rarely required unless cervical stenosis is encountered. The catheter should be primed with saline (or with the fluid to be instilled) to minimize the infusion of air and bubbles, which sometimes cause image artifacts and pain.

Practitioners have chosen different catheters for sonohysterography such as a rigid Schultze cannula or a rigid Rueben cannula.[15,16] Others have used a 5.5 Fr Soules intrauterine insemination catheter (Cook, Spencer, IN, USA). This flexible catheter is remarkably painless at its insertion. However, patients with a patulous and/or an incompetent cervix, or those with an enlarged uterus and synechiae are best examined with one of the following catheters: (1) Tampa catheter (5 Fr with a 2-ml balloon) set for hysterosonography (Ackrad Laboratories, Cranford, NJ, USA); (2) H/S Elliptosphere with a latex-free urethane (Ackrad Laboratories); (3) Goldstein sonohysterography catheter (Cook OB/GYN); and (4) size 8 Fr pediatric Foley.[2,5,8,13] The balloon is filled with 0.8–1.0 ml of fluid to avoid artifact. Because the filling of the balloon may cause discomfort, the patient should be made aware of the step, thus minimizing non-anticipated reaction. The preferred location for the placement of the balloon is within the endocervical canal.

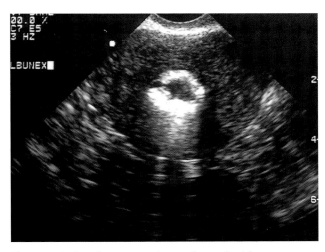

Figure 7.3 Sonohysterography performed with contrast (sonicated albumin microspheres, Albunex®) enhancement. Although endometrial 'halo' can be easily visualized, there is a sonographic impairment in the recognition of isoechoic (to the contrast) images.

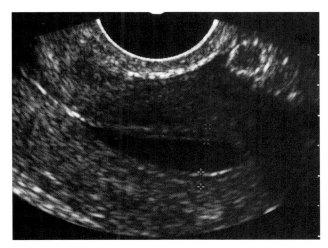

Figure 7.4 Normal sonohysterography.

(h) The speculum is carefully withdrawn to avoid dislodgment of the catheter, and the transvaginal probe is properly 'draped' with a condom before reinsertion into the vaginal canal and positioning at the vault. Although sonohysterography can be performed transvaginally and transabdominally, most physicians use the transvaginal approach.

(i) It is important to use a systematic technique for viewing the pelvis and to recreate a three-dimensional view of the uterus. This is achieved by gentle rotation of the probe, scanning from one cornu to the other in the sagittal axis, maintaining the ultrasound probe in touch with the uterus. The operator should keep a mental three-dimensional image of the uterus.

Several solutions have been used to obtain an adequate acoustic window including saline, Ringer's lactate, and 1.5% glycine solution.[1,2,8,17] Contrast agents, albumin microspheres (Albunex®) (*Fig. 7.3*), and suspension of galactose monosaccharide microparticles (Echovist®) may also intensify the ultrasonic acoustic properties of the uterus.

A 10–20 ml syringe with warmed injectable sterile saline is connected to the catheter. The initial infusion rate should not exceed 2–5 ml/min and it should be adjusted to a rate dictated by the patient's comfort and adequacy of the sonographic image. While the solution is being infused, the uterus is scanned longitudinally, fanning from cornu to cornu: every millimeter of the endometrial surface should be imaged. A volume of 2–10 ml of fluid is enough to distend most cavities and outline lesions, since only a small ribbon of fluid is needed. Patients who have adenomyosis and intrauterine adhesions may require several attempts at infusion because at times it is difficult to distend the cavity.

Proper technique in performing a sonohysterogram is imperative, since inadequate uterine distension may result in poor visualization and overzealous instillation may easily obscure uterine pathology.[6]

(j) Sequential images should be recorded on a combination of videotapes and still photographs to obtain permanent records.

(k) Prior to the completion of the procedure, the balloon is deflated and the lower portion of the uterus and cervical canal are re-examined for any further irregularities during an additional bolus injection of fluid.

(l) The patient should be allowed to rest for 5–10 minutes before discharge.

(m) If an endometrial biopsy is contemplated after the sonohysterography, 10 ml of 1% lidocaine could be used to distend the endometrial cavity to provide adequate anesthesia.[2]

The entire sonohysterography procedure lasts an average of 3–10 minutes. A normal sonohysterogram is shown in *Fig. 7.4*.

Indications

The indications for fluid-enhanced sonographic imaging of the uterine cavity in reproductive-aged women are summarized in *Table 7.1*.

Table 7.1 Indications for sonohysterography in the infertile woman.

Abnormal uterine bleeding
Before ART, infertility work-up and spontaneous
   recurrent abortions
Synechiae and 'second-look sonohysterography'
Polyps
Mapping uterine fibroids
Adenomyosis
Congenital uterine malformations
Abnormal hysterosalpingogram
Indirect assessment of tubal patency
Retained foreign bodies
Postabortal placental remnants
Triage for operative procedures

ART, assisted reproductive treatment.

Abnormal uterine bleeding

The evaluation of a patient with abnormal uterine bleeding is one of the most common indications for sonohysterography.[18–20] These patients necessitate the performance of sonohysterography independent of the menstrual calendar. However, a quantitative serum β-hCG should be obtained before the sonohysterography to exclude pregnancy.

The main diagnostic difficulty lies in distinguishing women with functional disorders from those with organic lesions. In the patient with abnormal uterine bleeding, sonohysterography can be used to differentiate the patient with a thin endometrial lining who may not require intervention from the patient with thickened endometrial echoes who demands further investigation.[1,2] Underlying causes for bleeding, such as endometrial hyperplasia as a result of chronic anovulation, endometrial polyps, submucous fibroids, and endometrial carcinoma, should be carefully considered. Sonohysterography showing an ill-defined endometrium with areas of asymmetry and/or focal thickening warrants hysteroscopy with directed biopsy.

Before assisted reproductive treatments for infertility

Sonohysterography may have a place in the initial work-up of an infertile woman. It has been estimated that intrauterine pathology is present in 5–10% of infertile couples and in up to 50% of those with recurrent pregnancy loss.[21–31] Sonohysterography can be used to determine the size and location of endometrial intracavitary growths, synechiae, and uterine malformations, and provides indirect evidence of tubal patency.[2,4,8,9,14,21,25] In addition, sonohysterography may play an important role in assisted reproductive treatments to maximize their success and minimize potential complications. Structural uterine abnormalities may play a key role in interfering with implantation,[3] and have been detected in up to 45% of women undergoing in vitro fertilization (IVF),[3,32] making screening sonohysterography highly valuable.

Lindheim and Sauer[33] have reported on the performance of prescreening sonohysterography in 50 patients before receipt of donated oocytes. Examinations were performed either in the follicular phase or after progesterone withdrawal. They found intrauterine pathology in 38% of the women studied. Furthermore, sonohysterography and hysterosalpingography (HSG) were concordant in 95.6% of the cases.

The authors incorporate sonohysterography as the first-line screening for the evaluation of the uterus before embryo transfer in patients undergoing in vitro fertilization, ovum donation, and IVF-surrogacy.[34]

The diagnosis and surgical correction of intrauterine defects in women with recurrent pregnancy losses significantly increases the rate of subsequent full-term deliveries.[29–31] Given the high rate of uterine anomalies and the potential benefits of surgical repair, it is important to evaluate accurately the uterine cavity in patients with recurrent pregnancy loss, using the methodology demonstrating the lowest rates of false-positive and -negative results. Keltz et al[28] detected uterine pathology by sonohysterography in 50% of their patients with recurrent pregnancy loss. They concluded that sonohysterography is a highly sensitive, specific, and accurate screening tool for the evaluation of uterine cavity defects associated with recurrent pregnancy loss, while offering several advantages over conventional HSG.

Synechiae

When adhesions are suspected (history of curettage, postabortal infection, multiple uterine surgery, etc.) catheters with balloons are preferable for sonohysterography, as they allow better distension of the cavity.[1,2,5] Failure to fully distend the cavity may prevent visualization of endometrial pathology. Filmy adhesions are seen as thin linear echogenicities (*Fig. 7.5*), whereas a thick adhesion shows a broad bridging band (*Fig. 7.6*). Sonohysterography provides a map of the adhesions that is helpful for guidance during operative hysteroscopy. Furthermore, there is good concordance with the hysteroscopic staging of adhesions as described by the American Society of Reproductive Medicine (formerly the American Fertility Society) and sonohysterographic findings.

Postoperative sonohysterography can be conducted as a less invasive 'second-look' procedure following operative hysteroscopies. 'Second-look sonohysterography' can be performed as early as 3 days after a hysteroscopic adhesiolysis procedure (*Fig. 7.7*) and 7 days after resection of submucosal myomas. Since most adhesions are formed 'de novo' and are filmy and avascular, blunt dissection can easily be carried out mechanically by the inflation of the uterine cavity with the sterile warm saline. In the great majority of patients where second-look sonohysterography is performed, the discomfort caused by the injection is minimal and well tolerated. Antibiotic prophylaxis and analgesics should be prescribed for all women undergoing second-look sonohysterography. The authors have not experienced complications; however, patient selection might be the determining factor for a successful postoperative sonohysterography. The authors have also found good correlation of postoperative sonohysterography with resectoscopic findings.

Polyps

Polyps are smooth marginated masses of homogeneous echotexture.[1,2,8] Although polyps start as sessile lesions, they may become pedunculated (*Fig. 7.8*).

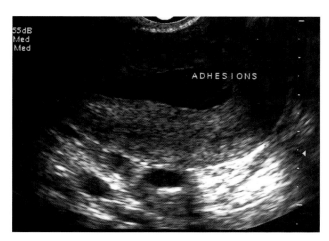

Figure 7.5 Sonohysterography demonstrating filmy adhesions within the fundal uterine region.

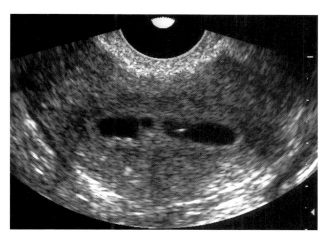

Figure 7.6 Broad bridging adhesion band is demonstrated by the sonohysterography in a patient who underwent two uterine curettages for an early second-trimester incomplete abortion.

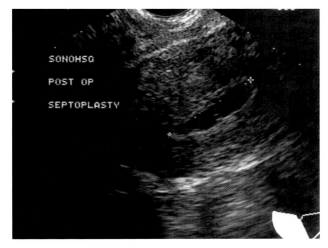

Figure 7.7 'Second-look sonohysterography' performed after a hysteroscopic resection of a large uterine septum. Study demonstrated successful septoplasty.

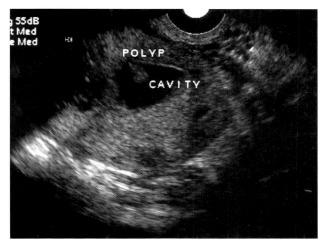

Figure 7.8 A smooth, homogeneous, pedunculated polyp is shown in the sonohysterography.

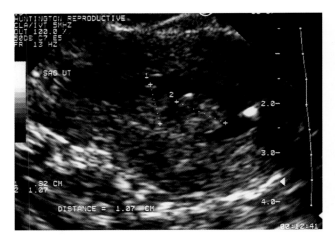

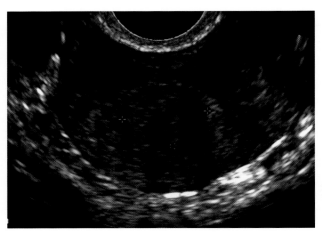

Figure 7.9 Sonohysterography demonstrates the presence of two polyps located in the posterior wall of the endometrial cavity.

Figure 7.10 Transvaginal sonography examination suggestive of an endometrial isoechoic and irregular lesion.

Imaging of polyps usually shows a distinct myometrial–endometrial interface, and rarely demonstrates an interruption in the endometrial lining. For these reasons, polyps may appear similar to endometrial hypertrophy or a myoma.

Polyps are usually hyperechoic. More importantly, if several polyps are suspected (*Fig. 7.9*), two pathologies may be present, such as fibroids and polyps, fibroids and adhesions, and polyps and endometrial hyperplasia. Indeed, Chung and Parsons[2] have shown that multiple forms of uterine pathology occurred in 11% of a series of patients examined before hysterectomy.

Small vessels and sinusoids can be imaged by color Doppler sonography in large polyps.

Fibroids

Uterine leiomyomata are the most common solid pelvic tumors occurring in women.[1,18,23,25] Pathology literature suggests that approximately 75% of carefully sectioned hysterectomy specimens, with procedures performed for all indications, contain fibroids. These were not all clinically significant lesions, but this finding indicates that the prevalence of fibroids is far greater than previously anticipated. Approximately 20–25% of women will develop fibroids at some time during their reproductive life. Furthermore, it has been estimated that 20–50% of women with clinically recognizable fibroids (palpable on bimanual examination) will have clinical symptoms, including 30% of the women with recurrent pregnancy losses. Although the actual incidence of infertility related to myomata

is difficult to estimate accurately, various studies estimate a range of 1.8–9.1%.[18,23,25,35,36] Despite the uncertainty regarding their impact on infertility, fibroids do have a well-documented association with other adverse reproductive events such as spontaneous abortion, premature labor, outlet obstruction, and abnormal fetal presentation.

Patients with clinical symptoms directly attributable to their myomata should be managed with an effective form of therapy associated with the lowest morbidity. Numerous clinical studies have concluded that to achieve a satisfactory postoperative result through hysteroscopic resection, at least half of the intramural lesion must be projecting into the uterine cavity. To determine the most effective surgical plan, each myoma must be carefully assessed in an attempt to define accurately its potential role regarding the patients' symptoms. This process of myoma mapping requires detailed information regarding the number, size, and location of each lesion, as well as determination of the extent of uterine cavity involvement. Since the endometrial cavity is a virtual space and fibroids may have a scattered distribution and projections into the cavity, a topographic determination of the lesion by TVS can be quite challenging (*Fig. 7.10*). Sonohysterography allows accurate delineation of the fibroid within the cavity, percentage of intracavitary growth and extension and postoperative recurrence rate. Sonohysterography helps the 'programming' of surgery (*Fig. 7.11*).

Fibroids are typically either isoechoic or hypoechoic relative to the surrounding myometrium. They will frequently be associated with an acoustic shadow resulting from attenuation of the ultrasound beam.

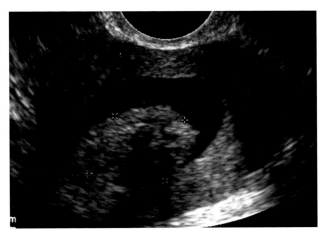

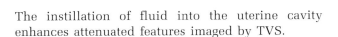

Figure 7.11 Sonohysterography performed in the same patient as shown in Fig. 7.10 precisely documenting a large posterior submucosal uterine fibroid.

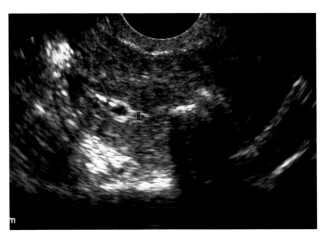

Figure 7.12 A very abnormal endometrial cavity shown by sonohysterography in a DES-exposed woman. Hysterosalpingogram and hysteroscopy examinations confirmed a very small 'T-shaped' malformation.

The instillation of fluid into the uterine cavity enhances attenuated features imaged by TVS.

Several investigators have compared sonohysterography with hysteroscopy and HSG.[2,4,12–14,16–18,25] Both sonohysterography and hysteroscopy had 100% sensitivity and specificity for fibroids, but sonohysterography is more accurate for measuring myomas.[36] In addition, sonohysterographic mapping of the fibroids (number, size, location, and the extent of intramural involvement) is superior to the determinations obtained with office hysteroscopy. The time required for the performance of the sonohysterography (< 15 min) is significantly shorter than that of the office hysteroscopy (20–26 min). Furthermore, patients tend to prefer sonohysterography to office hysteroscopy.

Adenomyosis

The ability to diagnose adenomyosis by ultrasonography has been substantially enhanced with the improvement of ultrasound imaging.[20,37–39] The sonographic scoring system reported by Hirai et al[37] in 1993 exhibits a sensitivity of 87% and 91%, and color Doppler imaging improved accuracy by an additional 5%.[38] While Goldstein[20] did not study the diagnostic accuracy of sonohysterography, he showed that sonohysterography improved the visualization of the aberrant glands of the basal layer and cysts with honeycomb pattern through the instillation of fluid into the uterine cavity. Sonohysterography accentuates the disruption that occurs between the subendometrial and myometrial junction, while aiding in the differential diagnosis of endometrial hyperplasia, which is often difficult to diagnose with TVS.

Congenital uterine malformation

In the patient with a uterine anomaly, it is essential to differentiate septate from bicornuate and uterus didelphys, because of different complications and different treatment approaches. HSG does not provide sensitive information about myometrial anatomy and consequently it does not differentiate between the above pathologies. However, TVS and sonohysterography may accomplish differentiation of bicornuate uterus from the septate uterus. These imaging techniques provide reliable information about the myometrium and the external contour of the uterus.[1,2] In the bicornuate uterus, a myometrial notching can be observed at the fundus, whereas in most septate uteri the external contour is smooth. Sonohysterography adds to the three-dimensional viewing of the cavity by permitting visualization of the presence or absence of communicating uterine horns.

The evaluation of the uterine cavity of prenatally DES-exposed women can be assessed accurately by sonohysterography (*Fig. 7.12*). It has also been suggested that sonohysterography be performed at the time of premarital and pre-pregnancy counseling in women known to have congenital kidney and/or upper urinary tract abnormalities.

Abnormal findings on hysterosalpingography

Sonohysterography is often useful after abnormal findings are encountered at HSG to help determine the nature, size, and location of intracavitary lesions. It also aids in distinguishing between a global and a localized process. Sonohysterography can readily expose intrauterine adhesions, septum, and other findings that would otherwise not be disclosed owing to the lack of a three-dimensional viewing of the uterus.[14]

Indirect assessment of tubal obstruction

Richman et al[40] have observed that a prolonged and overdistended uterine cavity with injection of hysterosalpingographic contrast could falsely suggest tubal obstruction. In addition, cornual spasms have been observed in the hysterosalpingographic examination that may be overcome by the less intrusive sonographic evaluation.

Retained foreign bodies

Sonohysterography may be of benefit to women who either give a history of a 'lost' IUD or when the string cannot be visualized during an examination. Sonohysterography is a valuable tool for locating a foreign body within the uterine cavity and to ascertain whether the IUD is embedded in the myometrium or is adjacent to it.[1,2,4,17] The enhancement of the imaging with fluid infusion or an examination during the menstrual period ('spontaneous sonohysterography') could spare the patient from undergoing a radiographic examination of the pelvis, and the IUD can be removed during the same office visit.

Bussey and Laing[41] described the use of sonohysterography for documentation and removal of a fragment of laminaria from the uterine cavity.

Postabortal placental remnant

Diagnosis of retained placenta after spontaneous or induced abortion necessitates the performance of curettage. Prolonged postabortion bleeding is the main clinical sign of placental remnant; however, the diagnosis of postabortal trophoblastic residua is at times inconclusive by conventional ultrasonography.[42,43] Rulin et al[42] found that when the ultrasonographic findings were negative for placental remnants there was no need to perform a dilation and curettage (D&C); nevertheless when the ultrasound was positive the predictive value of TVS was only 69%. The introduction of color Doppler imaging improved the diagnostic accuracy by demonstrating lacunar blood flow within the lesion.[43] Color Doppler blood sampling should be improved by sonohysterography location of the placental remnants (*Fig. 7.13*). The use of these techniques improves diagnostic accuracy and reduces unnecessary D&Cs, thus preventing

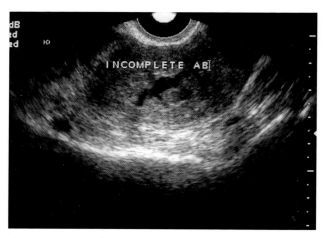

Figure 7.13 Sonohysterography performed in a woman who had abnormal bleeding following a D&C procedure. Endometrial irregularities are compatible with postabortal remnants. An additional uncomplicated procedure was required to evacuate postabortal trophoblastic tissue.

complications such as cervical laceration, hemorrhage, synechiae, and uterine perforation.

Triage for operative procedure

The information gathered from sonohysterography helps to determine whether endometrial biopsy, D&C, or diagnostic or operative hysteroscopy are needed.[5,20] It also aids in the selection of the type of hysteroscopic procedure and ascertains the hysteroscopic expertise required to remove the offending lesion.[5] Office operative sonohysterography with micrograsping forceps or loops to remove small pathologies might become possible in the near future.[6]

Comparisons with gold standards

Advantages

Although hysteroscopy and hysterosalpingography remain the 'gold standard' tests for the assessment of the uterine cavity, hysterosalpingography lacks specificity and hysteroscopy is both sensitive and specific, generally requiring performance in an operating room setting under local and/or general anesthesia.[1–5,18] These requirements and flaws increase the risks and the cost.[18] In addition, there are failed hysteroscopies owing to poor visualization caused by blood, inability to insert the hysteroscope, and inadvertent uterine perforation.

Randolph et al[14] demonstrated that there was agreement between sonohysterography and hysteroscopy findings in 53 of 54 cases evaluated, resulting in a calculated sensitivity for sonohysterography of 98% and a specificity of 100%. The sensitivity of sonohysterography was 98% and specificity was 92% when comparing the sonohysterography data to hysterosalpingography. In addition, several other investigations have reported similar findings.[2,4,12–14,16–18,25,36] Cincinelli et al[44] showed that sonohysterography is as sensitive and specific as hysteroscopy.

The adnexa may be simultaneously visualized and coexisting pathology can be evaluated during sonohysterography, whereas hysterosalpingography and hysteroscopy cannot provide direct imaging of the ovaries and adnexa.[1–5,9] In addition, the lack or the presence of fluid in the cul-de-sac after sonohysterography provides indirect evidence about tubal patency.

Lastly, sonohysterography is less expensive than hysterosalpingography (average cost ranges $100.00–1000.00) and hysteroscopy ($300.00–2000.00), as sonohysterography charges range from $200.00 to $600.00.[33]

Pitfalls and complications

Sonohysterography is a straightforward procedure, and the few potential side-effects and complications should be anticipated and discussed with the patient before the examination.

Difficulties in passing a catheter because of cervical stenosis (rare) may either require gentle dilation with a small dilator or the placement of an endocervical laminaria before the examination. Alternatively, the practitioner could take advantage of a 'spontaneous, menstrual-filled uterine cavity', which could provide an acoustic interface enabling the evaluation of the endometrial cavity.

Suboptimal visualization of the uterus could occur if the woman is experiencing pain or the uterus is oriented in a plane that is difficult to image. Occasionally, inadequate testing results from the presence of false passages.

An unstable cervix may require the placement of a single tooth tenaculum at the anterior cervical lip after the administration of 1% lidocaine ($\sim$ 1 ml) to minimize the patient's discomfort. Vaginal spotting and light bleeding are not uncommon.[1,2,15,45]

Severe pain, exacerbation of an undetected infection, and vasovagal responses are uncommon, but cramping can occur during fast saline infusion, especially if it has not been warmed (37°C).[2,13] The authors have encountered moderate vasovagal reactions on two occasions when the sonohysterography was performed at the time of initial visit. Perhaps heightened anxiety predisposes to these reactions. Interestingly, one patient had a large adenomyotic uterus which in itself would increase the release of prostaglandins and other 'stress' substances favoring reactions.

High placement of the catheter into the cavity and the inflation of the balloon can lead to the misdiagnosis of cervical pathology. In addition, flushing cervical mucus into the uterine cavity could potentially mimic synechiae. Overdistension of the cavity and a fast rate of saline infusion may cause pain and distort anatomical configuration. Incidental injection of air bubbles (the lack of priming the catheter) may obscure visualization of the uterine cavity.

Repeating sonohysterography after menses may demonstrate that the initial findings of a secretory polypoid-like endometrium does not indicate any pathology.

Dubinski et al[46] described a case of endometritis following sonohysterography, performed 2 weeks after an endometrial biopsy. Thus, it would seem prudent to limit the number of invasive uterine procedures during short time intervals. In addition, antibiotic coverage may be warranted if consecutive procedures were necessary.

If the patient has endometrial carcinoma, there is a theoretical risk of retrograde flushing of malignant endometrium. Studies have shown that lymphatic and venous intravasation of contrast medium do not alter 5-year survival rates in patients with endometrial cancer.[47] Therefore, it is believed that the same principles would apply for sonohysterography examinations.

To our knowledge, perforation of the uterus has never been reported with sonohysterography. If caution is exercised, most of the potential complications can be avoided.

Contraindications

Sonohysterography is a safe procedure, although a few contraindications should be noted. First, avoid the possibility of disrupting a normally implanted pregnancy. Although Sternberg[48] reported that there was no increase in adverse fetal effects if a hysterosalpingogram was inadvertently performed during pregnancy, it seems prudent to obtain a quantitative pregnancy test before the sonohysterogram. However, if sonohysterography is performed in the presence of a pregnancy, the investigator could feel somewhat reassured by Sternberg's report,[48] as well as the fact that with sonohysterography the embryo is not exposed to radiation. It is also important to avoid reactivation of pelvic inflammatory disease.

Conclusions

Sonohysterography is a relatively simple, quick, safe, inexpensive, and sensitive technique, which complements routine examinations in the evaluation of uterine disease. It assists in determining who needs further diagnostic or therapeutic intervention. Adherence to aseptic techniques and careful procedural evaluation are important to avoid infection. Gynecologists should consider making sonohysterography a routine part of their gynecological procedure as long as they possess education in ultrasound; otherwise they should use a skilled radiologist/ultrasonographer.

Some sonographers and gynecologists speculate that sonohysterography may replace diagnostic hysteroscopy and HSG. Some clinicians rely so much on sonohysterography that they begin treatment based on sonohysterography data; others believe that sonohysterography may become the procedure of choice for evaluating the endometrial cavity. While these authors respect and partially concur with all the previous statements, they believe that fluid enhancement for sonographic imaging of the uterine cavity in infertile women is the next step to a detailed history and physical examination and pelvic sonography. Sonohysterography will presents limitations, and because of them, clinicians should exercise their expertise and use sonohysterography either as the procedure of choice or to complement other investigations as dictated by the clinical situation.

Acknowledgment

The authors acknowledge Mr Gustavo S Serafini for editorial assistance in the preparation of this manuscript.

REFERENCES

1. Graham D, Chung SN. Office sonohysterography. *Adv Obstet Gynecol* 1997; **4**:137–159.
2. Chung PH, Parsons AK. A practical guide to using saline infusion sonohysterography. *Contemp Obstet Gynecol* 1997; **42**:21–34.
3. Ayida G, Chamberlain P, Barlow D, Kennedy S. Uterine cavity assessment prior to in vitro fertilization: comparison of transvaginal scanning, saline contrast hysterosonography and hysteroscopy. *Ultrasound Obstet Gynecol* 1997; **10**:59–62.
4. Hill A. Sonohysterography in the office: instruments and technique. *Contemp Obstet Gynecol* 1997; **42**:95–110.
5. Bradley LD, Andrews BJ. Saline infusion sonography for endometrial evaluation. *Female Patient* 1998; **23**:12–41.
6. Lindheim SR. Sonohysterography: nascent applications. *OBG Management* 1997; 46–55.
7. Nannini R, Chelo E, Branconi F, Tantini C, Scarselli GF. Dynamic echohysteroscopy: a new diagnostic technique in the study of female infertility. *Acta Eur Fertil* 1981; **12**:165–171.
8. Parsons AK, Lense JJ. Sonohysterography for endometrial abnormalities: preliminary results. *J Clin Ultrasound* 1993; **21**:87–95.
9. Maroulis GB, Parsons AK, Yeko TR. Hydrogenecography: a new technique enables vaginal sonography to visualize pelvic adhesions and other pelvic structures. *Fertil Steril* 1992; **58**:1073–1075.
10. Cullinan JA, Fleischer AC, Kepple DM, Arnold AL. Sonohysterography: a technique for endometrial evaluation. *Radiographics* 1995; **15**:501–514.
11. Schlief R, Deichert U. Hysterosalpingo-contrast sonography of the uterus and fallopian tubes: results of a clinical trial of a new contrast medium in 120 patients. *Radiology* 1991; **178**:213–215.
12. Fleischer AC, Vasquez JM, Cullinan JA, Eisenberg E. Sonohysterography combined with sonosalpingography: correlation with endoscopic findings in infertility patients. *J Ultrasound Med* 1997; **16**:381–384.
13. Goldstein SR. Saline infusion sonohysterography. *Clin Obstet Gynecol* 1996; **39**:248–258.
14. Randolph JR, Ying YK, Maier DB, Schmidt CL, Riddick DH. Comparison of real-time ultrasonography, hysterosalpingography, and laparoscopy/hysteroscopy in the evaluation of uterine abnormalities and tubal patency. *Fertil Steril* 1986; **46**:828–832.
15. Bonilla-Musoles F, Simon C, Serra V, Sampaio M, Pellicer A. An assessment of hysterosalpingosonography as a diagnostic tool for uterine cavity defects and tubal patency. *J Clin Ultrasound* 1992; **20**:175–181.
16. Syrop CH, Sahakian V. Transvaginal sonographic detection of endometrial polyps with fluid contrast augmentation. *Obstet Gynecol* 1992; **79**:1041–1043.

17. Van Roessel J, Wamsteker K, Exalto N. Sonographic investigation of the uterus during artificial uterine cavity distention. *J Clin Ultrasound* 1987; **15**:439–450.

18. Bernard JP, Lécuru F, Darles C, Robin F, de Bievre P, Taurelle R. Saline contrast sonohysterography as first-line investigation for women with uterine bleeding. *Ultrasound Obstet Gynecol* 1997; **10**:121–125.

19. Saidi MH, Sadler RK, Theis VD *et al*. Comparison of sonography, sonohysterography, and hysteroscopy for evaluation of abnormal uterine bleeding. *J Ultrasound Med* 1997; **16**:587–591.

20. Goldstein SR. Use of ultrasonohysterography for triage of perimenopausal patients with unexplained uterine bleeding. *Am J Obstet Gynecol* 1994; **170**:565–570.

21. Kelly AC. The uterine factor and fertility. *Infertil Reprod Med Clin North Am* 1991; **2**:391–407.

22. Gutmann JN. Imaging in the evaluation of female infertility. *J Reprod Med* 1992; **37**:54–61.

23. March CM. Hysteroscopy. *J Reprod Med* 1992; **37**:293–312.

24. Narayan R, Goswamy RK. Transvaginal sonography of the uterine cavity with hysteroscopic correlation in the investigation of infertility. *Ultrasound Obstet Gynecol* 1993; **3**:129–133.

25. Romano F, Cicinelli E, Anastasio PS, Epifani S, Fanelli F, Galantino P. Sonohysterography versus hysteroscopy for diagnosing endouterine abnormalities in fertile women. *Intl J Gynaecol Obstet* 1994; **45**:253–260.

26. Acién P. Uterine anomalies and recurrent miscarriage. *Infertil Reprod Med Clin North Am* 1996; **7**:689–719.

27. Alatas C, Aksoy E, Akarsu C, Yakin K, Aksoy S, Hayran M. Evaluation of intrauterine abnormalities in infertile patients by sonohysterography. *Human Reprod* 1997; **12**:487–490.

28. Keltz MD, Olive DL, Kim AH, Arici A. Sonohysterography for screening in recurrent pregnancy loss. *Fertil Steril* 1997; **67**:670–674.

29. Tho PT, Byrd JR, McDonough PG. Etiologies and subsequent reproductive performance of 100 couples with recurrent abortion. *Fertil Steril* 1979; **32**:389–395.

30. Harger J, Archer D, Marchese S, Muracca-Clemens M, Garver K. Etiology of recurrent pregnancy losses and outcome of subsequent pregnancies. *Obstet Gynecol* 1983; **62**:574–581.

31. Stray-Pedersen B, Stray-Pedersen S. Etiologic factors and subsequent reproductive performance in 195 couples with a prior history of habitual abortion. *Am J Obstet Gynecol* 1984; **148**:140–146.

32. Seinara P, Maccario S, Visentin L, DiGregario A. Hysteroscopy in an IVF-ER program. *Acta Obstet Gynecol Scand* 1988; **67**:135–137.

33. Lindheim SR, Sauer MV. Upper genital-tract screening with hysterosonography in patients receiving donated oocytes. *Intl J Gynecol Obstet* 1998; **60**:47–50.

34. Serafini P, Nelson J, Batzofin J. IVF-surrogates of donated oocytes. In: Sauer MV, ed. *Principles of Oocyte and Embryo Donation*. New York: Springer-Verlag, 1998: 313–322.

35. Fujkuda M, Shimizu T, Fukuda K, Yomura W, Shimizu S. Transvaginal hysterosonography for differential diagnosis between submucous and intramural myoma. *Gynecol Obstet Invest* 1993; **35**:236–239.

36. Cicinelli E, Romano F, Anastasio PS, Blasi N, Parisi C, Galantino P. Transabdominal sonohysterography, transvaginal sonography, and hysteroscopy in the evaluation of submucous myomas. *Obstet Gynecol* 1995; **85**:42–47.

37. Hirai M, Ookubo H, Inaba N *et al*. A study for the diagnosis of adenomyosis by TVS. *Chiba Med J* 1993; **69**:25.

38. Hirai M, Shibata K, Sagai H, Sekiya S, Goldberg BB. Transvaginal pulsed and color Doppler sonography for the evaluation of adenomyosis. *J Ultrasound Med* 1995; **14**:529–532.

39. Atzori E, Tronci C, Sionis L. Transvaginal ultrasound in the diagnosis of diffuse adenomyosis. *Gynecol Obstet Invest* 1996; **42**:39–41.

40. Richman TS, Viscomi GN, DeCherney A, Polan ML, Alcebo LO. Fallopian tubal patency assessed by ultrasound following fluid injection. *Radiology* 1984; **152**:507–510.

41. Bussey LA, Laing FC. Sonohysterography for detection of a retained laminaria fragment. *J Ultrasound Med* 1996; **16**:249–251.

42. Rulin MC, Bornstein SG, Campbell JD. The reliability of ultrasonography in the management of spontaneous abortion, clinically thought to be complete: a prospective study. *Am J Obstet Gynecol* 1993; **168**:12–15.

43. Tal J, Timor-Tritsch I, Degani S. Accurate diagnosis of postabortal placental remnant by sonohysterography and color Doppler sonographic studies. *Gynecol Obstet Invest* 1997; **43**:131–134.

44. Cicinelli E, Romano F, Anastasio PS, Blasi N, Parisi C. Sonohysterography versus hysteroscopy in the diagnosis of endouterine polyps. *Gynecol Obstet Invest* 1994; **38**:266–271.

45. Widrich T, Bradley LD, Mitchinson AR, Collins RL. Comparison of saline infusion sonography with office hysteroscopy for the evaluation of the endometrium. *Am J Obstet Gynecol* 1996; **174**:1327–1334.

46. Dubinsky TJ, Parvey R, Gormaz G, Maklad N. Transvaginal hysterosonography in the evaluation of small endoluminal masses. *J Ultrasound Med* 1995; **14**:1–6.

47. DeVore GR, Schwartz PE, Morris J. Hysterography: a 5-year follow-up in patients with endometrial carcinoma. *Obstet Gynecol* 1982; **60**:369–372.

48. Sternberg J. Irradiation and radiocontamination during pregnancy. *Am J Obstet Gynecol* 1970; **108**:490–513.

8 Sonosalpingography

Arthur C Fleischer, Anna K Parsons, Jaime M Vasquez and Jeanne A Cullinan

Sonosalpingography (SSG) is a technique which uses transvaginal sonography to evaluate tubal patency and morphology (*Fig. 8.1*). It involves the use of either saline and/or a contrast medium for assessment of tubal patency. Several multi-centered studies indicate that it is as accurate as the established techniques such as hysterosalpingography (HSG) for assessment of tubal patency.[1,2] This chapter will describe the current use of sonosalpingography as well as its limitations and future refinements.

Technique

Sonosalpingography utilizes transvaginal sonography (TVS) during instillation of either saline or contrast medium into the uterine lumen. It is best performed after sonohysterography, since sonohysterography is vital in delineating the endometrial surfaces for presence of synechiae or intraluminal lesions such as polyps or submucosal fibroids.[3,4] Another advantage of performing sonohysterography prior to sonosalpingography is that the fluid introduced by sonohysterography tends to surround the ovary, giving a hypoechoic background for assessment of the echogenic contrast which is expressed from a patent tube after intrauterine injection (*Fig. 8.2*).

The study must be performed in real time and recorded on videotape. The examiner is encouraged to apply gentle pressure with the probe while sonographically assessing the mobility of the uterus, ovary, and tube.

Saline can be used initially for assessment for tubal patency. However, if there is any doubt about tubal spill, contrast should be used. It is necessary to have a ballooned catheter to block egress of fluid from the uterine lumen during injection. After sonohysterography has been performed, the saline should be removed prior to instillation of positive contrast.

These authors found that in about 75% of the patients in a study series tubal patency could be assessed by repeated injections of 3–5 ml of sterile saline. However, contrast afforded accurate assessment of tubal patency in almost 92% of the patients.[5] Therefore, when there is no definite spillage or when the initial findings are equivocal, a positive contrast is needed to establish tubal patency.

Some investigators advocate the use of color Doppler sonography with saline instillation in order to best depict tubal patency.[6] This technique can also be used with contrast. Preliminary work suggests that three-dimensional and harmonic imaging greatly enhances sonographic depiction of the tube (A. Parsons, personal communication) (*Fig. 8.2d*).

Albunex® has been used for multiple applications, including evaluation of tubal patency. It provides an echogenic contrast to document tubal patency and spillage. The safety of Albunex® has been established in multiple studies, but its cost ($83/10 ml vial) makes selected use necessary. Albunex® consists of microbubbles suspended in human albumen. It must be stored and used properly for its best effect.

Normal and abnormal anatomy

Before contrast or saline is introduced, it is recommended that the sonographer identify the approximate location of the tube by identifying the ovary and endometrium that invaginates into the uterine cornua (see *Fig. 8.1b*). Once this scan plane is established, the practitioner can follow contrast spillage around the ovary, since the fimbriated end of the tube is near. In some cases, the contrast can be 'chased' by re-injection of 5–10 ml of saline to maximize tubal delineation.

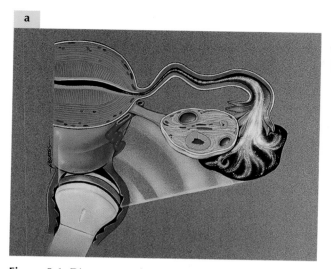
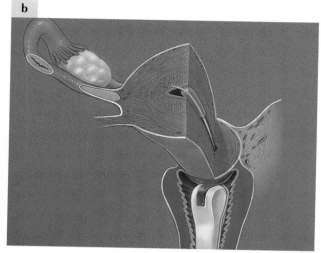

Figure 8.1 Diagrams and TVS images showing sonosalpingography. (a) Diagram showing positive (echogenic) contrast within and egressing from the left tube while being imaged with a transvaginal sonographic probe (drawing by Paul Gross). (b) Same subject as in (a) showing short axis image of uterine lumen and tubes (drawing by Paul Gross).

If there is pain during injection, this may be a sign of tubal obstruction, either intrinsic or extrinsic from adhesions. Spasm may be present and may cause transitory lack of filling of the proximal portion of the tube (*Fig. 8.3*).

With the use of saline or contrast, the normal tubal lumen is easily identified as thin (approximately 1 mm) serginious adnexal structures. The motion of saline and/or contrast also helps to identify the lumen, particularly when color Doppler sonography is used.

Hydrosalpinges appear as fusiform cystic structures on TVS (*Figs 8.4* and *8.5*). The contrast may dilute or bubbles may come out of suspension, making complete delineation difficult to recognize (see *Fig. 8.4*). If a hydrosalpinx is seen, patients may be given 200 mg doxycycline initially, then 100 mg po bid for 5 days for prophylaxis of pelvic inflammatory disease.

Comparison with hysterosalpingography

The large multi-centered study in Europe has indicated that sonosalpingography with Levovist® (which is a suspension of microbubbles in a galactose solution) is as accurate for assessment of tubal patency as hysterosalpingography (HSG).[1] In many cases, SSG is preferable in that it does not produce significant pain during the procedure and does not require fluoroscopic evaluation. However, one limitation of SSG is that it does not allow a confident diagnosis of salpingitis isthmica nodosa. If this condition is suspected, HSG is the preferred modality for delineation of anatomic detail.

Another problem that can occur with the use of Albunex® is difficulty in establishing tubal patency in patients with obstructing lesions such as cornual fibroids. Another limitation is that the contrast can

Figure 8.2 *(opposite)* Normal patent tubes. (a) TVS during Albunex® instillation showing entire tube. The Doppler range gate is on the isthmic portion of the tube and showed Doppler shift confirming patency. The ampullary portion of the tube (arrowhead) shows normal anatomic widening of the lumen. (b) Sequential images showing normal periovarian flow in a patient with a patent tube. (i) Initial TVS of an ovary containing a mature follicle with clear fluid surrounding it; (ii) 7 seconds later showing some pooling of echogenic contrast inferior to the ovary and contrast egressing from fimbriated end of tube (arrow); (iii) 40 seconds later showing fill in around the entire ovary; (iv) 2 minutes later showing nearly complete dissolution of contrast into surrounding fluid around the ovary. An adhesion between the ovary and bowel is outlined by surrounding anechoic fluid. (c) Bilaterally patent tubes. (i) Prior to sonohysterography, right ovary with a nearly mature follicle; (ii) after sonohysterography, saline pools around the right ovary; (iii) 'catfish' configuration of the tubal ostia as depicted in transverse section showing contrast in both proximal tubes; (iv) the right tube could be followed into its interstitial portion; (v) same as (iv) above, showing proximal left tube. (d) Three-dimensional color Doppler sonogram of normal tube obtained during Albunex® instillation using harmonic imaging.

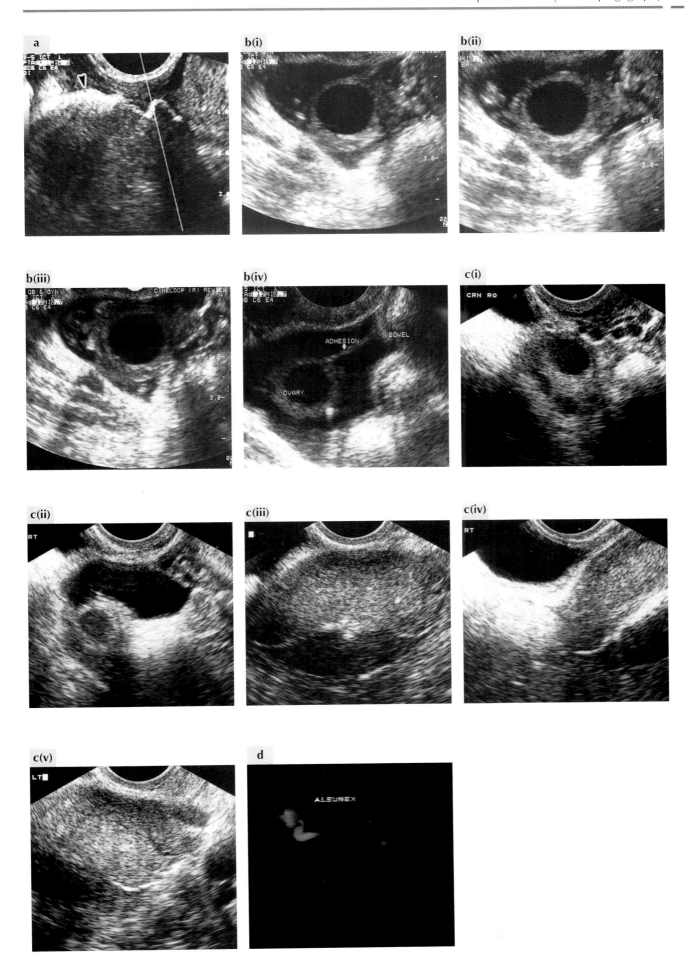

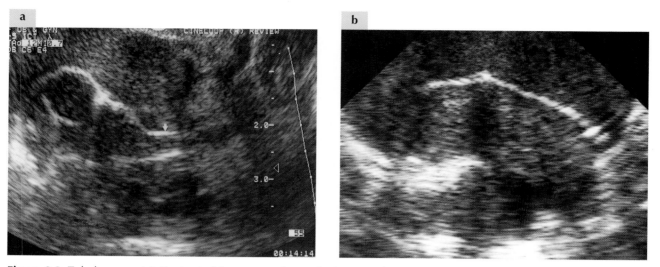

Figure 8.3 Tubal spasm. (a) Contrast did not extend past the interstitial portion of the tube (arrow) even after observation for 20 minutes. Follow-up scans at 30 and 45 minutes showed no tubal spillage. (b) Initial tubal spasm at tubal ostia which filled normally 10 minutes later.

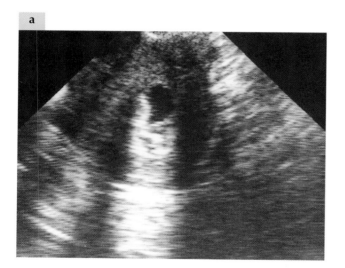

Figure 8.4 Tubal obstruction (extrinsic). (a) Initial distension of lumen without tubal spill. (b,c) Bilateral cornual fibroids (between cursors) probably caused this appearance.

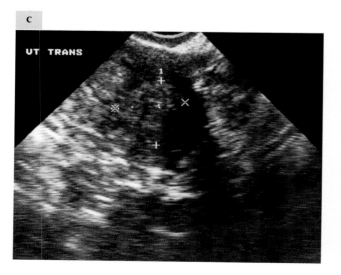

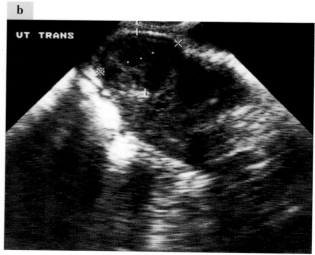

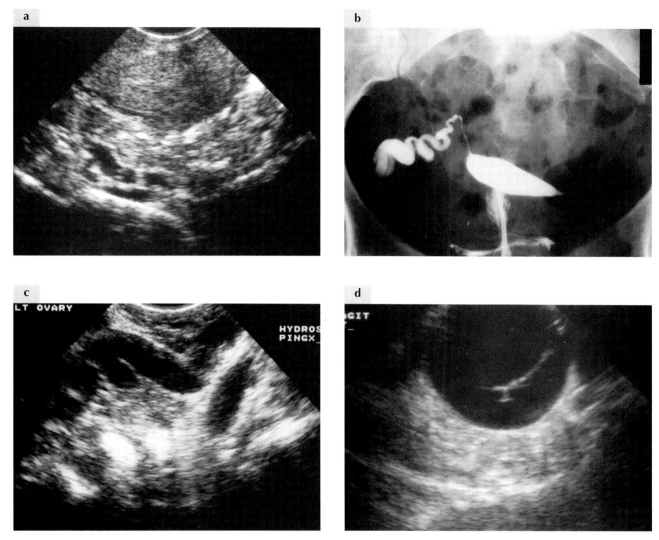

Figure 8.5 Hydrosalpinges as diagnosed on TVS without contrast. (a) TVS showing small hydrosalpinx. (b) HSG of same patient as in (a) showing small hydrosalpinx without intraperitoneal spill. (c) Unilateral distension of left tube seen prior to sonosalpingography. (d) Sactosalpinx of left tube seen prior to SSG.

become diluted in hydrosalpinges that contain a significant amount of fluid. Less than optimal echogenicity can result from improper storage of contrast or faulty administration of the contrast.

SSG findings

In patent tubes, contrast can be seen exiting the fimbriated end of the tube which usually surrounds and is adjacent to the ovary (see *Fig. 8.2*). Fibroids may obstruct flow within the tube, as can intraluminal processes owing to adhesions or previous surgery (see *Fig. 8.4*). True obstruction is associated

with lack of egress of saline or contrast from the fimbriated end of the tube after an appropriate length (15–20 minutes) of observation (see *Fig. 8.5*). Hydrosalpinges appear as fusiform structures which are fluid filled. Occasionally the tubal endosalpingeal folds can be recognized[7] (*Fig. 8.6*).

Investigators must be cautious in differentiating tubal obstruction from tubal spasm. In some patients, introduction of contrast may be associated with tubal spasm and a follow-up examination after the spasm relaxes may indicate tubal patency.

Some workers advocate the use of saline with color Doppler sonography. This technique provides

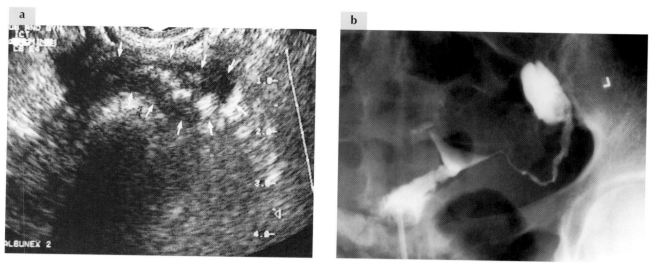

Figure 8.6 Hydrosalpinx with fimbrial obstruction. (a) Distended left tube (arrows) as shown on SSG. (b) Hysterosalpingography showing left hydrosalpinx and no intraperitoneal spill.

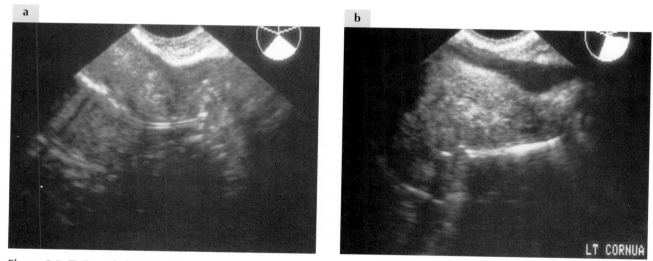

Figure 8.7 TVS-guided tubal dilatation. (a) Initial TVS showing catheter post-tubal ostia. (b) With extension of inner catheter into the isthmic portion of the left tube.

detection of motion of fluid or contrast within and out of the tube.[8] In our series, contrast was needed in about half of the cases in order to insure that the initial sonographic evaluation with saline for tubal patency was accurate.[5]

Summary

Sonosalpingography provides accurate assessment of tubal patency. In addition, the mobility and relative position of the tube and ovary can be assessed. The diagnostic accuracy of this technique is comparable to HSG and chromoperturbation and it can be performed in an office setting. SSG will become the initial study of choice for evaluation of tubal patency, with HSG reserved for specific conditions such as salpingitis isthmica nodosa. TVS can also be used for selective tubal dilatation, insuring proper location of the catheter tip (*Fig. 8.7*).

REFERENCES

1. Campbell S, Bourne TH, Tan SL, Collins WP. Hysterosalpingo contrast sonography (HyCoSy) and its future role within the investigation of infertility in Europe. *Ultrasound Obstet Gynecol* 1994; **4**:245–253.

2. Lerner J. *Sonographic Evaluation of Tubal Patency using Albunex®*. Madrid: Marban, 1977: 53.

3. Parsons A, Lense J. Sonohysterography for endometrial abnormalities: preliminary results. *Clin Ultrasound* 1993; **21**:87–95.

4. Cullinan J, Fleischer A, Kepple D, Arnold A. Sonohysterography: a technique for endometrial evaluation. *RadioGraphics* 1995; **15**:501-514.

5. Fleischer AC, Vasquez JM, Cullinan JA, Eisenberg E. Sonohysterography combined with sonosalpingography: correlation with endoscopic findings in infertility patients. *J Ultrasound Med* 1997; **16**:381–384.

6. Kupesic A. *Evaluation of Infertile Patients using Transvaginal Color Doppler and 3-D Imaging.* Madrid: Marban, 1997: 49.

7. Tessler F, Perrella L, Fleischer A, Grant E. Endovaginal sonographic diagnosis of Fallopian tube dilation. *Am J Roentgenol* 1989; **153**:523–525.

8. Stern J, Peters AJ, Coulam CB. Colour Doppler ultrasonography assessment of tubal patency: a comparison study with traditional techniques. *Fertil Steril* 1992; **58**:897–900.

9 Hysterosalpingography

John A Richmond

Introduction

Hysterosalpingography is a diagnostic procedure in which there is radiographic visualization of the endocervical canal, the endometrial cavity, and the lumina of the fallopian tubes by an injected radiopaque contrast medium. A wide variety of uterine and tubal abnormalities, which cause infertility and other reproductive problems, can be demonstrated by this procedure. A normal endometrial cavity on the hysterosalpingogram (HSG) obviates the need for hysteroscopy. When there has been radiographic demonstration of a lesion within the endometrial cavity, then the tandem use of the two procedures is recommended, with hysteroscopy as the treatment modality.[1,2] The American Society for Reproductive Medicine (formerly the American Fertility Society) has recognized hysterosalpingography and laparoscopy as complementary procedures in the diagnostic evaluation of the fallopian tubes and for determination of the appropriate surgical treatment and the prognosis in cases of distal tubal obstruction.[3]

There are many variations in the appearance of a normal HSG. The margins of the endocervical canal may be smooth or serrated, depending on the degree of prominence of the mucosal folds, the plicae palmatae.[4] The junction of the endocervical canal and endometrial cavity is commonly demarcated by only a localized narrowing, the internal os; but a well-defined narrow segment, representing a more prominent uterine isthmus, may exist above the internal os, between the endocervical canal and the endometrial cavity. The endometrial cavity is usually triangular in shape, or sometimes T-shaped, in the anteroposterior (AP) or frontal projection, and has an oblong shape in the lateral view (*Figs 9.1* and *9.2*). The contour of the endometrial cavity is smooth or slightly irregular and can be altered by uterine contractions during the course of an examination. Normal endometrium can occasionally produce polypoid filling defects in the contrast medium, which range in size from 5 mm to 10 mm

in diameter and can be seen throughout the endometrial cavity or confined to only one area[5] (*Figs 9.3* and *9.4*). This normal variation has no clinical implications and should not be confused with endometrial hyperplasia, which may result in a shaggy, irregular cavity contour and is found in patients with a history of amenorrhea and irregular menses. The polypoid filling defects of normal endometrium are not dissimilar to defects caused by small submucous leiomyomas or polyps, but the diffuse or regional pattern of involvement is unusual for these small mass lesions. Furthermore, the hysteroscopic appearance of this normal endometrial variation is distinct from that of submucous leiomyomas and polyps. However, unless abnormal uterine bleeding is present, hysteroscopic evaluation is unnecessary; and a diagnostic endometrial curettage is no longer warranted, now that the nature of this radiographic pattern has become better known.

The normal fallopian tube consists of a thin proximal portion, representing the interstitial segment and the isthmus, and a more distended distal portion, which represents the ampulla and its termination in the fimbria (see *Fig. 9.1*). The interstitial segment is approximately 1 cm in length and is contained within the wall of the uterus. The isthmus is the extrauterine segment of the thin portion of the tube. There is a gradual increase in the size of the lumen in the midportion of the tube, representing the transition from the isthmus to the ampulla. The ampulla contains longitudinal mucosal folds or rugae, the endosalpingeal plicae.

A normal HSG does not exclude the presence of significant pelvic adhesions, and laparoscopy may subsequently be required for further evaluation. However, there is evidence of a possible therapeutic effect of hysterosalpingography in patients with normal and patent fallopian tubes. In a recent study, 29% of 132 infertility patients became pregnant without laparoscopic intervention following a normal HSG with a water-soluble contrast medium.[6] It was recommended that laparoscopy not be

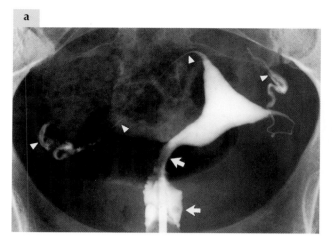

Figure 9.1 Normal HSG in a patient, gravida(G)3 para(P)0 spontaneous abortion(SAB)3, being evaluated for recurrent abortion. (a) Frontal view prior to spill of contrast medium from the fallopian tubes. The endocervical canal (lower arrow) has smooth margins. A well-defined uterine isthmus (upper arrow) leads to a triangular shaped endometrial cavity, formed by the fundus and lateral walls of the uterus. The thin proximal portion of each fallopian tube represents the interstitial segment and the isthmus (small triangles adjacent to the right tube only). The more distended distal portions of the tubes, the ampullae (laterally placed small triangles), contain thin, linear filling defects representing the mucosal folds, the endosalpingeal plicae. (b) Lateral view of the endometrial cavity (arrow), which is oblong shaped in this projection and formed by the anterior and posterior walls of the uterus.

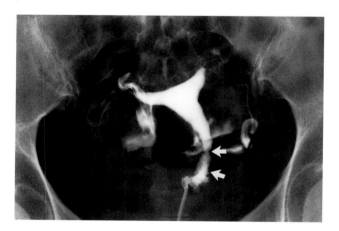

Figure 9.2 Normal HSG with a T-shaped endometrial cavity in a patient with secondary infertility. The endocervical canal (lower arrow) has slightly serrated margins caused by normal mucosal folds, the plicae palmatae. The internal os (upper arrow) is small and well defined. Free spill of contrast medium from the tubes is noted below the right cornu and at and slightly above the level of the internal os.

performed for at least 3 months following a normal HSG, because the pregnancy rate in the first 3 months was four times that of any subsequent 3-month period.

Abnormalities of the uterus

Congenital uterine (Müllerian duct fusion) anomalies are associated with an increased incidence of first and second trimester spontaneous abortion, premature labor, and fetal malpresentation. In a study of 186 pregnancies in 150 women with Müllerian duct fusion anomalies, 80% of all pregnancies required a cesarean section for fetal malpresentation; and septate and bicornuate uteri had the highest incidences of spontaneous abortion and premature infants.[7] In addition, vaginal septa are more commonly seen in association with uterine anomalies, and a transverse septum may obstruct one cervix of a uterus didelphys or the

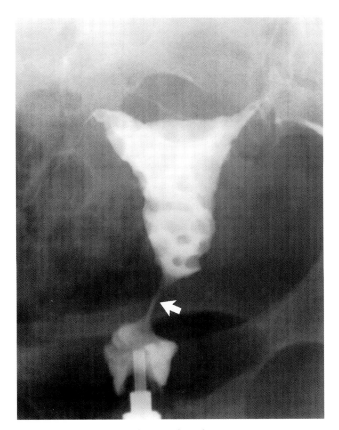

Figure 9.3 Variation of normal endometrium in a patient with primary infertility for 1 year and normal menstrual periods. There are small polypoid filling defects in the contrast medium throughout the endometrial cavity, with a larger defect at the fundus, all representing normal proliferative endometrium. Confirmed by hysteroscopic inspection and diagnostic curettage. Incidentally noted is a well demarcated uterine isthmus (arrow).

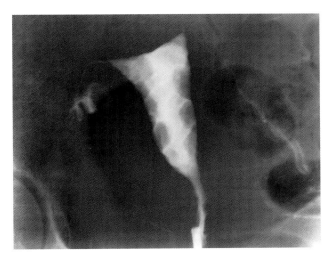

Figure 9.4 Variation of normal endometrium in a patient being evaluated for infertility. Multiple polypoid filling defects are seen along the lateral aspects of the endometrial cavity and near the fundus. Confirmed by hysteroscopic examination and diagnostic curettage.

cervix of a unicornuate uterus or other anomaly, causing a hematocolpos or hematometrium and associated pain. Furthermore, a uterine anomaly may coexist with one or more of a spectrum of other congenital anomalies included in the acronym of VATER or VACTERL (Vertebral, Anorectal, Cardiac, TracheoEsophageal, Renal, and Limb) association. Some of the vertebral anomalies that may be identified on the scout radiograph of the pelvis preceding hysterosalpingography include absence of the lower sacrum and coccyx, fusion of lower lumbar vertebrae, and lumbar hemivertebra. Neonatal conditions such as imperforate anus, rectal atresia, or esophageal atresia with tracheoesophageal fistula can be elicited by clinical history, and associated thoracic or lower abdominal surgical scars may be noted. Unilateral renal agenesis or renal ectopia may occur, and any patient with a uterine anomaly should be further evaluated with a renal ultrasound examination.

The American Society for Reproductive Medicine has developed a classification of uterine anomalies consisting of the following categories: agenesis or hypoplasia, unicornuate (with or without rudimentary horn), didelphys, bicornuate (complete or partial), septate (complete or partial), arcuate, and diethylstilbestrol (DES) deformity[3] (*Figs 9.5–9.7*). In addition to this classification, the communicating uterus is considered a separate type of anomaly, in which there is a localized communication between otherwise separate and duplicated endometrial cavities and endocervical canals.[8] The communicating uterus consists of either a septate or bicornuate uterus in combination with a duplicated or septate cervix and a septate or septum-free vagina (*Fig. 9.8*). Nine different types have been described, based on various combinations of uterine, cervical, and vaginal abnormalities. The localized communication occurs at the level of the uterine isthmus in eight types and between a patent endocervical canal and a blind ending endocervical sac in the ninth type. The hysterosalpingographer should have a thorough understanding of the preceding classifications.

Because septate and bicornuate uteri may have a similar radiographic appearance, an ultrasound examination to delineate the external uterine contour may be necessary to establish the correct diagnosis. On the HSG, an angle of divergence of the duplicated endometrial cavities ⩽ 75° has been shown to consistently correlate with a diagnosis of a septate uterus.[9] An ultrasound examination is recommended for further evaluation of patients with an angle >75° (see *Fig. 9.7*).

The initial diagnosis of DES exposure is rarely made from an HSG. Rather, women with known DES exposure are referred for hysterosalpingography

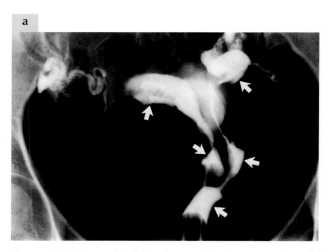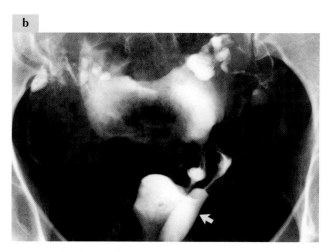

Figure 9.5 Uterus didelphys in a patient being evaluated for primary infertility and a suspected uterine anomaly. (a) A balloon catheter has been placed in a small anterior vagina (lower arrow), as the left cervix was obscured by a vaginal septum. A second balloon catheter has been placed in the right endocervical canal (middle arrow), and a partially distended left endocervical canal is noted at the same level (middle arrow). Slightly curved and oblong shaped, duplicated endometrial cavities (upper arrows) are demonstrated. The lower half of the left endometrial cavity is not distended owing to uterine contraction. (b) Asymmetric vaginas, opacified by drainage of contrast medium from the uterus didelphys after the balloon catheters had been removed. A small anterior vagina (arrow) and a larger posterior vagina are delineated.

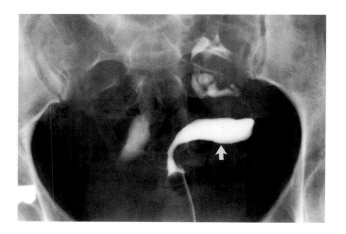

Figure 9.6 Unicornuate uterus in a patient being evaluated for a suspected uterine anomaly. A single oblong-shaped endometrial cavity (arrow) is seen on the left side of the pelvis and gives rise to the left fallopian tube. The presence or absence of a right rudimentary horn cannot be determined.

because of infertility and other reproductive problems. In a study of 267 DES-exposed patients, an abnormal endometrial cavity was demonstrated on the HSG in 69%, while 31% had normal cavities.[10] An abnormal cavity was much more likely to be seen in patients with vaginal epithelial or structural cervical changes. In a subsequent report based on 616 pregnancies in 327 DES-exposed women, the pregnancy outcome with respect to spontaneous abortion, ectopic pregnancy, and premature infants was significantly worse in those with radiographically abnormal cavities, compared with those with normal cavities.[11] Small size, T-shape, constrictions, irregular margins, and filling

defects were described as diagnostic features of the abnormal endometrial cavities (*Fig. 9.9*).

Intrauterine adhesions are usually caused by a previous curettage and are typically visualized on the HSG as irregular or linear filling defects in the contrast medium (*Fig. 9.10*). The extent and location of the adhesions usually determine the clinical significance. Adhesions in the lower endometrial cavity that obstruct the flow of contrast medium at the internal os will result in secondary amenorrhea and infertility (*Fig. 9.11*). This is not an uncommon hysterographic appearance in patients being evaluated for Asherman's syndrome and is usually caused

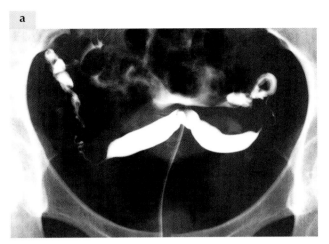
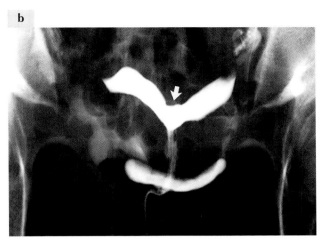

Figure 9.7 Bicornuate uterus in a patient being evaluated for primary infertility. The diagnosis was made by an ultrasound examination preceding the HSG. (a) An anteflexed V-shaped endometrial cavity is demonstrated, with the balloon catheter inflated in the lower cavity. The fallopian tubes are normal, and free spill of contrast medium is noted. (b) An angled view of the endometrial cavity, after deflation of the balloon, allows visualization of a collapsed endocervical canal and that portion of the lower cavity formerly occupied by the inflated balloon. The angle of divergence (arrow) is not optimally delineated but approximates 90°.

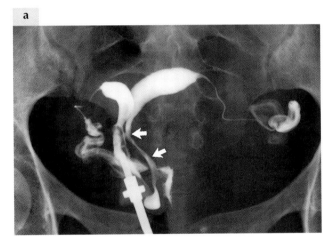
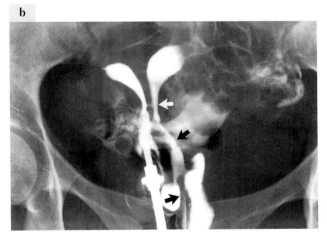

Figure 9.8 Communicating uterus, representing a septate uterus with a duplicated cervix, in a woman, G1 P0 SAB1, being evaluated for a uterine anomaly after two cervices and a vaginal septum had been discovered on a pelvic examination. A hysteroscopic excision of the uterine septum was subsequently performed. (a) A vacuum cannula has been attached to the right cervix, with its tip terminating in the right lower endometrial cavity. Injection of contrast medium demonstrates duplicated, oblong-shaped endometrial cavities and normal fallopian tubes. There is a localized communication (upper arrow) between the cavities at the level of the uterine isthmi, with drainage of contrast medium into a collapsed left endocervical canal (lower arrow). A small amount of leakage into the upper vaginas is also noted. (b) A slightly different projection demonstrates the close approximation of the endometrial cavities, consistent with a septate uterus. The localized communication is again noted (white arrow). The left endocervical canal (upper black arrow) overrides the vaginal septum (lower black arrow), which is the vertical defect outlined by leakage of contrast medium into the right and left vaginas.

by localized adhesions that can be treated successfully by hysteroscopic lysis. However, extensive involvement of the endometrial cavity may exist and should always be considered a possibility. Adhesions in the upper cavity may cause infertility by adversely affecting implantation of the fertilized ovum or by obstructing access to one or both fallopian tubes. Furthermore, successful hysteroscopic lysis of adhesions is more difficult in the upper cavity (CM March, personal communication).

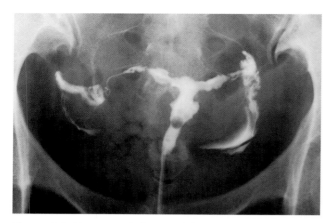

Figure 9.9 Upper genital tract deformity in a DES-exposed woman, G1 P0 SAB1. The endometrial cavity is T-shaped, with constrictions in the upper cavity. A small air bubble is incidentally noted in the lower cavity.

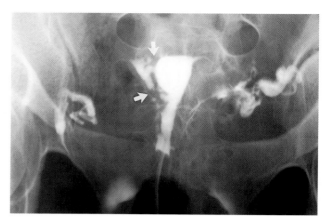

Figure 9.10 Mild intrauterine adhesions on the right side of the endometrial cavity, producing linear and irregular filling defects (arrows) from the lower cavity to the fundus. The patient, G3 elective abortion (EAB)2 SAB1, was being evaluated for secondary infertility. The diagnosis was confirmed at hysteroscopy.

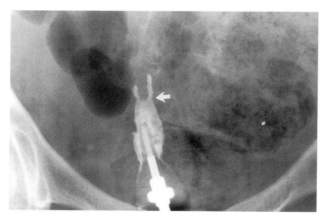

Figure 9.11 Asherman's syndrome in a woman, G3 P2 EAB1, with secondary amenorrhea for 10 months following the elective abortion. The endocervical canal is visualized, and there is obstruction to the flow of contrast medium at the level of the internal os (arrow). This is more commonly caused by adhesions confined to the lower endometrial cavity, but the possibility of diffuse involvement of the cavity should also be considered.

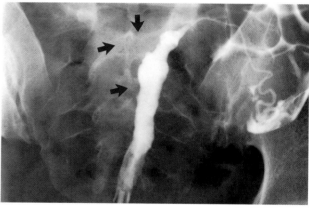

Figure 9.12 Intrauterine adhesions in the upper endometrial cavity, producing a deformity that mimics a unicornuate uterus. Nearly three-quarters of the upper cavity (approximated by arrows) has been obliterated by adhesions, preventing access to the right fallopian tube. The patient, G3 P2 SAB1, had secondary infertility for 6 years. Her most recent pregnancy, a cesarean section delivery of a normal infant, was complicated by a placenta accreta and uterine atony, requiring a curettage. This was presumably the source of the adhesions.

Intrauterine adhesions can constrict and deform the endometrial cavity and, occasionally, may mimic a uterine anomaly (*Fig. 9.12*). Another etiology of intrauterine adhesions is tuberculosis, which can spread from the fallopian tubes and cause cavity deformity or diffuse endometrial fibrosis that is radiographically indistinguishable from Asherman's syndrome (*Fig. 9.13*). However, there will be no history of a previous curettage, and the patient will present with infertility and either primary or secondary amenorrhea.

Small submucous leiomyomas and polyps produce round filling defects in the endometrial cavity and endocervical canal and may cause uterine bleeding. These lesions cannot be differentiated on the HSG, but can subsequently be specifically diagnosed and removed hysteroscopically. The optimal delineation

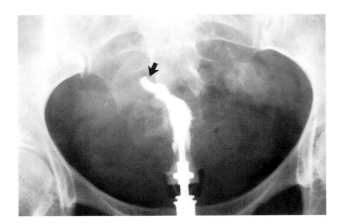

Figure 9.13 Advanced genital tuberculosis in a 29-year-old woman with primary infertility and primary amenorrhea, who had been treated for tuberculous meningitis in Mexico at age 16. The endocervical canal is visualized, and there has been almost complete obliteration of the endometrial cavity, except for a small remnant (arrow). The radiographic appearance of endometrial tuberculosis cannot be differentiated from Asherman's syndrome, but the clinical histories will differ. In this case, there was no previous curettage, but there was a history of active tuberculosis and primary amenorrhea.

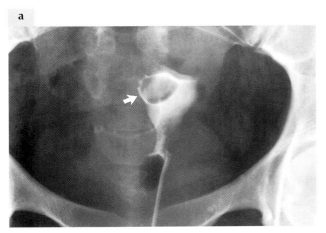
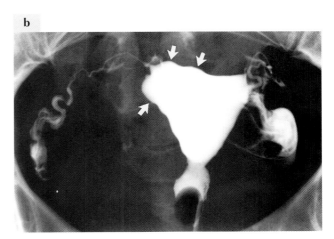

Figure 9.14 Polyp on the right side of the upper endometrial cavity in a patient, G1 P0 SAB1, being evaluated for secondary infertility. The lesion was removed at hysteroscopy. (a) A round filling defect, consistent with a submucous leiomyoma or a polyp, is demonstrated in the early phase of visualization of the cavity. (b) The filling defect becomes obscured by contrast medium in the fully distended cavity. There is associated enlargement of the right side of the upper endometrial cavity (arrows). This type of localized enlargement can also be caused by an intramural leiomyoma, with no filling defect to indicate a mass lesion.

of these small masses occurs with early filling of the endometrial cavity, as the lesions can be obscured in a fully distended cavity (*Fig. 9.14*). Larger filling defects are generally caused by submucous leiomyomas or intramural leiomyomas with submucous components, and there may be associated enlargement and distortion to the endometrial cavity (*Fig. 9.15*). These lesions can adversely affect implantation of the fertilized ovum and may obstruct access to a tubal ostium, as well as cause uterine bleeding. Intramural leiomyomas may displace, rotate, distort, and enlarge the endometrial cavity and, in some cases, cause asymmetrical enlargement of the cavity or enlargement of only the endocervical canal (*Fig. 9.16*). A large ovarian mass or pedunculated subserosal leiomyoma can also cause displacement and rotation, but will not distort the cavity or affect

its size (*Fig. 9.17*). Intramural leiomyomas do not cause fallopian tube obstruction but may stretch the proximal thin portion of the tube. A HSG will provide important information in the preoperative evaluation of a myomectomy candidate. A normal endometrial cavity should not be explored at the time of surgery, while the presence of a submucous leiomyoma might require additional hysteroscopic treatment. If advanced fallopian tube disease is demonstrated, a hysterectomy may be a more appropriate procedure.

Adenomyosis is most commonly manifested by small linear or diverticular projections of contrast medium, which extend from the endometrial cavity into the inner wall of the uterus. These small projections are usually localized or scattered and

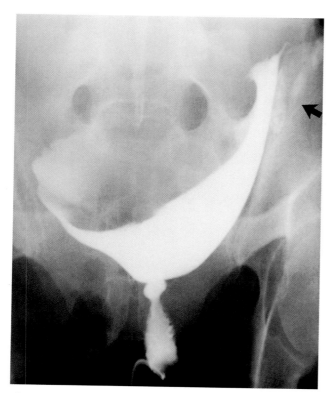

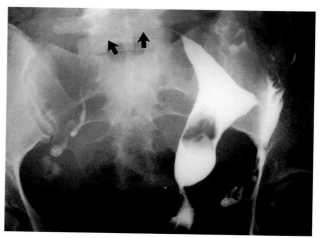

Figure 9.16 Intramural leiomyomas in a patient being evaluated for possible myomectomy. There is stretching of the interstitial segment and isthmus (arrows) of the right fallopian tube, but the tubes are otherwise normal. Associated enlargement of the endometrial cavity is noted, and there is a filling defect in the lower cavity, presumably representing a submucous leiomyoma. There was no surgical confirmation, as the patient desired a second opinion.

Figure 9.15 Large posterior and fundal submucous leiomyoma in a woman, G1 P0 SAB1, with a 20-week fibroid uterus on physical examination. The diagnosis was confirmed by a surgical myomectomy. The mass produces a large filling defect and causes enlargement of the endometrial cavity. Access to the right fallopian tube is blocked by the mass. A patent left fallopian tube (arrow) was demonstrated but is not well seen on this angled view.

presumably have no clinical significance. However, moderate to severe adenomyosis can result in extensive, branching channels of contrast medium throughout a thickened uterine wall (*Fig. 9.18*). A segment of the contour of the endometrial cavity may be obliterated by this process, and proximal tubal obstruction can occur when a cornu is severely affected. Occasionally, the overgrowth of uterine muscle associated with adenomyosis can produce a filling defect in the endometrial cavity that is indistinguishable from a submucous leiomyoma.[12] Clinically, the overgrowth of uterine muscle causes enlargement of the uterus, and menometrorrhagia and dysmenorrhea are common. Although small in number, the most severe cases of adenomyosis demonstrated by hysterosalpingography have been in women with primary infertility. If significant adenomyosis is discovered on a HSG in a patient being considered for a myomectomy, the uterus should be examined by magnetic resonance imaging to determine the predominant cause of uterine enlargement and possibly avoid unnecessary surgery or an unplanned hysterectomy.[13]

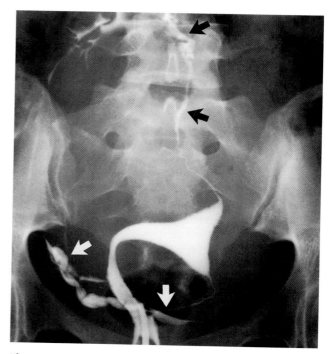

Figure 9.17 Large pedunculated, subserosal leiomyoma in a patient with a 20-week size mass on physical examination and who subsequently underwent a myomectomy. There is rotation of a normal endometrial cavity toward the left side of the pelvis, and normal fallopian tubes (black and white arrows) are displaced and draped over the mass. A similar appearance could be caused by a large ovarian mass.

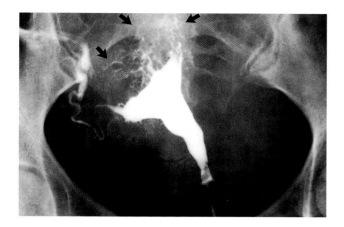

Figure 9.18 Adenomyosis, predominantly involving the fundus, in a 46-year-old patient, G0, with heavy vaginal bleeding for 1 year and a 12-week fibroid uterus on pelvic examination. The diagnosis was made on the basis of the HSG, which demonstrates branching channels of contrast medium (arrows) extending into an enlarged fundal area. This appearance might be confused with intravasation into uterine veins. In this case, the branching channels persisted after injection of contrast medium had ceased, whereas veins would disappear, owing to replacement of the contrast medium by non-opacified blood. The left fallopian tube was not visualized, possibly related to involvement of the left cornu by adenomyosis. A subsequent ultrasound study demonstrated an enlarged, globular uterus with distinct masses consistent with leiomyomas in the lateral walls of the lower uterus, but no distinct mass in the fundus.

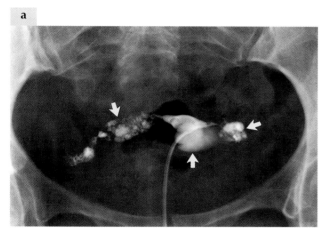

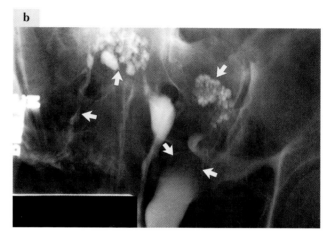

Figure 9.19 Severe bilateral SIN in a 37-year-old patient with primary infertility and an ultrasound diagnosis of a left hydrosalpinx. A left salpingectomy was subsequently performed, and severe pelvic endometriosis and a left ovarian cyst were discovered at the time of surgery. Approximately 1.5 years after the HSG, a right salpingectomy was performed for an ectopic tubal pregnancy. (a) Spot radiograph with the balloon catheter in an anteflexed endometrial cavity. Multiple diverticular collections of contrast medium (upper arrows) are demonstrated adjacent to the proximal portions of the fallopian tubes. A saccular collection of contrast medium (lower arrow) represents the distal portion of a left hydrosalpinx. (b) Angled view obtained after deflation of the catheter balloon, with better delineation of the lower cavity. Numerous diverticula (upper arrows) are again seen, consistent with severe SIN. A normal right ampulla (middle arrow) is noted, and there is free spill from the right tube. There is an area of apparent discontinuity (lower arrows) between a non-distended segment of proximal left ampulla and the hydrosalpinx below. This appearance is related to dilution of the contrast medium by retained fluid in the hydrosalpinx.

Fallopian tube abnormalities

Salpingitis isthmica nodosa (SIN) is a condition predominantly involving the interstitial segment and isthmus of the fallopian tube, in which the endothelial lining penetrates into the muscularis. If the depth of penetration is sufficient, nodular thickenings are produced along the serosal surface of the tube, which may be observed during laparoscopy. This entity may represent a manifestation of tubal infection or may be related to an acquired, non-inflammatory process similar to adenomyosis. SIN is demonstrated on the HSG by nodular diverticula or irregular tracks of contrast medium adjacent to the thin portion of the tube (*Fig. 9.19*). The degree of tubal involvement varies considerably and, more commonly, both tubes are affected. The diagnosis can be revealed only by the HSG, if the depth of penetration of the endosalpinx is insufficient to cause external thickening or the tubal involvement is confined to the interstitial segment (*Fig. 9.20*). The incidence of SIN in patients undergoing hysterosalpingography is approximately 4%, based on a review of 1194 HSGs.[14] SIN is considered a tubal factor in infertility, because it usually coexists with radiographic evidence of chronic or healed salpingitis in the ampullary portion of the tube. This may reflect a selection bias of predominantly examining patients with infertility. On the other hand, SIN has been shown to be an etiologic factor in proximal tubal obstruction.[15] Furthermore, SIN is a significant factor in the incidence of ectopic tubal pregnancy.[16,17]

The radiographic findings caused by pelvic inflammatory disease (PID) are manifested primarily in the ampulla and at the fimbriated end, although occasionally an obstruction can be produced in the interstitial segment or proximal isthmus. These

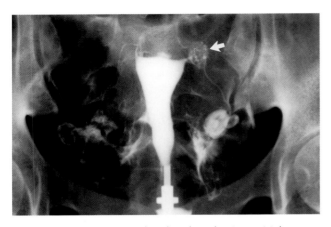

Figure 9.20 SIN (arrow) localized to the interstitial segment of the left fallopian tube. The HSG is otherwise normal.

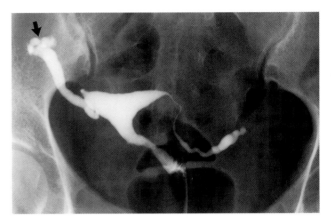

Figure 9.21 Severe pelvic inflammatory disease in a 27-year-old woman with primary infertility. There is obstruction and contour irregularity (arrow) at the distal end of the right fallopian tube, and the left tube is obstructed in the mid-ampulla. The ampullary mucosal folds have been destroyed bilaterally. The right ampulla is rigid, suggesting a thickened wall. The radiographic findings indicate a poor surgical prognosis.

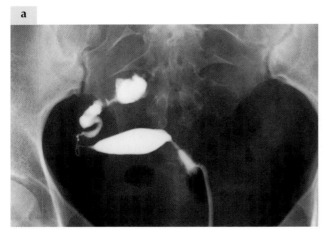

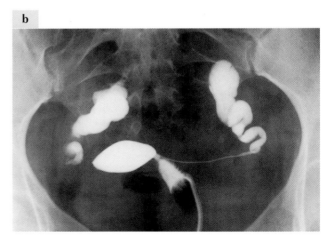

Figure 9.22 Pelvic inflammatory disease in a 24-year-old woman with primary infertility. There are bilateral hydrosalpinges with moderate dilatation of the ampullae and clubbing at the distal end of the left tube and a slightly irregular contour at the end of the right tube. Some mucosal fold preservation is noted in the distal left ampulla, but no mucosal folds can be seen in the right ampulla. (a) AP view of an anteflexed endometrial cavity and a right hydrosalpinx, with transient peristaltic activity in the midampulla. There is non-visualization of the left tube, with the patient in the supine position. (b) After the patient had been rotated into a prone position and additional contrast medium injected, there is now complete filling of the left tube, demonstrating a hydrosalpinx.

include ampullary dilatation and elongation, tubal rigidity, loss of the mucosal folds, clubbing or contour irregularity at the fimbriated end, and distal obstruction (*Figs 9.21* and *9.22*). In addition, there is a lack of normal peristalsis in the ampulla. The fluid in a hydrosalpinx occasionally produces a radiographic discontinuity of the tube owing to dilution of the contrast medium (see *Fig. 9.19*). Previous reports have indicated that the preservation of the mucosal folds in the ampulla and the degree of tubal distension are important prognostic factors in the pregnancy rate following tubal surgery.[18,19]

Subsequent studies have utilized a combination of the HSG and laparoscopic findings to predict preoperatively the success of distal tubal microsurgery with respect to pregnancy and ectopic pregnancy rates.[20,21] The term pregnancy rate was 60% following a fimbrioplasty in patients with fimbrial conglutination and tubal patency, while patients receiving a salpingostomy for distal obstruction and ampullary distension of > 25 mm had a term pregnancy rate of 22% and an ectopic pregnancy rate of 12%[20] (*Figs 9.23* and *9.24*). Although favorable prognostic factors, such as non-distension or slight distension of the

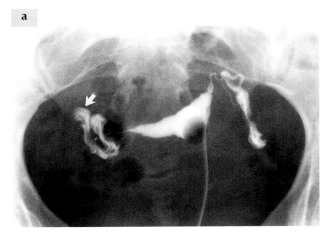
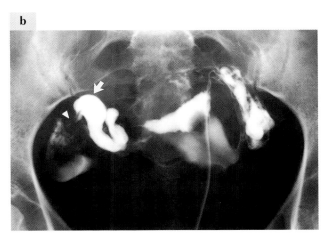

Figure 9.23 Conglutination of the fimbria of the right fallopian tube in a 35-year-old woman, G2 P0 EAB2, being evaluated for secondary infertility. (a) Spot radiograph, demonstrating normal appearing fallopian tubes and no distension in the distal right ampulla (arrow). (b) The right tube is narrowed at the fimbriated end (small triangle), but there is free spill from the tube. The right ampulla has become distended, predominantly in its distal portion (arrow), owing to the adherent fimbria. The radiographic findings indicate a favorable prognosis for a right fimbrioplasty.

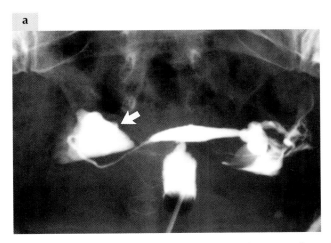
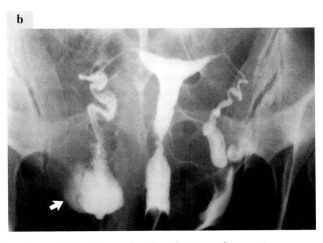

Figure 9.24 Right hydrosalpinx in a patient being evaluated for primary infertility and with a history of a previous appendectomy. At laparoscopy, the right fallopian tube was initially obscured by adhesions. Following lysis of the peritubal adhesions, a right hydrosalpinx was identified. It was elected not to open the right tube, owing to the size of the hydrosalpinx. (a) The endometrial cavity is anteflexed. The right tube terminates in a saccular collection of contrast medium (arrow), and the right ampulla is not adequately visualized. (b) The angled view demonstrates a normal appearing right ampulla, making it difficult to determine if the sacculation (arrow) at the distal end of the tube represents loculated spill or a localized distal hydrosalpinx.

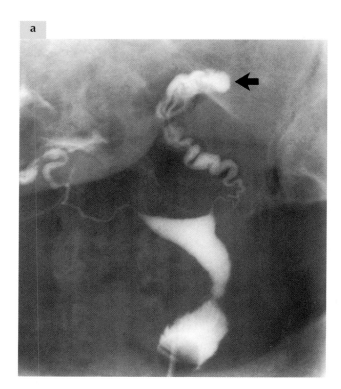

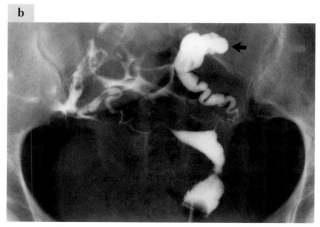

Figure 9.25 Lower abdominal and pelvic adhesions in a 34-year-old woman with primary infertility and a history of a previous appendectomy and peritonitis. There is obstruction to a non-distended left fallopian tube and evidence of left peritubal adhesions on the HSG. At laparoscopy, the left tube and ovary were encased in massive adhesions, and no attempt was made to free up the left tube. The right tube was normal and patent. (a) The right tube is normal, and free spill is noted. The left fallopian tube is directed superiorly toward the lower abdomen, suggestive of peritubal adhesions, and there is obstruction at the distal end of the tube (arrow). The left tube is otherwise normal in caliber and appearance. (b) With further injection of contrast medium, the left tube begins to dilate and simulate a small hydrosalpinx. This illustrates the importance of obtaining a radiograph of early tubal filling, so that the degree of distension of an obstructed tube can be assessed accurately, and overdistension of an obstructed tube is not misinterpreted.

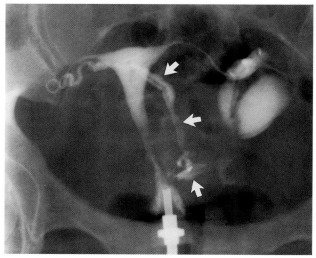

Figure 9.26 Pelvic inflammatory disease in a patient, G1 P1, with secondary infertility. A small to moderate left hydrosalpinx is present, with some mucosal fold preservation. Although the caliber of the right tube and the mucosal pattern of the right ampulla are normal, there are multiple signs of cul-de-sac and right peritubal adhesions. The ampulla (upper arrows) of the right tube is stretched and directed into the midline of the cul-de-sac, and there is beginning loculated spill (lower arrow) at the distal end of the right tube. The right tubal morphology is indicative of a good surgical prognosis, but this could be negated by severe adhesions.

ampulla and good preservation of mucosal folds, may be demonstrated on the HSG, these can be negated by severe pelvic adhesions[21] (*Figs 9.25* and *9.26*).

Pelvic adhesions may be caused by PID, endometriosis, ruptured appendicitis, or previous surgery. Obviously, the capability to diagnose adhesions on the HSG is limited compared with direct visualization of the pelvis by laparoscopy. Nonetheless, there are some radiographic signs or combinations of signs that are strong indicators of adhesions. Loculated spill of contrast medium is the most reliable sign, and this commonly occurs in the

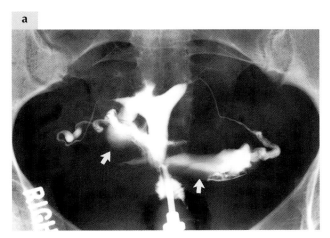
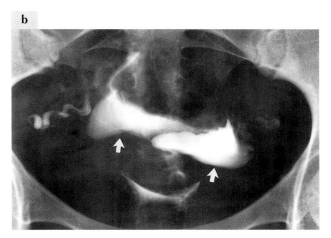

Figure 9.27 Cul-de-sac adhesions in a woman with primary infertility. (a) The fallopian tubes are normal. However, the bilateral spill of contrast medium (arrows) may be loculated. (b) The vacuum cannula has been removed, and the contrast medium has drained from the uterus. After the patient had been rotated into right and left lateral decubitus and prone positions, there is persistent loculation of the spill from both tubes, consistent with cul-de-sac adhesions.

cul-de-sac of Douglas (*Fig. 9.27*). In some instances, it may be difficult to distinguish loculated spill from a distal hydrosalpinx (see *Fig. 9.24*). The medial direction of the distal end of one or both tubes toward or into the midline of the cul-de-sac is an important sign, particularly if both tubes are involved (see *Fig. 9.26*). Stretching of the ampulla is a good sign, but is not frequently seen. A vertically oriented tube, with its distal end directed superiorly toward the lower abdomen, can indicate peritubal adhesions (see *Fig. 9.25*). This diagnosis becomes more reliable when the distal end of the tube is near or above the level of the pelvic inlet. It should be kept in mind that an adjacent mass lesion can alter the position of the fallopian tube or cause stretching of the ampulla, and this should be excluded before attributing these findings to adhesions. In a retrospective analysis of 100 HSGs in which peritubal adhesions were diagnosed on the basis of five specific signs (convoluted fallopian tube, loculated spill, ampullary dilatation, peritubal halo effect, and vertical tube), a correct diagnosis was verified by laparoscopy in 75% of the cases.[22] This report emphasized the importance of making a concerted effort to detect evidence of peritubal adhesions based on specific radiographic signs.

The radiographic spectrum of tubal alterations caused by tuberculosis has been reported previously in a study of 75 patients.[23] A non-specific, bilateral hydrosalpinx can be seen in the early stage of involvement, which is radiographically indistinguishable from hydrosalpinges caused by PID. With progression of the disease, one or more of the following characteristic features may be produced

that warrant a presumptive diagnosis of tuberculosis: marked narrowing and irregular contour of the ampulla, obstruction in the midportion of the tube (either the proximal ampulla, the zone of transition between the isthmus and ampulla, or the distal isthmus), multiple strictures, and distension and straightening ('pipestemming') of the isthmus and interstitial segment (*Fig. 9.28*). Occasionally the obstructed tubes appear to be identical to a bilateral tubal ligation. In addition, calcified lymph nodes or small, non-specific calcifications or plaques related to tuberculosis may be seen on the scout radiograph of the pelvis. In rare instances, a tubointestinal fistula has been demonstrated on the HSG.[24] As mentioned previously, the disease may progress from the tubes and produce deformity or complete fibrosis of the endometrial cavity (see *Fig. 9.13*). It is important to confirm the diagnosis by a positive endometrial biopsy for granulomas or a positive endometrial or menstrual culture, because tuberculosis is treated by a combined drug regimen and not surgical intervention. If the endometrial cavity has been obliterated, an endocervical curettage might yield granulomas or a positive culture. Hysterosalpingography is an excellent screening procedure for pelvic tuberculosis, as was emphasized in a previous report.[25]

Previous tubal surgery can be evaluated by hysterosalpingography, if a pregnancy has not been achieved within a reasonable time period following the surgical procedure. This would include fimbrioplasty and salpingostomy for distal tubal obstruction, salpingostomy for ectopic pregnancy, and tubal re-anastomosis (*Fig. 9.29*).

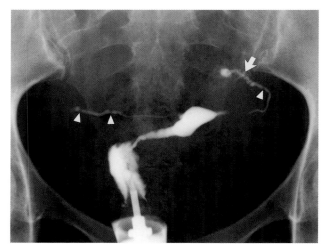

Figure 9.28 Genital tuberculosis in a woman with primary infertility. The right fallopian tube is obstructed in the zone of transition between the isthmus and ampulla, or possibly in a narrowed proximal ampulla. The left tube is blocked near the mid-ampulla, with narrowing and an irregular contour to the proximal ampulla (arrow). Scattered strictures (small triangles) are noted in both tubes. The unusual sites of obstruction, the narrowing of the ampullae, and the strictures are a combination of radiographic signs indicative of advanced tubal tuberculosis. Owing to uterine flexion caused by leiomyomas, the endometrial cavity could not be entered for biopsy. However, an endocervical curettage was positive for granulomas, confirming the diagnosis.

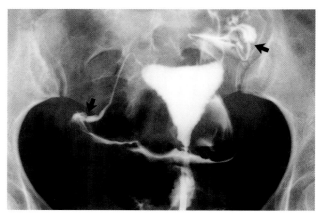

Figure 9.29 Bilateral tubal re-anastomosis in a woman who had not conceived within 6 months of the surgical procedure. The anastomotic sites (arrows) are well delineated, and bilateral tubal patency is demonstrated. Short ampullary segments are noted.

Performing hysterosalpingography

The selection of a particular cannula or catheter for hysterosalpingography should be based on criteria that will contribute to a successful examination, namely patient comfort, ease of use by the examiner, and providing a satisfactory seal to the cervix or uterus to prevent leakage of contrast medium. A disposable balloon catheter, the H/S Catheter Set (Ackrad Laboratories, Cranford, NJ, USA), effectively meets these criteria and is recommended as the primary technique in carrying out the procedure. The H/S catheter is available in sizes 5 and 7 French. Because of the small caliber of the catheter, it is easy to pass through a small external os, which would be found in most nulliparous women and those with cervical stenosis. More importantly, a small external os allows the inflated balloon to be retained in the endocervical canal without leakage of contrast medium from the cervix. Although the cervix is not usually the focus of an infertility investigation, it is desirable to include the endocervical

canal in the examination, particularly in evaluation of suspected intrauterine adhesions or a congenital uterine anomaly. In most parous women the catheter cannot be retained in the endocervical canal and must be passed into the endometrial cavity, with the inflated balloon positioned just above the internal os. An excellent alternative technique that can be used in women with a large external os or in whom an H/S catheter cannot be passed into the endometrial cavity is a vacuum cannula, the VUC-Instrument (AB Vacuum Extractor, Gothenburg, Sweden).[26] This is a reusable device in which the acorn tip of the cannula is inserted into the endocervical canal and held in place by a vacuum applied to a plastic cup placed against the cervix. The vacuum cannula must be disassembled, carefully cleansed in soap and water, and then sterilized in solution after each procedure. The use of either the H/S catheter or the vacuum cannula permits the removal of the speculum prior to the injection of contrast medium.

A water-soluble, iodinated contrast medium provides excellent delineation of the endometrial cavity and the fallopian tubes and is diagnostically far superior to an oil-based medium, which obscures important mucosal detail. In addition, the water-soluble medium is readily absorbed into the vascular system from an obstructed tube or from loculated and free spill within the peritoneal cavity, while an oily medium may be retained in a hydrosalpinx or by adhesions in the pelvis and then further enhance adhesion formation as a foreign body. The possible therapeutic use of an oily medium during laparoscopy has been suggested, based on a meta-analysis which indicated a significantly higher pregnancy rate following the use of oil-based media for hysterosalpingography compared with water-soluble media.[27]

Prior to the procedure, the examining physician should obtain a brief clinical history using the following questions.

Drug or food allergy? Hysterosalpingography is contraindicated in any patient who has had a severe respiratory or cardiac reaction to injected contrast medium, and assessment of the endometrial cavity and fallopian tubes should be by other means, such as hysteroscopy and laparoscopy. The occurrence of unpleasant side-effects of nausea and vomiting or mild allergic reactions consisting of hives and pruritis are commonly associated with the intravenous injection of water-soluble media, but are virtually non-existent during hysterosalpingography. However, if there are any risk factors, such as asthma or a food or drug allergy, the use of a non-ionic contrast medium is suggested. This is based on a study of 337 647 patients in whom there was a 12.66% incidence of allergic reactions and 0.22% incidence of severe reactions to intravenous use of high-osmolar ionic media compared with respective incidences of 3.13% and 0.04% for low-osmolar non-ionic media.[28]

Dates of last menstrual period? Hysterosalpingography should be performed during the proliferative phase of the menstrual cycle, after the menstrual flow has stopped and before the expected time of ovulation, to avoid irradiating an early pregnancy. The referring physician may schedule a certain date within this time frame, or the patient may be scheduled within 10 days of the onset of her menses and after the expected end of flow. A small amount of spotting does not particularly interfere with obtaining a satisfactory HSG, as long as there is no associated uterine cramping or significant blood clot in the endometrial cavity. In the patient with amenorrhea or irregular menses, a negative pregnancy test should be obtained immediately prior to the procedure.

Previous tubal infection? The development of acute salpingitis is the most important complication following the procedure, and this usually occurs in the patient with abnormal fallopian tubes related to previous infection. It has been shown that a prophylactic course of doxycycline, 100 mg twice daily for 5 days, is effective in reducing this complication.[29] If there is a history of previous salpingitis or any other risk factors, the referring physician should begin treatment 2 days prior to hysterosalpingography. Additionally, it is incumbent on the referring physician to ensure that any patient found to have pelvic tenderness on physical examination has received a course of doxycycline therapy that results in the resolution of the tenderness prior to a scheduled HSG. If a patient has abnormal fallopian tubes on the HSG, indicative of healed or chronic salpingitis, and is not on prophylactic antibiotic therapy, then treatment should begin following the procedure with an initial 200 mg dose. Whether on prophylactic therapy or not, each patient should be instructed to contact her physician for intravenous antibiotic treatment if symptoms of pelvic pain and fever develop after the HSG.

Previous lower abdominal and pelvic surgery? The surgical history can frequently be correlated with abnormalities demonstrated on the HSG, such as an outpouching of contrast medium caused by a cesarean section scar, evidence of peritubal adhesions associated with an appendectomy, or a proximal tubal obstruction related to a salpingectomy. If the examiner is unaware of a previous salpingectomy, the examination may be unduly prolonged in an effort to visualize a tube that has been removed.

Obstetrical history? The size of the external os may be a factor in the selection of a particular catheter or cannula for performing the procedure. A previous curettage following a spontaneous abortion may result in endometrial adhesions on the HSG.

This preliminary interview will provide information that relates to the safety and appropriate timing of the procedure and that will be useful in the interpretation of the HSG. It should be considered an integral part of the examination.

A scout radiograph of the pelvis is routinely obtained for determination of appropriate radiographic technique. This may reveal a pertinent finding such as fibroid calcification, tuberculous lymph node calcification, a soft tissue mass, a lumbar or sacral anomaly representing a component of the VACTERL association, retained oily contrast medium from a previous HSG, Falope rings, or a retained fragment of a contraceptive device.

Hysterosalpingography is performed using sterile technique. A volume of 20 ml of water-soluble contrast medium is drawn into a syringe, which is then attached to the H/S catheter via connecting tubing. This amount of contrast medium allows for variations in the size of the endometrial cavity and is sufficient for most examinations. Many patients require < 10 ml, but the volume needed for those with cavities enlarged by leiomyomas can range from 30 ml to > 100 ml. Contrast medium is injected through the connecting tubing and the H/S catheter to eliminate air from the system, before placement of the catheter. This is an important step, because an introduced air bubble may simulate a small mass lesion in the endometrial cavity or may obstruct the flow of contrast medium in a cornu and prevent tubal filling. Air bubbles are usually easily recognized as migratory filling defects, which commonly disintegrate into smaller bubbles and remain in the fundal area or pass through the fallopian tubes.

The comfort of the patient is an important part of the procedure, because this will lessen the possibility of uterine or tubal spasm. The use of an antiprostaglandin synthesis inhibitor approximately 1 hour in advance of hysterosalpingography is beneficial in this regard, particularly in an apprehensive patient. The placement of the speculum is the most uncomfortable part of the examination for many patients, particularly nulliparous women; therefore, the use of the narrow Pederson speculum is recommended for most patients, and the speculum and the vagina should be well lubricated. Secretions should be sponged from the upper vagina, so that the surface of the cervix is dry. A tenaculum is unnecessary and should not be used when the H/S catheter or the vacuum cannula is employed in the procedure. Rarely, a tenaculum or ring forceps may be required initially to retract a severely anteverted or retroverted cervix for successful placement of the catheter. The distal portion of the catheter is passed through the external os, and the balloon is inflated in the endocervical canal. If the inflated balloon cannot be retained in the endocervical canal or is expelled from the cervix before the examination is completed, then the catheter must be passed into the uterus. The catheter is contained within a sheath except for its distal portion, which can usually be guided into the uterus. However, passage through the internal os may be difficult. In this circumstance, the sheath can be advanced beyond the distal end of the catheter and into the endocervical canal to straighten the cervix, and this maneuver may allow subsequent successful passage of the catheter. If this does not work, the distal portion of the catheter may be controlled by the use of ring forceps, which will increase the force of insertion and allow the catheter to be torqued and passed in different directions. This will usually result in successful placement of the catheter, with the inflated balloon positioned just above the internal os. The speculum is then removed, while the sheath is held in a fixed position in the vagina to protect the catheter from being dislodged from the cervix or uterus. The removal of the speculum contributes significantly to the comfort of the patient and allows her to change position easily during the course of the examination. The patient should be instructed to relax and not to tense the abdomen or 'bear down', as this may expel the catheter from the cervix into the vagina.

Hysterosalpingography should only be performed using image-intensified fluoroscopy to monitor the flow of contrast medium. This will allow the proper timing of spot radiographs to visualize optimally the endometrial cavity and the fallopian tubes. In addition, an appropriate volume of contrast medium will be injected to ensure complete tubal filling and demonstration of tubal patency, and obstructed tubes will not be overdistended. The amount of fluoroscopic time required should be no more than 20 seconds in most instances, and sometimes considerably less. A slow steady injection of contrast medium is made, and the first spot radiograph is obtained during early filling of the endometrial cavity. Filling defects caused by small mass lesions are optimally delineated at this time (see *Fig. 9.14*). If the uterus is flexed so that the fundal and lateral margins are not adequately visualized, the fluoroscopy may be temporarily suspended and an overhead angled view obtained (see *Fig. 9.24*). There is no discomfort associated with the filling of the endocervical canal and the endometrial cavity with contrast medium. A second spot radiograph is taken after the endometrial cavity is fully distended and both fallopian tubes are visualized to the level of the distal ampullae, prior to the spill of contrast medium (see *Fig. 9.1a*). This will ensure optimal visualization of tubal detail, because segments of the tubes may subsequently become obscured by intraperitoneal spill. Usually two spot radiographs are all that is necessary, but an additional oblique view may be helpful if a tube is obscured by an overlying, distended endometrial cavity or if the segments of a tube are superimposed. It is very important that the examination progress in a timely and uninterrupted fashion, once the cavity is fully distended and the tubes begin to fill. The patient may develop cramping at this time, and the examination may become adversely affected by uterine or tubal spasm. It is not necessary to demonstrate free spill at fluoroscopy, but most of the tubal lengths should have been visualized. Small amounts of contrast medium should continue to be injected, particularly just before each overhead exposure is made. This will keep the endometrial cavity and the fallopian tubes fully distended by counteracting mild uterine contraction and tubal peristalsis, and free spill or tubal obstruction will be demonstrated. Overhead radiographs are obtained in the antero-posterior and lateral projections, so that the entire contour of the endometrial cavity is delineated. An overhead angled view is necessary when the uterus is flexed. If the uterus is anteflexed 90°, the X-ray tube should be angled 40° cephalad with the patient in the supine position. This will provide good visualization of the fundal and lateral margins of the endometrial cavity and, in some instances, the delineation of the fallopian tubes will be considerably improved (see *Fig. 9.24*). If the degree of flexion is < 90°, a tube angulation between 25° and 40° is used, depending on the estimated severity of the anteflexion. When the uterus is retroflexed or anteflexed > 90°, the X-ray tube is angled caudally. The direction of tube angulation is reversed from the preceding instructions, if the patient is in a prone position. The angled view makes the use of a tenaculum to straighten the uterus unnecessary.

If there is a predominant flow of contrast medium through one tube and minimal filling or non-visualization of the opposite tube, then fluoroscopy should be discontinued after a spot radiograph of the filled tube has been obtained. The patient is then rotated into a lateral decubitus position, so that the non-visualized tube is in a dependent position. Additional contrast medium is injected, and an overhead lateral exposure is made. Next, the patient is placed in a prone position, and after injection of contrast medium, an overhead posteroanterior radiograph is obtained. The non-filling tube will frequently be visualized by this technique (see *Fig. 9.22*). The importance of the prone position in this regard has been reported previously.[30] If there is persistent non-visualization of a tube, this is most likely related to cornual or tubal spasm and not obstruction. Cornual spasm can be recognized by an incompletely distended cornu. The possibility of a non-visualized tube representing a proximal obstruction is unlikely but should be considered. A proximal tubal obstruction is more commonly represented by a well-distended interstitial segment or distended proximal isthmus and interstitial segment, assuming that no leakage of contrast medium from the cervix has occurred, resulting in incomplete tubal filling. This is similar in appearance to a visualized tubal remnant from a previous tubal fulguration or salpingectomy.

Conclusion

Hysterosalpingography should be approached with an emphasis on imaging detail, in order to provide as much information as possible concerning the status of the endometrial cavity and the fallopian tubes. Occasionally, an unexpected or unusual radiographic finding will be demonstrated (*Fig. 9.30*).

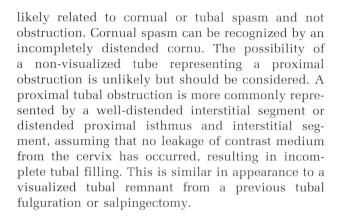

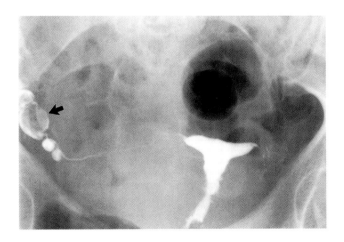

Figure 9.30 Ectopic pregnancy, producing a filling defect (arrow) in the distal ampulla of the right fallopian tube, prior to spill of contrast medium. The initial diagnosis was suspected on the basis of the HSG. A positive pregnancy test was obtained the following day, which led to the laparoscopic removal of a 5–6 week fetus from the right tube. A history of a left salpingectomy for an ectopic pregnancy (ECT) had been revealed by the patient, G3 P0 SAB2 ECT1, prior to hysterosalpingography, and her last menstrual period had occurred within the previous 10 days. In reviewing the HSG with the patient after the procedure had been completed, it was learned that the 'period' had lasted longer than usual.

REFERENCES

1. Snowden EU, Jarrett JC, Dawood MY. Comparison of diagnostic accuracy of laparoscopy, hysteroscopy, and hysterosalpingography in evaluation of female infertility. *Fertil Steril* 1984; **41**:709–713.
2. Fayez JA, Mutie G, Schneider PJ. The diagnostic value of hysterosalpingography and hysteroscopy in infertility investigation. *Am J Obstet Gynecol* 1987; **156**:558–560.
3. American Fertility Society. The American Fertility Society classifications of adnexal adhesions, distal tubal occlusion, tubal occlusion secondary to tubal ligation, tubal pregnancies, Müllerian anomalies, and intrauterine adhesions. *Fertil Steril* 1988; **49**:944–955.
4. Asplund J. The uterine cervix and isthmus under normal and pathological conditions: a clinical and roentgenological study. *Acta Radiol* 1952; **91**(suppl):3–76.
5. Slezak P, Tillinger KG. Hysterographic evidence of polypoid filling defects in the uterine cavity. *Radiology* 1975; **115**:79–83.
6. Cundiff G, Carr BR, Marshburn PB. Infertile couples with a normal hysterosalpingogram: reproductive

outcome and its relationship to clinical and laparoscopic findings. *J Reprod Med* 1995; **40**:19–24.

7. Stein AL, March CM. The outcome of pregnancy in women with Mullerian duct anomalies. *J Reprod Med* 1990; **35**:411–414.

8. Toaff ME, Lev-Toaff AS, Toaff R. Communicating uteri: review and classification with introduction of two previously unreported cases. *Fertil Steril* 1984; **41**:661–679.

9. Reuter KL, Daly DC, Cohen SM. Septate versus bicornuate uteri: errors in imaging diagnosis. *Radiology* 1989; **172**:749–752.

10. Kaufman RH, Adam E, Binder GL, Gerthoffer E. Upper genital tract changes and pregnancy outcome in offspring exposed in utero to diethylstilbestrol. *Am J Obstet Gynecol* 1980; **137**:299–308.

11. Kaufman RH, Noller K, Adam E *et al*. Upper genital tract abnormalities and pregnancy outcome in diethylstilbestrol-exposed progeny. *Am J Obstet Gynecol* 1984; **148**:973–984.

12. Marshak RH, Eliasoph J. The roentgen findings in adenomyosis. *Radiology* 1955; **64**: 846–851.

13. Togashi K, Nishimura K, Itoh K *et al*. Adenomyosis: diagnosis with MR imaging. *Radiology* 1988; **166**:111–114.

14. Creasy JL, Clark RL, Cuttino JT, Groff TR. Salpingitis isthmica nodosa: radiologic and clinical correlates. *Radiology* 1985; **154**:597–600.

15. Fortier KJ, Haney AF. The pathologic spectrum of uterotubal junction obstruction. *Obstet Gynecol* 1985; **65**:93–98.

16. Majmudar B, Henderson PH, Semple E. Salpingitis isthmica nodosa: a high-risk factor for tubal pregnancy. *Obstet Gynecol* 1983; **62**:73–78.

17. Persaud V. Etiology of tubal ectopic pregnancy. *Obstet Gynecol* 1970; **36**:257–263.

18. Özaras H. The value of plastic operations on the fallopian tubes in the treatment of female infertility. *Acta Obstet Gynecol Scand* 1968; **47**:489–500.

19. Young PE, Egan JE, Barlow JJ, Mulligan WJ. Reconstructive surgery for infertility at the Boston Hospital for Women. *Am J Obstet Gynecol* 1970; **108**:1092–1097.

20. Donnez J, Casanas-Roux F. Prognostic factors of fimbrial microsurgery. *Fertil Steril* 1986; **46**:200–204.

21. Mage G, Pouly JL, Bouquet de Jolinière J, Chabrand S, Riouallon A, Bruhat MA. A preoperative classification to predict the intrauterine and ectopic pregnancy rates after distal tubal microsurgery. *Fertil Steril* 1986; **46**:807–810.

22. Karasick S, Goldfarb AF. Peritubal adhesions in infertile women: diagnosis with hysterosalpingography. *Am J Roentgenol* 1989; **152**:777–779.

23. Ekengren K, Rydén ABV. Roentgen diagnosis of tuberculous salpingitis. *Acta Radiol* 1950; **34**:193–214.

24. Silva PD, Richmond JA, Lobo RA. Diagnosis and management of a tuberculous, tuboappendiceal fistula. *Am J Obstet Gynecol* 1988; **159**:440–441.

25. Klein TA, Richmond JA, Mishell DR. Pelvic tuberculosis. *Obstet Gynecol* 1976; **48**:99–104.

26. Malmström T. A vacuum uterine cannula. *Obstet Gynecol* 1961; **18**:773–776.

27. Watson A, Vanderkeckhove P, Lilford R, Vail A, Brosens I, Hughes E. A meta-analysis of the therapeutic role of oil-soluble contrast media at hysterosalpingography: a surprising result? *Fertil Steril* 1994; **61**:470–477.

28. Katayama H, Yamaguchi K, Kozuka T, Takashima T, Seez P, Matsuura K. Adverse reactions to ionic and nonionic contrast media. *Radiology* 1990; **175**:621–628.

29. Pittaway DE, Winfield AC, Maxson W, Daniell J, Herbert C, Wentz AC. Prevention of acute pelvic inflammatory disease after hysterosalpingography: efficacy of doxycycline prophylaxis. *Am J Obstet Gynecol* 1983; **147**:623–626.

30. Spring DB, Boll DA. Prone hysterosalpingography. *Radiology* 1980; **136**:235–236.

10 Scrotal abnormalities associated with infertility

Carol B Benson

Male factors are the primary cause of infertility in 20–30% of couples and play a contributing role in another 20–25%.[1–3] Male factors include a variety of disorders that interfere with the production or transport of normal sperm; scrotal abnormalities account for almost half of these disorders.[1,2]

Ultrasound with Doppler is the imaging modality of choice for evaluating the male partner of an infertile couple. It is safe because it uses no ionizing radiation. Scans can be performed rapidly and are relatively inexpensive. Sonography of the scrotum is performed with linear or curvilinear transducers of high frequencies, in the range 7–15 MHz. The transducer is placed directly on the skin and the scrotum is scanned in longitudinal and transverse planes. Color Doppler is performed at similar or slightly lower frequencies than gray scale imaging and is used to assess blood flow in the testicle, epididymis, and scrotal wall.

Varicocele

A varicocele is formed by dilatation of the pampiniform plexus of veins that courses along the spermatic cord. Many cases result from incompetent venous valves, allowing reflux and stasis of blood in the involved veins.

Varicoceles are associated with infertility and abnormal semen analysis,[1,4–6] although the exact relationship and the pathophysiology are not clearly understood. It has been postulated that stasis in dilated veins in the scrotum causes temperature elevation, which interferes with production of normal sperm. The prevalence of varicocele is higher among males of infertile couples than in the general population. In particular, varicoceles are found in 40% of men with infertility as compared

with 13% of healthy men and 26% of men seeking vasectomy.[5,7] Furthermore, after varicocelectomy, approximately half the patients demonstrate improvement in seminal parameters.[6]

The sonographic diagnosis of a varicocele is made when there is a cluster of dilated veins in the scrotal wall, with diameters of > 2 mm (*Fig. 10.1*), or when there is at least one dilated vein with a diameter of $\geq$ 3 mm.[1,5,8] The dilated vessels appear as serpiginous tubular structures, most commonly posterior, lateral, and inferior to the testicle; approximately 25% are bilateral. Flow can usually be identified in these veins with pulsed or color

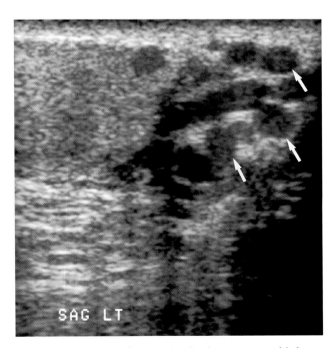

Figure 10.1 Varicocele. Longitudinal sonogram of left hemiscrotum demonstrating several dilated veins (arrows) inferior to the testicle.

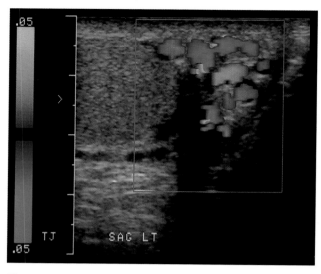

Figure 10.2 Varicocele. Color Doppler sonogram of left varicocele demonstrating flow with color in dilated veins inferior to the left testicle.

Doppler (*Fig. 10.2*), and reflux through incompetent valves can often be elicited by the Valsalva maneuver.[9]

Testicular abnormalities

Testicular abnormalities associated with infertility and abnormal sperm production include testicular atrophy, cryptorchidism, testicular neoplasms, orchitis, microlithiasis, testicular infarction, and trauma.[2,5,8–10] Each of these entities will be discussed.

Testicular atrophy

Testicular atrophy results from a variety of abnormalities or insults. Testicular atrophy is often present with chromosomal abnormalities such as Klinefelter

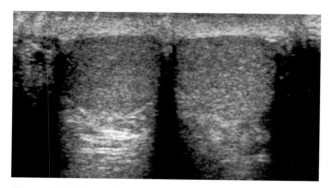

Figure 10.3 Normal testicles. Transverse sonogram of testicles demonstrating side-by-side comparison on a single image. The testicles are symmetric in size and echotexture, both with homogeneous echogenicity.

(47XXY) or Y chromosome deletions.[29] Previously normal testicles may become atrophic following orchitis, undiagnosed torsion, or cryptorchidism.[2,10]

The normal testicle measures approximately 5×3×3 cm. On ultrasound the two normal testicles are similar in size with homogeneous echotexture of moderate echogenicity (*Fig. 10.3*). With increasing age, the average size of the testicles gradually decreases, but the echogenicity remains homogeneous and symmetric.

Atrophic testicles are smaller than normal, with homogeneous echotexture that is hypoechoic when compared with a normal testicle. Diminished blood flow is usually found with Doppler (*Fig. 10.4*). When the atrophy is unilateral, the contralateral normal testicle should be used for comparison during the sonographic examination. Comparison is particularly helpful for assessing echogenicity and blood flow in the affected testicle.

Atrophic testicles should have homogeneous echotexture. If a mass is identified within the testicular parenchyma, it should be considered suspicious for tumor, regardless of its presence in a diffusely abnormal testicle.

Cryptorchidism

Cryptorchidism is a congenital abnormality in which there is failure of descent of the testicle into the scrotum prior to birth. As a result the hemiscrotum on the side with the undescended testis is empty. In some infants, descent occurs in the first few months after birth, but in most cases the testicle remains undescended until surgically affixed in the scrotum. Cryptorchidism affects about 1% of infants older than 3 months[11] and 0.2–0.8% of 1 year olds.[10] It is commonly bilateral.[11,12]

Men with a history of cryptorchidism are at risk for developing oligospermia, azoospermia, and testicular atrophy, regardless of the timing of surgical repair.[5,10] Among men with abnormally low sperm counts, 15% of cases can be attributed to cryptorchidism.[10] In addition to abnormal spermatogenesis, cryptorchid testicles are at increased risk for developing germ cell tumors, with higher risk the later in life orchiopexy is performed. Furthermore, in a patient with unilateral cryptorchidism, the contralateral, normally descended testicle is also at elevated risk for testicular cancer, when compared with men with normally descended testicles.[12]

In adults with untreated cryptorchidism, the undescended testicle can be located by sonography in 60–80% of cases, usually along the spermatic

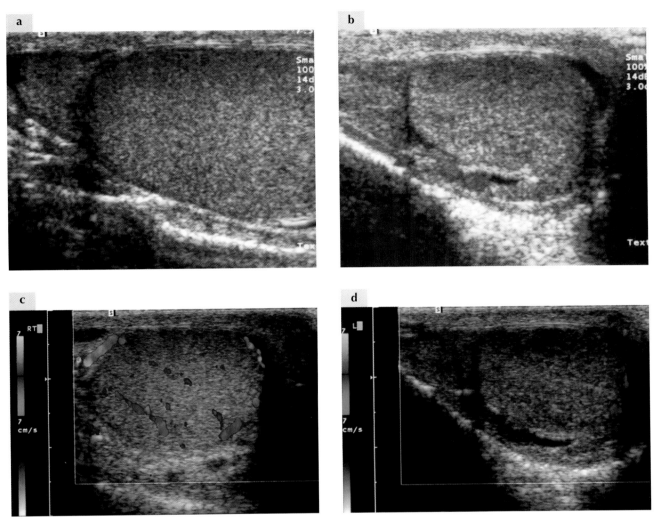

Figure 10.4 Unilateral testicular atrophy. (a) Longitudinal sonogram of normal testicle demonstrating homogeneous echogenicity. (b) Longitudinal sonogram of atropic, contralateral testicle demonstrating decreased size and echogenicity when compared with the normal side. (c) Color Doppler sonogram of normal testicle demonstrating intratesticular flow. (d) Color Doppler sonogram of atrophic testicle demonstrating diminished flow on that side as compared with the normal side.

cord or in the inguinal region. Intra-abdominal undescended testes may require CT, MRI, or surgical exploration for their detection.[12]

Sonographically, the undescended testicle in an adult is typically quite small, with homogeneously decreased echogenicity when compared with a normal testicle (*Fig. 10.5*). The epididymis can often be seen capping the cryptorchid testicle, and may be almost as big as the atrophic testicle. A mass lesion in a cryptorchid testicle is likely to be malignant and should be treated as such.

Testicular neoplasms

The presence of a testicular neoplasm can cause endocrinologic abnormalities and diminished sperm

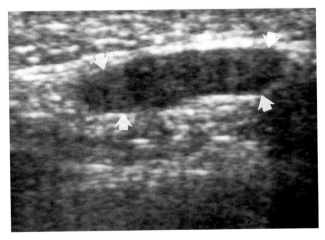

Figure 10.5 Undescended testicle. Longitudinal sonogram of left groin demonstrating small, hypoechoic testicle (arrows) that is cryptorchid.

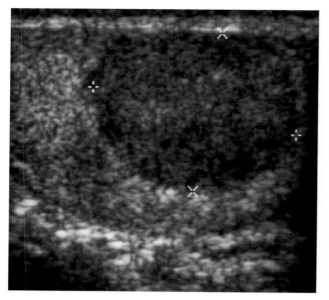

Figure 10.6 Testicular tumor. Sonogram of left testicle demonstrating intratesticular mass (calipers) that proved to be a primary germ cell tumor of the testicle.

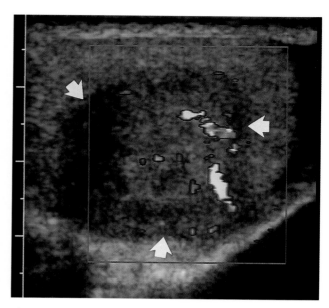

Figure 10.7 Testicular tumor. Color Doppler sonogram of testicular tumor demonstrating increased flow in the mass (arrows) as compared with the surrounding testicular parenchyma.

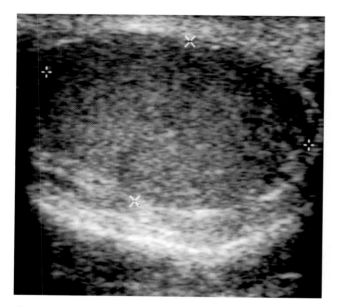

Figure 10.8 Testicular lymphoma. On this longitudinal sonogram, the left testicle is enlarged (calipers) with heterogeneous echotexture and poorly defined areas of decreased echogenicity owing to infiltration by lymphoma.

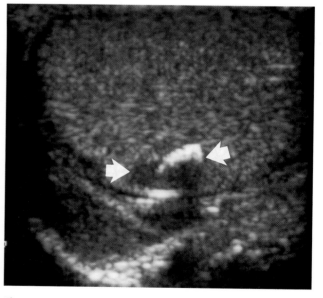

Figure 10.9 Burned out testicular tumor. Testicular sonogram demonstrating dense calcification associated with a hypoechoic mass (arrows) within the testicle that proved to be a burned out testicular tumor. The patient had metastatic tumor in the retroperitoneum.

production.[1,2,5,10,13] This explains the increased incidence of testicular tumors in men with infertility, as compared with normally fertile men.[14]

Malignant testicular tumor

Most testicular tumors are malignant, and of these, most are primary germ cell tumors. Less common malignancies include malignant Leydig or Sertoli cell tumors, metastatic tumors, and leukemia and lymphoma involving the testicle.

Testicular cancers often appear sonographically as well-defined intratesticular masses (*Fig. 10.6*). Many are hypoechoic compared with normal testicular parenchyma. Heterogeneity, cystic areas, and calcification are common. The lesions may have irregular margins, and the tumor may be multicentric. Aggressive, large tumors may have extended into the epididymis or scrotal wall by the time of discovery.[9,15–18] Blood flow in and around testicular tumors is usually increased compared with the normal parenchyma (*Fig. 10.7*).[19,20]

Non-germ-cell primary testicular malignancies and some metastatic tumors appear as well-defined intratesticular masses, indistinguishable from germ cell tumors.[21,22] In other cases of metastases, as well as many cases of testicular leukemia and lymphoma, the testicular involvement is infiltrative rather than focal. In these cases, poorly defined areas of altered echogenicity are seen within the testicle with margins that gradually fade into normal testicular parenchyma (*Fig. 10.8*). The involved testicle is usually enlarged.[17–19] Blood flow is typically increased with these malignancies, whether focal or infiltrative.[19,22]

Burned out testicular tumors are germ cell tumors that have regressed in the testicle, but viable metastatic disease may be found outside the scrotum. Patients with this malignancy most often present with retroperitoneal germ cell tumors. On ultrasound, regressed germ cell tumors are small intratesticular masses with dense calcification (*Fig. 10.9*). In some cases, only a thick calcification will be identified.[16,23] At pathology, these lesions are made up of fibrosis and calcifications with no viable tumor cells.[23]

Benign testicular tumors

Approximately 5% of testicular tumors are benign, arising from Leydig or Sertoli cells in the testicle. These tumors may alter the normal endocrinologic balance, affecting sperm production.[13]

Leydig and Sertoli cell tumors appear as intratesticular masses and are indistinguishable from malignant testicular tumors. Like testicular cancers, these benign tumors have increased blood flow compared with the surrounding testicular parenchyma.[19]

Benign testicular tumors cannot be reliably distinguished from malignant testicular tumors by ultrasound or Doppler imaging.

Orchitis

Infection involving the testicle may result from an ascending infection of the genitourinary tract or from hematogenous spread of disease. Ascending infections usually begin in the epididymis, and, when severe, spread to involve the testicle. Sonography in these cases demonstrates thickening of the epididymis and poorly defined areas of decreased echogenicity in the adjacent testicle. Blood flow in the testicle and epididymis is markedly increased (*Fig. 10.10*).[24]

Orchitis from hematogenous organisms is usually caused by tuberculosis or mumps virus. On ultrasound, the involved testicle is typically enlarged and diffusely hypoechoic. Unlike epididymo-orchitis, where testicular changes are usually focal, the changes with mumps or tuberculous orchitis are often homogeneous and diffuse. Testicular blood flow is increased in the involved testicle, but the increase may be less marked with tuberculous orchitis than

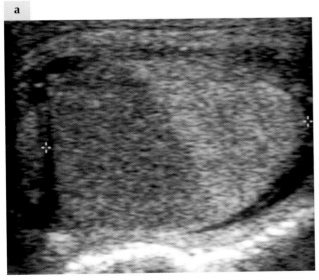
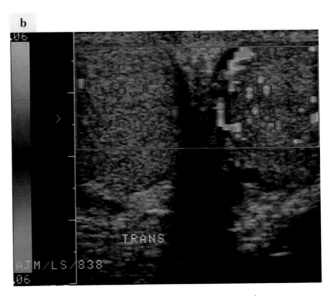

Figure 10.10 Orchitis. (a) Longitudinal sonogram of right testicle demonstrating decreased echogenicity in the upper pole of the right testicle (calipers) owing to orchitis. (b) Color Doppler sonogram in a different patient with left-sided orchitis demonstrating increased flow throughout the left testicle as compared with the right.

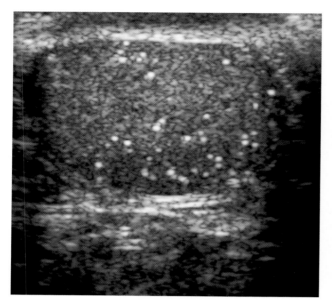

Figure 10.11 Microlithiasis. Longitudinal sonogram of testicle demonstrating multiple punctate calcifications throughout.

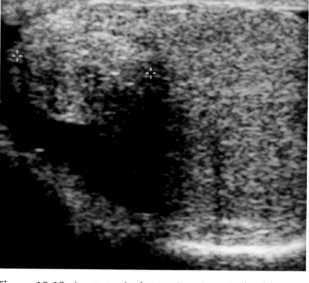

Figure 10.12 Acute testicular torsion. Longitudinal sonogram of right hemiscrotum demonstrating mass (calipers) superior to testicle that causes acoustic shadowing and represents the twisted cord and epididymis.

with other infections.[24] Testicular atrophy may result, despite successful eradication of the infectious agent.

Microlithiasis

Testicular microlithiasis is characterized by multiple tiny calcifications scattered throughout the testicular parenchyma (*Fig. 10.11*). There may be several calcifications or many, and the process is usually bilateral.[25–27] Microlithiasis is thought to be associated with increased risk of testicular cancer.[26] It has also been implicated as a cause of infertility and abnormal spermatogenesis.[16]

Testicular infarction

The most common cause of testicular infarction is testicular torsion. Torsion occurs when the testicle twists on its vascular pedicle, such that blood flow to and from the testicle is occluded. Patients at highest risk for torsion are those with 'bell-clapper' deformities. This congenital abnormality relates to the encapsulation of the testicle by the tunica vaginalis. The tunica vaginalis lines the inside of the scrotum and is reflected over the testicle except at the bare area, where the testicle is attached to the scrotal wall. Vessels and tubules enter and leave the testicle across this bare area. If the bare area is abnormally small, a bell-clapper deformity is present, and the testicle is at risk for twisting on its narrow stalk.[28]

Testicular torsion commonly occurs in adolescent boys, but occasionally affects younger boys or men. Patients typically present with acute onset of scrotal pain. It is not uncommon to elicit a history of prior, similar, less severe episodes of scrotal pain that had resolved spontaneously.

With acute torsions, most testicles can be saved if surgery is performed within 4–6 hours of the acute event. Many can still be saved up to 15 hours after the torsion occurred. From 15 to 24 hours afterwards, the salvage rate declines rapidly, and after 24 hours salvage is rare.[28,39]

Missed torsions are those in which the testicle is not viable by the time surgery is performed. In such cases, the patient is left with one testicle and is at risk for future problems of infertility and diminished sperm production. Furthermore, the bell-clapper deformity is often bilateral and, therefore, patients who have had torsion of one testicle are at risk for torsion of the other. The patient could ultimately lose both testicles to torsion and become completely sterile, if surgical correction of the remaining testicle is not performed at the time of surgery for the first torsion.

On ultrasound, in the first 4–6 hours after torsion occurs, the testicle may appear normal in size and echogenicity, but the twisted pedicle will appear as a complex mass with shadowing, located superior or lateral to the testicle (*Fig. 10.12*). This complex mass may mimic a thickened epididymis. Absent or markedly diminished flow in the testicle and

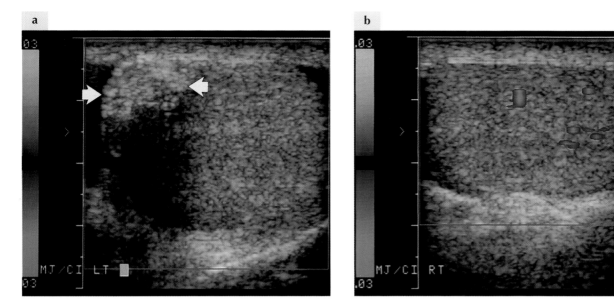

Figure 10.13 Acute testicular torsion. (a) Color Doppler sonogram of torsed testicle demonstrating absent flow in the testicle and epididymis. The heterogeneous mass of the twisted cord and epididymis (arrows) is located superior to the testicle. (b) Color Doppler sonogram of normal testicle for comparison demonstrates flow within the testicular parenchyma.

epididymis is diagnostic for torsion and is easily confirmed by comparing flow with color Doppler in the symptomatic side to flow in the contralateral, normal testicle (*Fig. 10.13*).

As the interval of time since torsion increases, the testicle swells, becomes hypoechoic, and eventually appears heterogeneous with cystic areas. Flow remains absent in the testicle, but becomes increased in the scrotal wall in association with wall thickening.[28–32]

Occasionally, a focal intratesticular infarction will occur either spontaneously or in association with epididymitis. In such cases, patients present with scrotal pain that may mimic acute torsion. On ultrasound, some testicular infarcts are wedge-shaped, hypoechoic defects extending to the periphery of the testicle. Other infarcts may appear as focal intratesticular masses, indistinguishable from a testicular neoplasm. Acutely, these lesions are avascular. With time, the infarcts develop heterogeneous echotexture and eventually become smaller to form an intratesticular scar.[9]

Trauma

Serious trauma to the scrotum can result in testicular rupture, fracture, or contusion. Severe disruption of the testicular parenchyma is often treated with orchiectomy, because surgical repair is impossible. In such cases, patients are left with one rather than two testicles, and are at risk for infertility.

After scrotal trauma, the patient may be quite tender and physical examination of the testicle may not be possible. Ultrasound is used to assess the integrity of the testicle and its capsule. With testicular rupture, the capsule of the testicle is disrupted and testicular parenchyma and blood are seen extending from the testicle into the scrotal sac (*Fig. 10.14*). A

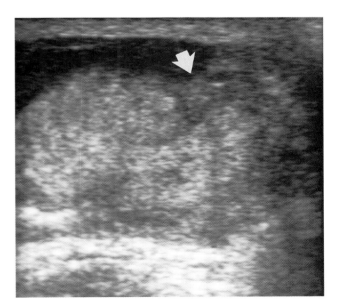

Figure 10.14 Testicular rupture. Longitudinal sonogram of testicle rupture from trauma demonstrating disruption of capsule (arrow) with protrusion of testicular parenchyma and blood outside the capsule.

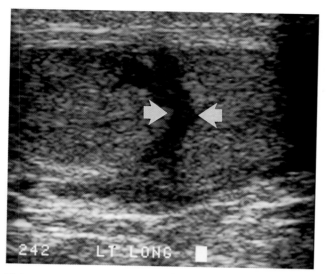

Figure 10.15 Testicular fracture. Longitudinal sonogram demonstrating a hypoechoic fracture (arrows) through the midpole of the testicle.

testicular fracture appears as an irregular, hypoechoic band crossing the testicle, within an intact tunica albuginea (*Fig. 10.15*). Cystic areas caused by

hemorrhage may be seen in the fracture band. A testicular contusion appears as an irregular, hypoechoic mass within the testicle that may mimic a tumor. The contusion will change rapidly with time, usually developing cystic changes within a week of the acute trauma. Contusions eventually decrease in size and become a parenchymal scar.[9] Because these lesions may mimic a testicular tumor, close sonographic follow-up is warranted until the lesion has decreased in size significantly or resolved.

Summary

In summary, sonography and Doppler are useful tools for evaluating men with abnormal semen analyses. Varicoceles are easily diagnosed and abnormalities of the testicles can be found. In many cases, surgical or medical intervention to treat the abnormalities identified by ultrasound can lead to improved seminal parameters, increasing the chance of conception in a previously infertile couple.

REFERENCES

1. Jarow JP. Role of ultrasonography in the evaluation of the infertile male. *Semin Urol* 1994; **12**:274–282.
2. De Kretser DM. Male infertility. *Lancet* 1997; **349**:787–790.
3. Templeton A. Infertility – epidemiology, aetiology and effective management. *Health Bull* 1995; **53**:294–298.
4. Curtis P, Nicholas OA, Berger L, Shaw RW. The ultrasound diagnosis and clinical significance of varicocele. *Ultrasound Obstet Gynecol* 1995; **6**:186–190.
5. Kim ED, Lipshultz LI. Role of ultrasound in the assessment of male infertility. *J Clin Ultrasound* 1996; **24**:437–453.
6. Jarow JP, Ogle SR, Eskew LA. Seminal improvement following repair of ultrasound detected subclinical varicoceles. *J Urol* 1996; **155**:1287–1290.
7. Hirsch AV. Can we be more confident about identifying a varicocele by clinical examination or by ultrasound? *Ultrasound Obstet Gynecol* 1995; **6**:166–167.
8. Honig SC. Use of ultrasonography in the evaluation of the infertile man. *World J Urol* 1993; **11**:102–110.
9. Benson CB, Doubilet PM, Richie RP. Sonography of the male genital tract. *Am J Roentgenol* 1989; **153**:705–713.
10. Abyholm T. Azoospermia and oligozoospermia; etiology and clinical findings. *Arch Androl* 1983; **10**:57–65.
11. Berkowitz GS, Lapinski RH, Dolgin SE, Gazella JG, Bodian CA, Holzman IR. Prevalence and natural history of cryptorchidism. *Pediatrics* 1993; **92**:44–49.
12. Friedland GW, Chang P. The role of imaging in the management of impalpable undescended testis. *Am J Roentgenol* 1988; **151**:1107–1111.
13. Sokol RZ. The diagnosis and treatment of male infertility. *Curr Opin Obstet Gynecol* 1995; **7**:177–181.
14. Nashan D, Behre HM, Grunert HJ, Nieschlag E. Diagnostic value of scrotal sonography in infertile men: report of 658 cases. *Andrologia* 1990; **22**:387–395.
15. Feld R, Middleton WD. Recent advances in sonography of the testis and scrotum. *Radiol Clin North Am* 1992; **30**:1033–1051.
16. Doherty FJ. Ultrasound of the nonacute scrotum. *Semin Ultrasound CT MR* 1991; **12**:131–156.
17. Benson CB. The role of ultrasound in diagnosis and staging of testicular cancer. *Semin Urol* 1988; **6**:189–202.
18. Langer JE. Ultrasound of the scrotum. *Semin Roentgenol* 1993; **28**:5–18.
19. Luker GD, Siegel MJ. Pediatric testicular tumors: evaluation with gray-scale and color Doppler US. *Radiology* 1994; **191**:561–564.
20. Horstman WG, Melson GL, Middleton WD, Andriole GL. Testicular tumors: findings with color Doppler US. *Radiology* 1992; **185**:733–737.

21. Benson CB, Deligdish C, Loughlin KR. Sonographic detection of testicular plasmacytoma. *J Clin Ultrasound* 1987; **15**:353–356.

22. Mazzu D, Jeffrey RB, Ralls PW. Lymphoma and leukemia involving the testicles: findings on gray-scale and color Doppler sonography. *Am J Roentgenol* 1995; **164**:645–647.

23. Comiter CV, Benson CB, Capelouto CC *et al*. Nonpalpable intratesticular masses detected by sonography. *J Urol* 1995; **154**:1367–1369.

24. Kim SH, Pollack HM, Cho KS, Pollack MS, Han MC. Tuberculous epididymitis and epididymo-orchitis: sonographic findings. *Urology* 1993; **150**:81–84.

25. Backus ML, Mack LA, Middleton WD, King BF, Winter TC, True LD. Testicular microlithiasis: imaging appearances and pathologic correlation. *Radiology* 1994; **192**:781–785.

26. Patel MD, Olcott EW, Kerschmann RL, Callen PW, Gooding GAW. Sonographically detected testicular microlithiasis and testicular carcinoma. *J Clin Ultrasound* 1993; **21**:447–452.

27. Janzen DL, Mathieson JR, Marsh JI *et al*. Testicular microlithiasis: sonographic and clinical features. *Am J Roentgenol* 1992; **158**:1057–1060.

28. Tumeh SS, Benson CB, Richie JP. Acute diseases of the scrotum. *Semin Ultrasound CT MR* 1991; **12**:115–130.

29. Middleton WD, Middleton MA, Dierks M, Keetch D, Dierks S. Sonographic prediction of viability in testicular torsion: preliminary observations. *J Ultrasound Med* 1997; **16**:23–27.

30. Pryor JL, Watson LR, Day DL *et al*. Scrotal ultrasound for evaluation of subacute testicular torsion: sonographic findings and adverse clinical implications. *J Urol* 1994; **151**:693–697.

31. Wilbert DM, Schaerfe CW, Stern WD, Strohmaier WL, Bichler KH. Evaluation of the acute scrotum by color-coded Doppler ultrasonography. *J Urol* 1993; **149**:1475–1477.

32. Fitzgerald SW, Erickson S, DeWire DM *et al*. Color Doppler sonography in the evaluation of the adult acute scrotum. *J Ultrasound Med* 1992; **11**:543–548.

11 Role of transrectal ultrasound in male infertility

Ewa Kuligowska and Helen M Fenlon

Introduction

Infertility, defined as the inability to conceive after 1 year of unprotected intercourse, affects 15% of couples in the USA.[1-3] A male factor is responsible in up to 50% of cases. Conditions resulting in male infertility include congenital and developmental anomalies (cryptorchidism, Kleinfelter's syndrome, agenesis of the vas deferens, seminal vesicles and ejaculatory ducts), varicoceles, endocrinopathies, distal duct obstruction (including cysts and calculi of the vas deferens, seminal vesicles and ejaculatory ducts), inflammatory and infective conditions (mumps orchitis, syphilis, and bacterial infections involving the testes, epididymis, vas deferens, seminal vesicles, ejaculatory ducts and prostate), and ejaculatory dysfunction.

Adequate clinical management of male infertility depends on the accurate identification and diagnosis of a variety of causative conditions that can be broadly classified as correctable or non-correctable.[4,5] Abnormalities that cause testicular failure and impaired spermatogenesis cannot be surgically corrected, whereas obstructive processes involving the sperm transport system are potentially curable.[4] A combination of thorough clinical evaluation and seminal analysis helps differentiate patients with irreversible defects from those with distal duct obstruction that may be amenable to surgical or radiologic intervention. Oligospermia, defined as a reduction in the number of spermatozoa in the ejaculate ($< 10^6$ spermatozoa per ml), is present in 80% of infertile men, while azoospermia, defined as total absence of spermatozoa in the ejaculate, is present in 15–20% of patients.[3] Patients with testicular failure or impaired spermatogenesis have azoospermia or oligospermia with normal ejaculate volumes (> 1 ml), because most of the ejaculate volume is produced by the seminal vesicles. Patients with azoospermia or severe oligospermia and low ejaculate volumes

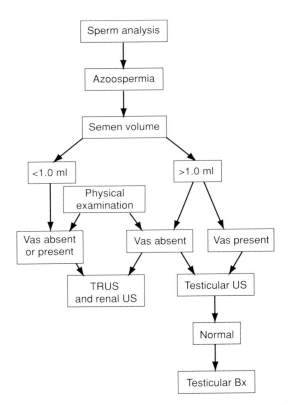

Figure 11.1 Proposed algorithm for the investigation of infertile male patients.

(< 1 ml), in the absence of retrograde ejaculation, should be investigated for distal duct abnormalities including agenesis or hypoplasia of the vas deferens, seminal vesicles, and ejaculatory ducts, distal ductal obliteration by fibrosis and calcification, and distal duct obstruction by calculi or cysts (*Fig. 11.1*).[2,3]

Traditional evaluation of the distal male reproductive tract has been limited until recently by an inability to directly and non-invasively visualize the distal portions of the vas deferens, seminal vesicles, ejaculatory ducts and prostate.[4–11] Clinical examination provides little or no anatomic information regarding the distal ductal system.[2] Vasography, although effective in delineating distal ductal structures, is invasive and may result in iatrogenic damage to the vas deferens.[2,4,5] Non-invasive imaging modalities, including computerized tomography, magnetic resonance imaging and transrectal ultrasound (TRUS), are increasingly used to evaluate infertile male patients. MR imaging with dedicated endorectal coils is effective in demonstrating the distal male reproductive system, but its use is limited by considerations of cost and availability.[11] CT provides only limited visualization of the distal ducts and is rarely indicated. TRUS is the most widely accepted of the cross-sectional imaging techniques and has almost totally replaced vasography in many institutions.[4–10]

Technique of TRUS

TRUS should be performed with a dedicated high frequency endorectal transducer (7.5–9 MHz).[4,5] No patient preparation is required. Patients are examined in the left lateral decubitus position with the transducer inserted in the rectum (*Fig. 11.2*). The terminal vas deferens, seminal vesicles, ejaculatory ducts and prostate are examined in a systematic manner in both axial and sagittal planes and measurements are recorded in three dimensions. Careful attention is paid, not only to the dimensions of the distal ductal structures, but also to the internal architecture and echotexture of the vas deferens and seminal vesicles.[4] In addition, renal ultrasound should be performed to detect potential associated renal anomalies.

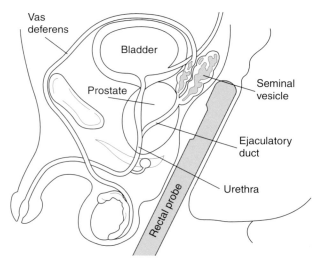

Figure 11.2 Diagrammatic representation of the distal male reproductive system in the sagittal plane with an ultrasound transducer inserted in the rectum.

Accurate interpretation of TRUS examinations requires familiarity with the normal sonographic appearances of the distal male reproductive tract, recognition of a variety of pathologic variations that may occur, and a knowledge of the embryologic basis of disease.

Embryology

By the fourth week of embryonic life, the wolffian (mesonephric) duct bends forward to join the ventral portion of the cloaca, which subsequently differentiates into the urogenital sinus. About the same time, the ureter develops as an outgrowth from the posteromedial aspect of the wolffian duct, 4–6 cm cephalad to its insertion into the urogenital sinus. The segment of the wolffian duct lying between its opening into the urogenital sinus and the ureteral bud is known embryologically as the combined nephric duct. This becomes progressively absorbed into the urogenital sinus and by the seventh week forms the bladder trigone. With downward migration of the combined nephric duct to reach the urogenital sinus, both the ureteral bud and wolffian ducts migrate inferiorly and finally achieve independent openings into the urogenital sinus.[11–13]

From this point onwards, the orifices of the wolffian duct and ureteral bud migrate apart with the ureteral orifice moving upward and laterally and the wolffian duct orifice moving downward and medially. As a result, the wolffian duct, later becoming the vas deferens, will cross over the ureter. This process of separation and rotation is complete by the eighth week. By the twelfth week, the ureteral orifice and the wolffian duct acquire their final location.[11–13]

From the fifth to sixth week of embryonic life, the seminal vesicles develop as lateral outgrowths at the caudal end of each wolffian duct and migrate to lie posterior to the developing bladder and inferolateral to the vas deferens and ureter. Although initially a simple saccular structure, each seminal vesicle develops, with time, complex internal convolutions corresponding to the folds of the excretory epithelium. The most caudal portion of each wolffian duct develops into paired ejaculatory ducts.[11–13]

The wolffian duct, therefore, gives rise to the renal collecting system, ureter, bladder trigone, vas deferens, seminal vesicles, ejaculatory ducts, epididymis, paradidymis and appendix epididymis. Thus, the complex associations of congenital anomalies of the distal male reproductive tract and urinary tract can be explained by their communal embryological derivation from the wolffian duct. The nature and severity of such anomalies is related to the stage at which developmental arrest or insult occurs in utero.[11–13]

The Müllerian ducts are induced by the wolffian ducts during the fifth fetal week. The Müllerian ducts migrate caudally and fuse in the midline with an outgrowth of the urogenital sinus to form the prostatic utricle, which has no further function. The Sertoli cells of the developing testes secrete Müllerian regression factor, which promotes Müllerian duct involution. The only remnants of the Müllerian duct in the developing male fetus are the prostatic utricle and the appendix of the testis.[11–13]

Normal anatomy

Vas deferens

The vas deferens are paired tubular structures that pass from the scrotum into the pelvis through the inguinal canal. At the internal ring, they curve laterally, then pass medially and downward into the pelvis towards the base of the bladder (*Fig. 11.3*). On

axial TRUS imaging, the distal portion of each vas deferens is seen passing posteromedial to the ipsilateral seminal vesicle and has a mean diameter of 3–5 mm. The tortuous and dilated terminal 5 cm of each vas is known as the ampulla, which has an external diameter of approximately 5–8 mm (*Fig. 11.4*).[4–10]

Seminal vesicles

Normal seminal vesicles are paired, saccular, elongated organs lying above the prostate and posterior to the bladder (see *Fig. 11.3*). Normal seminal vesicles are hypoechoic to prostate with multiple fine internal echoes corresponding to the folds of the excretory epithelium. Laterally, the seminal vesicles diverge in the perivesical fat, while medially they converge to join with the ampulla of the vas deferens to form the ejaculatory ducts, producing the typical 'bow-tie' appearance on axial TRUS images (see *Fig. 11.4*).[4–10]

Seminal vesicles may vary in size, shape and degree of distension. They are, however, usually symmetric and measure no more than 5–10 cm in length and 2–5 cm in width, with an estimated mean volume of approximately 15 ml. Caution is advised, however, in measuring seminal vesicle volume in only two dimensions, as a seemingly small vesicle may extend a long way cephalad behind the bladder and thus have a normal volume.[6]

Ejaculatory ducts

The confluence of the vasal ampullae and seminal vesicles to form paired ejaculatory ducts is normally identified at the level of the prostatic capsule or just within the substance of the prostate. The intraprostatic course of each duct within a fibromuscular envelope is usually visible on TRUS and is identified as a fine curvilinear hypoechoic structure (see *Fig. 11.4*). The lumen of the ejaculatory duct should not exceed 2 mm in maximum width. On sagittal TRUS images, the course of each ejaculatory duct can normally be traced down to a focal area of hyperechogenicity corresponding to the verumontanum. Small echogenic foci, representing concretions in the periurethral glands at the level of the verumontanum, provide a useful sonographic landmark for the junction of the ejaculatory ducts and the urethra.[4–10]

It is worth mentioning that careful attention should be paid on TRUS, not only to the dimensions of the distal ductal structures, but also to their echotexture and internal architecture. The normal vas deferens and seminal vesicles are hypoechoic to normal

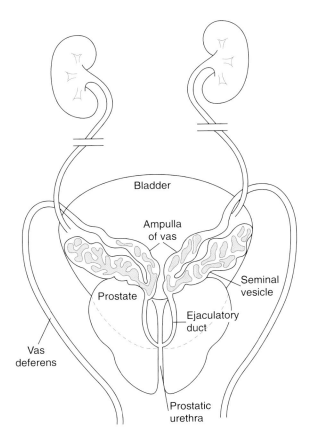

Figure 11.3 Diagrammatic representation of the normal anatomy of the distal male reproductive system (normal coronal view).

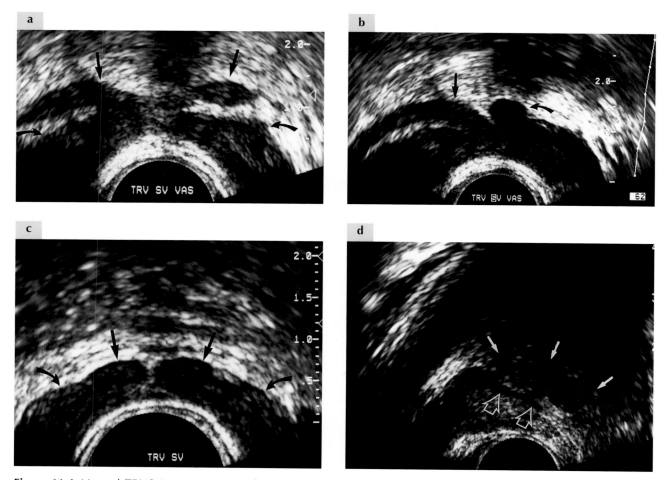

Figure 11.4 Normal TRUS Anatomy. (a) Axial view demonstrates the typical 'bow-tie' appearance of the normal distal vas deferens (straight arrows) and seminal vesicles (curved arrows) bilaterally. Note normal fine internal echotexture corresponding to normal tubular epithelium. (b) Axial oblique view obtained caudal to (a) demonstrates a normal vas deferens on the right (straight arrow) and a normal vasal ampulla (curved arrow) on the left. (c) Axial view obtained caudal to (b) demonstrates the confluence of the vasal ampulla (straight arrows) with the seminal vesicles (curved arrows) to form the ejaculatory ducts more inferiorly (not shown). (d) Sagittal view demonstrates a normal right ejaculatory duct (open arrows) which is identified as a curvilinear hypoechoic structure coursing through the substance of the prostate (straight arrows).

prostate. If they are isoechoic or hyperechoic compared with the prostate, obliteration of the lumen by fibrosis or calcification should be suspected. In the presence of diffuse fibrosis or calcification, the normal internal convolutions of the seminal vesicles and vas deferens, corresponding to normal tubular epithelium, cannot be identified on TRUS.[4,5]

Pathology

Vas deferens

Congenital abnormalities of the vas deferens are the most common finding on TRUS in males with azoospermia and low ejaculate volumes.[4–10]

Congenital absence or agenesis of the vas deferens is reported in 1–2.5% of most series of infertile men and accounts for 4.4–17% of cases of azoospermia.[3,4,14] Agenesis of the vas may be partial or complete, unilateral or bilateral, and is frequently associated with absence or hypoplasia of the distal two-thirds of the epididymis (*Fig. 11.5*). The combination of low ejaculate volume, azoospermia, normal testicular size and consistency and nonpalpable vas deferens on physical examination is diagnostic of this entity.[5–10]

True vasal agenesis is always associated with an ipsilateral seminal vesicle anomaly, as the two structures share a common embryological derivation from the wolffian duct.[4,5,] The combination of a sonographically absent or atrophic seminal vesicle in a patient in whom the vas deferens cannot be felt

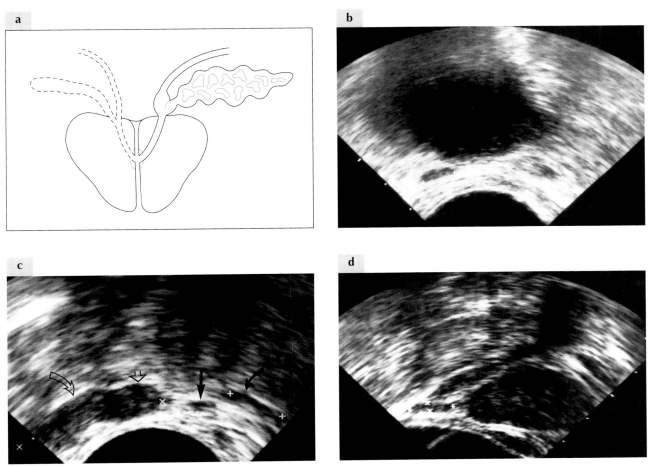

Figure 11.5 Absence and hypoplasia of the vas deferens. (a) Diagrammatic representation of the distal ducts demonstrating unilateral absence of the vas deferens, seminal vesicles and ejaculatory ducts. (b) Axial view demonstrates complete absence of the vas deferens bilaterally associated with bilateral rudimentary seminal vesicles (cursors). (c) Axial view demonstrates unilateral hypoplasia of the seminal vesicle (curved solid arrow) and vas deferens (straight solid arrow) on the left with normal vas deferens (open arrowhead) and seminal vesicles (curved open arrow) on the right. (d) Sagittal view in another patient demonstrates a rudimentary seminal vesicle on the right (cursors).

on that side is conclusive evidence of vasal agenesis. In the extremely rare condition of vasal atrophy secondary to infection or obstruction, the distal vas deferens and ampulla may be absent sonographically, but the proximal vas may be palpable and a normal ipsilateral seminal vesicle may be identified on TRUS. Likewise, because of their common embryologic origin, agenesis of the vas deferens is always associated with absence of the ipsilateral ejaculatory duct.[4,5]

The spectrum of TRUS findings in patients with vas agenesis ranges from complete absence of the vas to persistence of a vestigial remnant, identified as a diminutive, isoechoic or hyperechoic oval structure, measuring 3 mm in diameter posterior to the bladder (see *Fig. 11.5*). On TRUS, vasal hypoplasia is recognized as unilateral or bilateral reduction in size of

the vas deferens. As clinical palpation of the vas deferens may be difficult, particularly when there is thickening of the spermatic cord, TRUS should be routinely performed when vasal agenesis is suspected (in all patients with low volume azoospermia) to confirm or refute the clinical diagnosis and to detect other associated distal ductal anomalies. Where unilateral vasal agenesis or hypoplasia is detected, a search for a contralateral duct abnormality is mandatory to account for infertility in patients with azoospermia and low ejaculate volumes.[4,5]

There are a number of interesting associations of vasal agenesis. In addition to seminal vesicle and ejaculatory abnormalities, 16–43% of patients with vasal agenesis have renal anomalies including renal agenesis, crossed fused ectopia or an ectopic pelvic kidney, more common on the left side.[4–16]

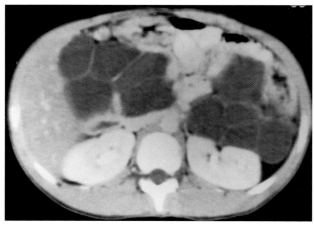

Figure 11.6 A 27-year-old male with cystic fibrosis and bilateral absence of the vas deferens and seminal vesicles on TRUS (not shown). There is diffuse replacement of the pancreas by multiple cysts as shown on an enhanced CT image through the upper abdomen.

Sonographic evaluation of the scrotum may demonstrate absence or hypoplasia of the distal two-thirds of the epididymis. Vasal aplasia syndromes may occur as part of the clinical spectrum of cystic fibrosis (*Fig. 11.6*).[17–21] Males with cystic fibrosis have bilateral vasal agenesis and recognizable cystic fibrosis gene mutations. Up to 82% of patients with congenital bilateral absent vas deferens have at least one detectable cystic fibrosis gene mutation. Of patients with unilateral absence of the vas deferens, cystic fibrosis mutations are found only in patients with partial occlusion of the single formed vas. Despite the presence of gene mutations, most patients with vasal agenesis do not demonstrate significant symptoms of cystic fibrosis and 75% have normal sweat tests. Interestingly, patients with unilateral or bilateral vasal agenesis who also have renal anomalies will not typically demonstrate mutations on cystic fibrosis gene analysis.[17]

Other vasal abnormalities that may be identified on TRUS in infertile male patients include increased echogenicity representing occlusion of the vas by fibrosis or calcification (*Fig. 11.7*), obstructing cysts of the vas deferens (*Fig. 11.8*), and vas deferens calculi (*Fig. 11.9*). The TRUS findings in patients with vasal occlusion by fibrosis or calcification range from subtle alterations in echotexture to frank calcification. Similar textural changes are usually present in the seminal vesicles and ejaculatory ducts. The pathogenesis of such diffuse distal ductal fibrosis or calcification is unclear. A congenital etiology is likely in patients with diffuse, bilateral, and symmetrical textural abnormalities, but some cases may be secondary to chronic indolent infection. Cysts and calculi of the vas deferens are most commonly seen in the terminal ampullary portion. Ampullary cysts and calculi frequently produce dilatation of the proximal vas deferens, as well as obstruction of the ipsilateral seminal vesicle. Occasionally, ampullary cysts may reach sufficient size to cause both ipsilateral and contralateral ductal obstruction.[4–10]

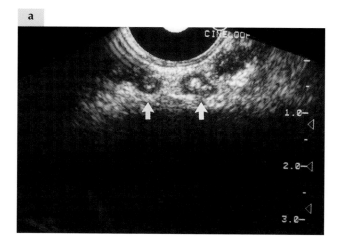
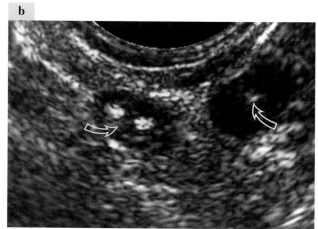

Figure 11.7 Vas deferens calcification or fibrosis. (a) *Axial view demonstrates diffuse increased echogenicity of the vas deferens bilaterally (arrows) owing to calcification or fibrosis. (b) *Magnified axial view in another patient demonstrates increased echogenicity of the vas deferens (curved arrows) owing to calcification or fibrosis. Note obliteration of the lumen and absence of the normal internal architecture of the vas deferens by echogenic material. [*By convention, images acquired during the initial years of the study were displayed with the transducer at the top of the image. More recent images are displayed with the transducer seen inferiorly.]

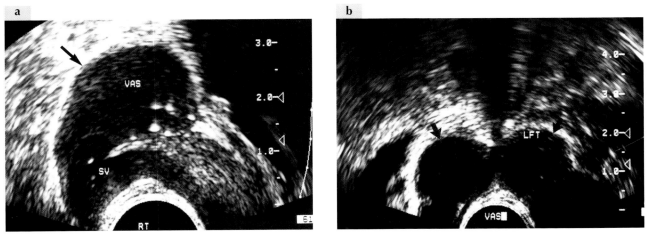

Figure 11.8 Vas deferens cysts. (a) Sagittal view demonstrates a cyst of the right vas deferens (arrow). (b) Axial view demonstrates bilateral vas deferens cysts (arrows).

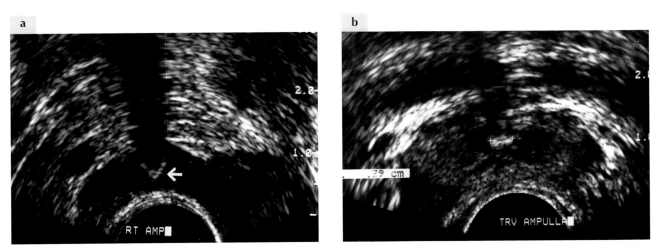

Figure 11.9 Distal ductal calculi. (a) Seminal vesicle calculus. Axial view demonstrates a large stone in the right seminal vesicle with posterior acoustic shadowing (arrow). (b) Vas deferens calculus. Axial view demonstrates a 4 mm calculus in the right vasal ampulla (cursors).

Seminal vesicles

The seminal vesicles arise as saccular dilatations of the vas deferens (distal wolffian duct) near its junction with the urogenital sinus. Eighty per cent to 90% of the ejaculate volume is elaborated by the seminal vesicles. Congenital anomalies and obstructive pathology of the seminal vesicles will result in a diminished ejaculate volume, low pH, and reduced fructose levels in the seminal fluid.

Abnormalities of the seminal vesicles associated with infertility include seminal vesicle agenesis and hypoplasia, obliteration of the lumen of the seminal vesicles by calcification and fibrosis (*Fig. 11.10*), and obstruction secondary to cysts (*Fig. 11.11*) and calculi.[22–32] As stated previously, seminal vesicle abnormalities occur in all patients with agenesis of the

vas deferens (see *Fig. 11.5*), where the seminal vesicle may be totally absent, atrophic, or hypoplastic (< 30% normal volume). Seminal vesicles are considered normal when > 25 mm in length, hypoplastic when > 16 mm but < 25 mm in length, atrophic when < 16 mm in length, and absent when no tissue is identified.[16] Although there may be complete absence of the seminal vesicle histologically, a diminutive, rudimentary fibrotic vestige may be seen on TRUS posterior to the bladder (see *Fig. 11.5*).

Occlusion of the seminal vesicles by calcification or fibrosis is thought to be congenital in origin, although, rarely, calcification and fibrosis may occur secondary to chronic infection (seminal vesiculitis). This is the most difficult diagnosis to make on TRUS in infertile male patients, as only subtle alterations in echotexture may be present. In addition to

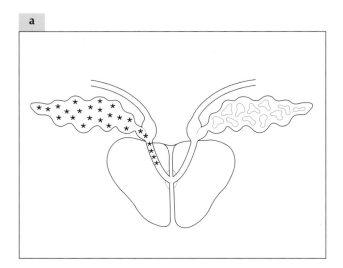

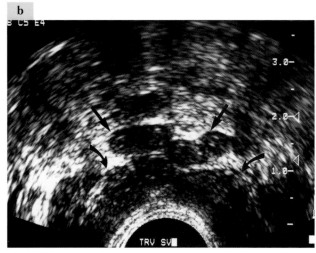

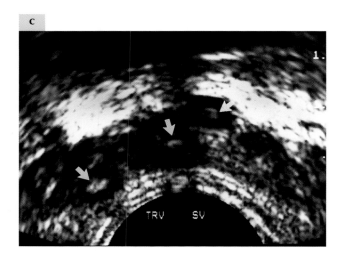

Figure 11.10 Seminal vesicle fibrosis or calcification. (a) Diagrammatic representation of the distal male reproductive system demonstrating echogenic material (fibrosis or calcification) in the right seminal vesicle and ipsilateral ejaculatory duct. (b) Axial view demonstrates subtle increase in echogenicity of the vas deferens (straight arrows) and seminal vesicles (curved arrows) bilaterally corresponding to fibrosis or calcification. (c) Axial view in another patient demonstrates diffuse obliteration of the lumen of the vas deferens and seminal vesicles by fibrosis or calcification (arrows).

increased echogenicity and lack of normal internal convolutions, the seminal vesicle may be either diminished or increased in size. Frequently, similar textural abnormalities are identified in the ipsilateral vas deferens and contralateral ductal system. Chronic seminal vesiculitis also predisposes to seminal vesicle calculus formation, probably as a result of chronic urinary reflux from the prostatic urethra. Calculi may also form as a result of concretions of static fluid and cellular debris in an obstructed seminal vesicle.

Seminal vesicle cysts are rare, are generally owing to a discontinuity between the seminal vesicle and ejaculatory duct, and are more commonly congenital than acquired (see *Fig. 11.11*). Congenital seminal vesicle cysts are commonly associated with anomalies of the ipsilateral wolffian duct (kidney, ureter, or bladder trigone). Such associated anomalies include ipsilateral renal dysgenesis (present in 80–90% of cases), duplication of the renal collecting system, ectopic insertion of the ureter, and ectopic location of the kidney.[4,6,22–32] The association of seminal vesicle cysts and ipsilateral renal and ureteric anomalies may be explained by an abnormally cephalic origin of the ureteric bud from the wolffian duct. With a high origin of the ureteric bud from the wolffian duct, the developing ureter may fail to meet and stimulate the differentiation of the nephrogenic blastema. Alternatively the more cephalic ureter may reach the nephrogenic blastema but terminate ectopically into a wolffian duct derivative (bladder, seminal vesicle). The likelihood of renal anomalies increases as the origin of the ureteric bud becomes more cephalic.

Seminal vesicle cysts are also described in patients with adult polycystic kidney disease (see *Fig. 11.11*). Unlike most other causes of seminal vesicle cysts, cystic transformation of the seminal vesicles in adult polycystic kidney disease is usually bilateral.[26] Even in the absence of a history of adult polycystic kidney disease (only 60% of patients will report a relevant family history), bilateral seminal vesicle cysts

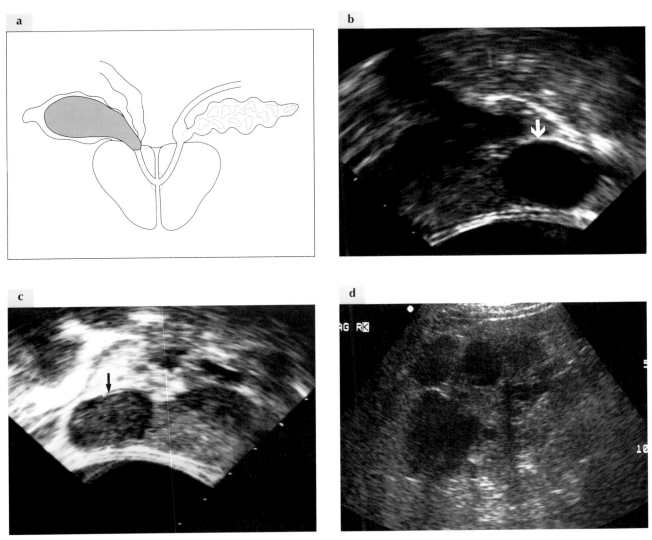

Figure 11.11 Seminal vesicle cysts. (a) Diagrammatic representation of the distal male reproductive system demonstrating a right seminal vesicle cyst with obstruction of the ipsilateral vas deferens. (b) Sagittal view demonstrates a simple cyst of the left seminal vesicle (arrow). (c) A hemorrhagic cyst (arrow) of the contralateral seminal vesicle is demonstrated on a sagittal view. (d) Sagittal view of the right kidney demonstrates multiple cortical cysts in a patient with bilateral seminal vesicle cysts (not shown) and adult polycystic kidney disease. Similar findings were present in the left kidney.

should suggest the presence of polycystic kidneys and prompt a full renal evaluation. Seminal vesicle cysts should be differentiated from cystic dilatation secondary to obstruction of the ejaculatory ducts, as the former may benefit from percutaneous aspiration while the latter is best treated by transurethral resection.

Ejaculatory ducts

Ejaculatory duct obstruction may occur secondary to extrinsic compression of the duct by periurethral and prostatic cysts (utricular and Müllerian duct cysts), because the orifices of the ducts enter into a cyst (ejaculatory duct cyst, ejaculatory duct diverticulum, wolffian duct cyst), secondary to occlusion by calcification or fibrosis, obstruction by calculi, or because of agenesis or hypoplasia of the duct itself (*Figs 11.12* and *11.13*).[4–10,33] Most cases of ejaculatory duct obstruction are associated with proximal dilatation of the seminal vesicles and vas deferens, except agenesis, hypoplasia, and atrophy which are frequently accompanied by atrophic changes or agenesis more proximally.

Sagittal TRUS images demonstrate the intraprostatic course of the ejaculatory duct as a thin hypoechoic curvilinear structure extending from the vasal ampulla to the verumontanum which, in turn, is

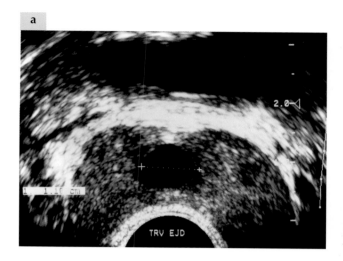

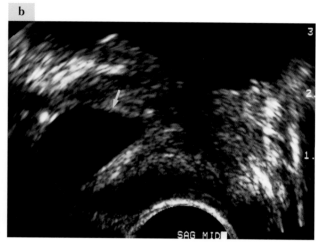

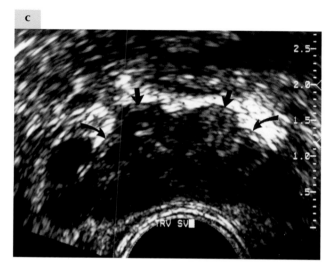

Figure 11.12 Ejaculatory duct cyst with proximal obstruction. (a) Axial view demonstrates an 11 mm ejaculatory duct cyst (cursors). (b) Sagittal view demonstrates the typical elongated appearance of an ejaculatory duct cyst (arrow). (c) Axial view obtained cranial to (b) demonstrates gross proximal dilatation of both vas deferens (straight arrows) and seminal vesicles (curved arrows).

identified as a focal area of increased echogenicity (see *Fig. 11.4*).[4–10] The lumen of the ejaculatory duct may be visible, but should not exceed 2 mm in maximum dimension. Cysts, calcification, fibrosis, and calculi are best appreciated on sagittal images.[4–6] Hyperechoic foci at the verumontanum are a normal finding, are not significantly associated with infertility, and should not be mistaken for ejaculatory duct calcification or calculi. Echogenic foci within the prostate and adjacent to the ejaculatory ducts, however, can produce ejaculatory duct obstruction and are more likely to be associated with infertility.[34]

Prostatic and periurethral cysts

A variety of intraprostatic and periurethral cysts, clearly identifiable on TRUS, may result in proximal obstruction of the male reproductive tract (see *Fig. 11.14*).[6,8–11,35] These cysts may be classified according to their location and the presence of spermatozoa within the cystic fluid.[4–6] Midline cysts, without

spermatozoa, are likely to be utricular cysts. Such cysts are considered embryologic remnants of an incompletely regressed Müllerian duct system (Müllerian duct cysts). The normal utricle is no more than a 6 mm dimple on the surface of the verumontanum. In 10% of males, however, the utricle is larger and extends in a cephalad direction over a variable distance. A tense utricular cyst may cause ejaculatory duct obstruction by extrinsic compression. Large and persistent utricular cysts are associated with various congenital anomalies, including proximal hypospadias, posterior urethral valves, prune belly syndrome, imperforate anus, and Down's syndrome.[6]

Midline intraprostatic cysts containing sperm are of wolffian duct origin, otherwise known as ejaculatory duct cysts. Although not strictly 'midline', but paramedian, these cysts appear to have a midline location on TRUS. These cysts frequently contain spermatozoa. More peripherally located degenerative prostatic cysts do not contain spermatozoa and

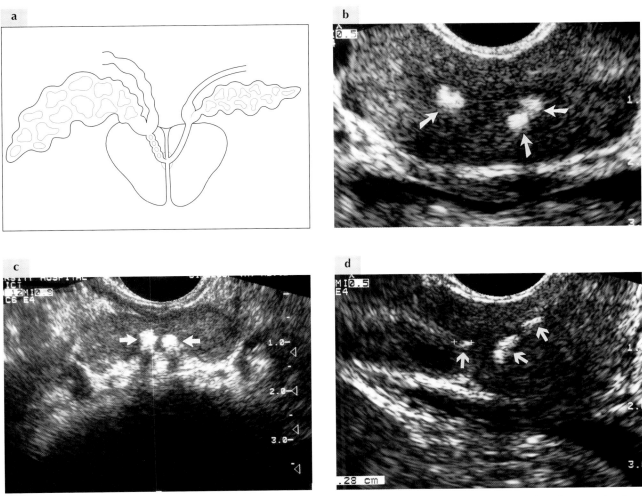

Figure 11.13 Ejaculatory duct calculi and calcification. (a) Diagrammatic representation of the distal male reproductive system demonstrating multiple ejaculatory duct calculi with proximal obstruction of the ipsilateral seminal vesicle and ejaculatory duct. (b)* Axial view demonstrates a single calculus in the right ejaculatory duct and two on the left (arrows). (c)* In another patient, axial TRUS image demonstrates bilateral calculi in the ejaculatory ducts with posterior acoustic shadowing (arrows). (d)* Diffuse calcification of the ejaculatory duct (arrows) is differentiated from ejaculatory duct calculi on TRUS by the absence of posterior acoustic shadowing. [*According to previous convention, the transducer is displayed at the top of these images.]

are called prostatic retention cysts. Although a frequent finding in normal fertile males, they are more commonly observed in infertile patients, suggesting that such cysts are not simply incidental TRUS findings. In general, however, these degenerative prostatic cysts rarely reach sufficient size to compress the adjacent ejaculatory ducts.[35]

The sonographic appearance of these midline and paramedian cysts is variable. Although cysts are clearly demonstrated on TRUS, it is often not possible to classify such cysts on the basis of the sonographic findings alone (see *Figs 11.12* and *11.14*). A small midline cyst close to the verumontanum is most likely an enlarged utricle or utricular cyst (Müllerian duct cyst). Cysts along the line of the ejaculatory duct are likely to be of wolffian or ejaculatory duct origin. A useful distinguishing feature is that ejaculatory duct cysts assume an elongated, oval appearance on sagittal images (see *Fig. 11.12*). The definitive method of differentiating the various types of prostatic cysts is direct needle aspiration under ultrasound guidance and analysis of the aspirate for sperm.

Management

Although representing only a small proportion of all infertile male patients, patients with certain congenital and acquired ductal anomalies can be cured with

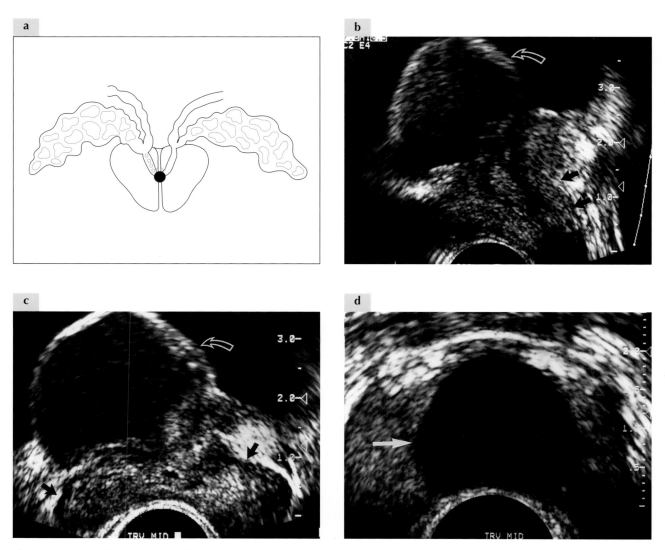

Figure 11.14 Midline cysts. (a) Diagrammatic representation of the distal male reproductive system demonstrating a midline cyst with bilateral proximal duct obstruction. Sagittal (b) and axial (c) views demonstrate a large midline cyst (curved arrows) extending above the prostate (straight arrows) and protruding into the urinary bladder. Note multiple internal echoes indicating the presence of spermatozoa. (d) In another patient, a 2 cm midline cyst is demonstrated on an axial view (arrow).

surgical intervention.[33,36–40] Suitability for surgery and the optimum operative approach, however, demand precise delineation of the nature and level of the abnormality. In general, distal ductal anomalies can be classified as surgically correctable or non-surgically correctable depending on the level and nature of obstruction. Surgically correctable causes of infertility are confined to lesions involving the distal two-thirds of the ejaculatory ducts, including ejaculatory duct cysts, calculi, fibrosis, and calcification. Agenesis or occlusion of the ductal system above this level is, by definition, non-surgically correctable and fertility can only be achieved by in vitro fertilization following epididymal aspiration (*Fig. 11.15*).[33]

Congenital bilateral agenesis of the vas deferens is, by definition, non-surgically correctable. However,

patients with vasal agenesis may be treated successfully with microscopic epididymal sperm aspiration and in vitro fertilization.[35–37] On the basis of physical examination alone, up to one-third of cases of bilateral vasal agenesis will be missed. TRUS is indicated in all patients with low volume azoospermia to detect vasal agenesis and identify associated anomalies. Scrotal ultrasound is recommended prior to epididymal sperm aspiration, as 30% of patients with vasal agenesis will have hypoplasia of the distal two-thirds of the epididymis. The side with the longest epididymal remnant should be selected for surgery.

If a midline cyst or lower ejaculatory duct calculus is identified, the optimum surgical approach is simple transurethral resection of the distal portion of the ejaculatory ducts (see *Fig. 11.15*). If TRUS fails to

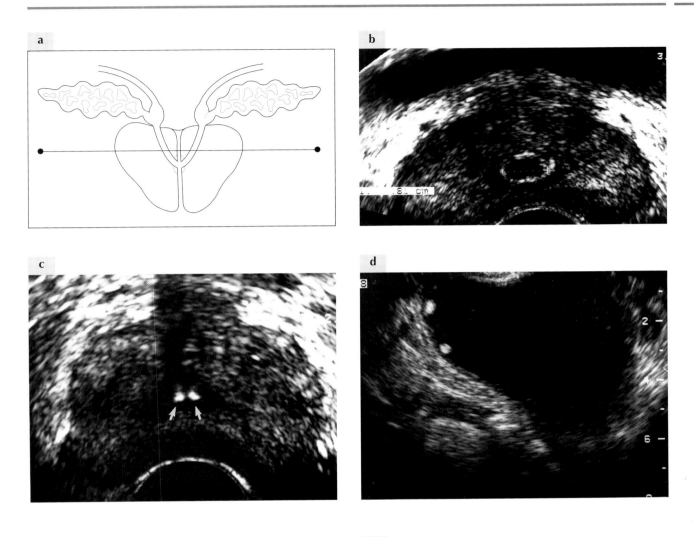

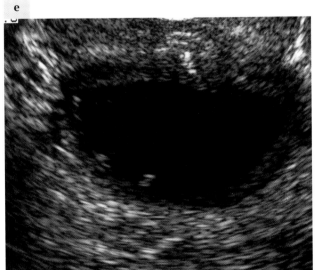

Figure 11.15 (a) Diagrammatic representation of the distal male reproductive system. The horizontal line demarcates surgically correctable from non-surgically correctable lesions based on their location. Lesions below the line causing ejaculatory duct obstruction are amenable to surgical correction by transurethral resection of the verumontanum or ejaculatory ducts. Ductal obstruction or occlusion above this level is not amenable to surgical correction. (b) An 8 mm distal ejaculatory duct cyst (cursors) that was successfully treated by transurethral resection of the ejaculatory ducts. (c) Distal ejaculatory duct calculi are demonstrated on an axial view. Again, because the calculi were located in the lower ejaculatory ducts, the patient was successfully treated with transurethral resection of the ejaculatory ducts. (d) and (e) TRUS guided cyst aspiration. (d) *Sagittal view demonstrates a large seminal vesicle cyst with multiple internal echoes corresponding to spermatozoa and mural calcification. (e) *Axial view demonstrates partial decompression of the cyst during TRUS-guided needle aspiration. Aspiration yielded spermatozoa for in vitro fertilization. [*Again, according to previous convention, the transducer is displayed at the top of these images.]

define a midline obstructing cyst or stone but shows diffuse ejaculatory duct obliteration by calcification or fibrosis with proximal dilatation, more extensive surgery is required. This involves incisions in the prostatic floor from just distal to the bladder neck to the verumontanum, lateral to the midline, sufficiently deep to enter the ejaculatory ducts from their origin posterolaterally to their termination in the prostatic urethra.[36–40]

Ejaculatory duct cysts that extend above the level of the prostate and cysts of the seminal vesicles and vas deferens can be treated effectively with TRUS-guided needle aspiration (see *Fig. 11.15*).[4,5] Cyst aspiration may be therapeutic in two ways: firstly, decompression of the cyst may help relieve proximal ductal obstruction; and, secondly, such cysts may contain spermatozoa which can be used for in vitro fertilization.

Conclusion

There are many possible etiologies for male infertility. A systematic, logical, and thorough evaluation of infertile male patients is mandatory to distinguish patients with correctable defects from those with non-correctable abnormalities. TRUS is a safe and effective method of demonstrating the distal male reproductive system that helps to identify patients appropriate for surgical or radiologic intervention and to eliminate further unnecessary investigation and intervention in patients who are unlikely to benefit. This chapter outlines the embryologic basis for anomalies of the distal male reproductive system, describes the normal anatomy and pathologic variations that may be seen on TRUS in infertile male patients, and highlights the contribution of TRUS in dictating appropriate patient management.

REFERENCES

1. de Kretser DM. Male infertility. *Lancet* 1997; **349**:787–790.

2. Templeton A. Infertility: epidemiology, aetiology, and effective management. *Health Bull (Edinburgh)* 1995; **53**:294–298.

3. Abyholm T. Azoospermia and oligozoospermia: etiology and clinical findings. *Arch Androl* 1983; **10**:57–61.

4. Kuligowska E, Baker CE, Oates RD. Male infertility: role of transrectal US in diagnosis and management. *Radiology* 1992; **185**:353–360.

5. Kuligowska E. Transrectal ultrasonography in diagnosis and management of male infertility. In: Jaffe R, Pierson RA, Abramowicz JS, eds. *Imaging in Infertility and Reproductive Endocrinology*. Philadelphia, PA: JB Lippincott, 1994:217–229.

6. Carter S St C, Shinohara K, Lipshultz LI. Transrectal ultrasonography in disorders of the seminal vesicles and ejaculatory ducts. *Urol Clin North Am* 1989; **16**:773–788.

7. Abbitt PL, Watson L, Howards S. Abnormalities of the seminal tract causing infertility: diagnosis with endorectal sonography. *Am J Roentgenol* 1991; **157**:337–339.

8. Jarow JP. Role of ultrasonography in the evaluation of the infertile male. *Semin Urol* 1994; **12**:274–282.

9. Jarow JP. Transrectal ultrasonography of infertile men. *Fertil Steril* 1993; **60**:1035–1039.

10. Honig SC. Use of ultrasonography in the evaluation of the infertile man. *World J Urol* 1993; **11**:102–110.

11. Parsons RB, Fisher AM, Bar-Chama N, Mitty HA. MR imaging in male infertility. *Radiographics* 1997; **17**:627–637.

12. Tanagho EA. Embryologic basis for lower ureteral anomalies: a hypothesis. *Urology* 1976; **7**:451–464.

13. Moore KL. *The Developing Human: Clinically Oriented Embryology* 3rd edn. Philadelphia, PA: WB Saunders, 1991:365–382.

14. Jequier AM, Ansell ID, Bullimore NJ. Congenital absence of the vasa deferentia presenting with infertility. *J Androl* 1985; **6**:15–18.

15. Pereira JK, Chait PG, Daneman A. Bilateral persisting mesonephric ducts. *Am J Roentgenol* 1993; **160**: 367–369.

16. Trigaux JP, Van Beers B, Delchambre F. Male genital tract malformations associated with ipsilateral renal agenesis: sonographic findings. *J Clin Ultrasound* 1991; **19**:3–10.

17. Mulhall JP, Oates RD. Vasal aplasia and cystic fibrosis. *Curr Opin Urol* 1995; **5**:316–319.

18. Augarten A, Yahav Y, Kerem BS *et al*. Congenital bilateral absence of the vas deferens in the absence of cystic fibrosis. *Lancet* 1994; **344**:1473–1474.

19. Mickle J, Milunsky A, Amos JA, Oates RD. Congenital unilateral absence of the vas deferens: a heterogenous disorder with two distinct subpopulations based upon etiology and mutational status of the cystic fibrosis gene. *Hum Reprod* 1995; **10**:1728–1735.

20. Oates RD, Amos JA. The genetic basis of congenital bilateral absence of the vas deferens and cystic fibrosis. *J Androl* 1994; **15**:1–8.

21. Chillon M, Casals T, Mercier B *et al*. Mutations in the cystic fibrosis gene in patients with congenital absence of the vas deferens. *N Engl J Med* 1995; **332**: 1475–1480.

22. Asch MR, Toi A. Seminal vesicles: imaging and intervention using transrectal ultrasound. *J Ultrasound Med* 1991; **10**:19–23.

23. Ejeckam GC, Govatsos S, Lewis AS. Cyst of seminal vesicle associated with ipsilateral renal agenesis. *Urology* 1984;**24**:372–374.

24. King BF, Hattery RR, Lieber MM, Berquist TH, Williamson B, Hartman GW. Congenital cystic disease of the seminal vesicles. *Radiology* 1991; **178**:207–211.

25. Heaney JA, Pfister RC, Meares EM. Giant cyst of the seminal vesicle with renal agenesis. *Am J Roentgenol* 1987; **149**:139–140.

26. Weingardt JP, Townsend RR, Russ PD, Rogers PT, Fitzgerald SW. Seminal vesicle cysts associated with autosomal dominant polycystic kidney disease detected by sonography. *J Ultrasound Med* 1995; **14**:475–477.

27. Walls WJ, Lin F. Ultrasound diagnosis of seminal vesicle cyst. *Radiology* 1975; **114**:693–694.

28. Kenney PJ, Leeson MD. Congenital anomalies of the seminal vesicles: spectrum of computed tomographic findings. *Radiology* 1983; **149**:247–251.

29. Adjiman M. Dysfunction of the seminal vesicle and male infertility. *Prog Reprod Biol Med* 1985; **12**:158–161.

30. Malatinsky E, Labady F, Lepies P, Zajac R, Jancar M. Congenital anomalies of the seminal ducts. *Intern Urol Nephrol* 1987; **19**:189–194.

31. Lucon AM, Nahas WC, Wroclawski ER, Borrelli M, Moreira de Goes P, Menezes de Goes G. Congenital cyst of the seminal vesicle. *Eur Urol* 1983; **9**:362–363.

32. Gevenois PA, Van Sinoy ML, Sintzoff SA *et al.* Cysts of the prostate and seminal vesicles: MR imaging findings in 11 patients. *Am J Roentgenol* 1990; **155**:1021–1024.

33. Meacham RB, Hellerstein DK, Lipshultz LI. Evaluation and treatment of ejaculatory duct obstruction in the infertile male. *Fertil Steril* 1993; **59**:393–397.

34. Poore RE, Jarow JP. Distribution of intraprostatic hyperechoic lesions in infertile men. *Urology* 1995; **45**:467–469.

35. Hamilton S, Fitzpatrick JM. Ultrasound diagnosis of a prostatic cyst causing acute urinary retention. *J Ultrasound Med* 1987; **6**:385–387.

36. Namiki M. Recent concepts in the management of male infertility. *Int J Urol* 1996; **3**:249–255.

37. Costabile RA. Infertility – is there anything we can do about it? *J Urol* 1997; **157**:158–159.

38. Sokol RZ. The diagnosis and treatment of male infertility. *Curr Opin Obstet Gynaecol* 1995; **7**:177–181.

39. Madgar I, Seidman DS, Levran D *et al.* Micromanipulation improves in-vitro fertilization results after epididymal or testicular sperm aspiration in patients with congenital absence of the vas deferens. *Human Reprod* 1996; **11**:2151–2154.

40. Schlegel PN, Girardi SK. Clinical review 87: in vitro fertilization for male factor infertility. *J Clin Endocrinol Metab* 1997; **82**:709–716.

12 Impotence

Carol B Benson

Introduction

Impotence, or erectile dysfunction, is defined as the inability to generate or maintain an erection adequate for vaginal intercourse. If the male member of a couple is impotent, the couple will be unable to have intercourse, and thus will be unable to conceive.

Erectile dysfunction is classified as psychogenic when it results from psychological factors, and as organic when a physiologic abnormality is present. Organic causes of impotence include anatomic abnormalities of the penis, hemodynamic abnormalities, either arterial or venous, and neurological abnormalities. Among men seeking medical attention for erectile dysfunction who have previously had normal function, an organic cause can be identified in 50–90% of cases.[1,3]

Ultrasound and Doppler are the imaging modalities of choice for evaluating erectile dysfunction;[1,3–8] ultrasound is used to assess the soft tissues of the penis, and Doppler imaging to assess arterial and venous blood flow. Occasionally, other imaging studies such as cavernosography and magnetic resonance imaging may be necessary for a full evaluation.

The normal penis and erectile function

In order to be able to diagnose abnormalities of the penis that lead to impotence, an understanding of the normal anatomy and physiology of the penis and its erectile function is required. The penis comprises three columns of spongy tissues, the two corpora cavernosa located side by side on the dorsal aspect of the penis and the corpus spongiosum located in the midline on the ventral side of the penis. The corpus spongiosum contains a small amount of sinusoidal tissue and the urethra.

The corpora cavernosa contain spongy cavernosal sinusoidal tissue which is collapsed in the non-erect state. Smooth muscle lines the walls of the sinusoids and, in the non-erect state, the muscles are contracted. The two corpora cavernosa are encapsulated by a fibrous sheath called the tunica albuginea. When an erection develops, the cavernosal sinusoids fill with blood and expand to stretch the tunica albuginea until the penis is tense and rigid.

The blood supply to each corpus cavernosum is via the cavernosal artery, a branch of the penile artery, which is in turn a branch of the internal pudendal artery. The cavernosal artery travels through the middle of the cavernosal sinusoids and gives off small perpendicular branches, called helicine branches, that deliver blood to the sinusoids. Venous drainage from the corpus cavernosum is via small veins that perforate the tunica albuginea to drain into the deep dorsal vein or into cavernosal veins at the base of the penis.

The development of an erection begins with a burst of motor nervous activity from parasympathetic nerves in the second, third, and fourth sacral nerves. The parasympathetic motor activity causes the smooth muscles of the sinusoids to relax and causes the cavernosal arteries to dilate. This leads to a rapid influx of blood to fill the opening sinusoids. As the sinusoids expand, the tunica albuginea is stretched to the point where it occludes the perforating draining veins. This venous occlusion keeps the blood from leaving the corpora cavernosa and maintains the erection.[9]

Organic impotence

Erectile dysfunction will occur if there is scarring of the sinusoids of the corpora cavernosa or the tunica albuginea.[10,11] This can result from prior penile trauma, prior priapism, or prior intracavernosal injections. Scarring prevents normal expansion of the sinusoids and the corpora. As an erection develops, there is traction and pulling at the site of scarring that can cause pain and rapid detumescence. In less severe cases, an erection may develop, but the scarring causes penile curvature. Too much curvature may make vaginal intercourse impossible.

Arterial impotence results when there is arterial insufficiency such that the arterial inflow is inadequate to fill the cavernosal sinusoids, and an erection cannot be generated. With insufficient arterial inflow, the sinusoids do not expand enough to stretch the tunica albuginea to occlude the draining veins. Thus, despite arterial inflow, the veins continue to drain blood from the corpora cavernosa.[5,9] Patients at risk for arterial insufficiency include those with atherosclerosis, diabetes, and vasculitis, and smokers.[12,13]

Venous incompetence occurs in patients when the cavernosal draining veins are not adequately occluded despite normal arterial inflow and sinusoidal filling. Patients typically report the ability to generate an erection, but inability to maintain it long enough for sexual function.[4,14] Venous incompetence may be an isolated abnormality or may be found in conjunction with arterial insufficiency.

Sonography of the penis

Normal

Sonography of the penis is performed with high frequency linear transducers in the range 5–10 MHz. The transducer is placed directly on the penis and transverse and longitudinal images are obtained. The tissues of the corpora of the penis have homogeneous echotexture. The three corpora are seen as rounded structures on transverse view, two on the dorsal side of the penis and one on the ventral side (*Fig. 12.1*). The urethra is not visible in the corpus spongiosum unless it is distended with fluid. The walls of the cavernosal arteries may be seen as two bright dots within each corpus cavernosum on transverse view and parallel echogenic lines on longitudinal view (*Fig. 12.2*). The tunica albuginea may be visible as a thin white line around each corpus.[10]

When the penis is erect, the corpora are enlarged and pressed together at the midline. They lose their homogeneous echotexture and become speckled in appearance, because the filled sinusoids are anechoic and their walls are echogenic. The cavernosal arteries are more prominent, because the

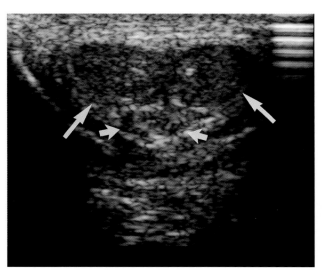

Figure 12.1 Normal penis. Transverse sonogram demonstrates the two rounded corpora cavernosa (arrows) on the dorsal side of the penis, and the smaller corpus spongiosum on the ventral side of the penis (short arrows).

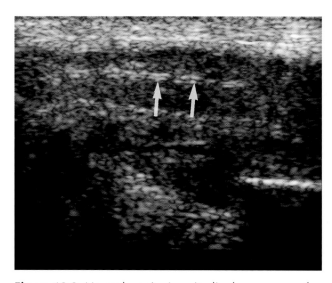

Figure 12.2 Normal penis. Longitudinal sonogram of corpus cavernosum in the non-erect state demonstrating echogenic walls of collapsed cavernosal artery (arrows).

arteries are dilated and surrounded by fluid (*Fig. 12.3*).

Cavernosal scarring

Cavernosal scarring appears as echogenic plaques within the corpora cavernosa. The plaques usually have an irregular shape and are often multiple. If the surrounding sinusoids are expanded with an erection, the plaques are more prominent on sonography (*Fig. 12.4*).

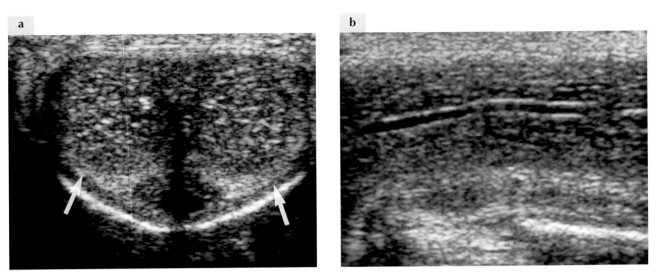

Figure 12.3 Normal erect penis. (a) Transverse sonogram demonstrating expansion of the corpora cavernosa (arrows) with blood. The corpora now have a speckled appearance owing to filling of the sinusoids. (b) Longitudinal sonogram of dilated cavernosal artery (calipers) within blood-filled sinusoids.

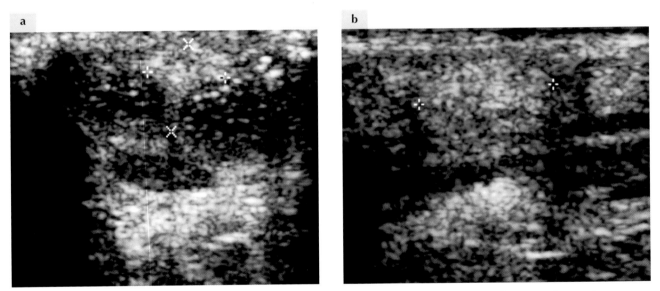

Figure 12.4 Cavernosal scarring. (a) Transverse sonogram of erect penis with echogenic plaque (calipers) due to scarring. (b) Longitudinal sonogram demonstrates echogenic plaque (calipers) within the corpus cavernosum.

Scarring of the tunica albuginea and Peyronie's disease

Scarring of the tunica albuginea causes focal thickening of the echogenic capsule of the corpus cavernosum. When the scar is calcified, it is termed Peyronie's disease. Tunical scarring is most commonly located in the midline between the two corpora cavernosa, but can occur anywhere along the tunica albuginea. Peyronie's plaques are brightly echogenic with acoustic shadowing (*Fig. 12.5*).[1,15,16]

Doppler of the penis

Normal

Arterial flow to the penis can be evaluated with color and pulsed Doppler in conjunction with the use of pharmacologic agents to generate an erection. The vasoactive pharmacologic agents and doses that are used include 10–15 µg prostaglandin E_1 and 30–50 mg papaverine.[1] These drugs cause sinusoidal smooth muscle relaxation and cavernosal arterial dilatation when they are injected into the corpora

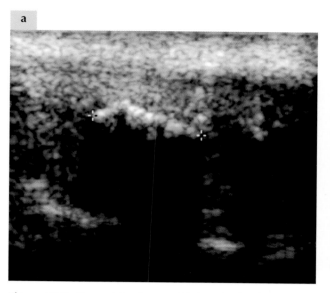
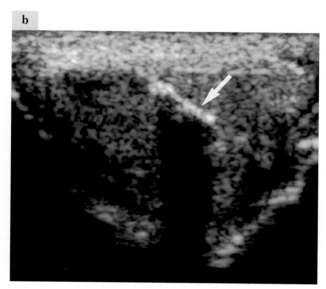

Figure 12.5 Peyronie's disease. (a) Longitudinal sonogram of midline of penis demonstrating calcified Peyronie's plaque (calipers). (b) Oblique transverse sonogram demonstrates calcified plaque (arrow) between the corpora cavernosa.

cavernosa. Prior to injection, some examiners place a simple tourniquet around the base of the penis. The pharmacologic agent is then injected directly into one corpus cavernosum using a small gauge needle. A single injection acts on both corpora because there are communications across the intercavernosal septum. After 2 minutes the tourniquet, if used, is removed, and the cavernosal arteries are assessed by Doppler imaging.

Doppler waveforms of the cavernosal arteries are best obtained by scanning longitudinally on the dorsal side of the penis. Color Doppler may occasionally be useful in localizing the arteries. Waveforms are obtained every 2–3 minutes until the peak systolic velocity exceeds 35 cm/s[4,17–19] or the peak systolic velocity plateaus. Maximum tumescence is usually obtained 8–10 minutes after injection, but may take as long as 20 minutes in anxious patients.[1,5,20–23] At this point, the end-diastolic velocity in the cavernosal arteries is measured.

During the development of an erection in a normal man, the peak systolic velocity rapidly increases to > 35 cm/s. The arterial waveform has a low resistance pattern with high end-diastolic flow (*Fig. 12.6*), because the resistance in the cavernosal sinusoids is low owing to relaxation of the sinusoidal smooth muscles. Once a full erection is obtained, the sinusoids are filled and the cavernosal arterial waveform develops a high resistance pattern with sharp systolic peaks and diminished, absent, or reversed end-diastolic flow (*Fig. 12.7*). The peak systolic velocity may fall

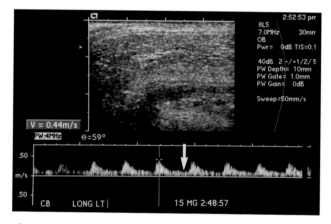

Figure 12.6 Normal cavernosal arterial waveform during development of an erection. Longitudinal sonogram with Doppler waveform below demonstrates normal peak systolic velocity (caliper) of 44 cm/s and low resistance pattern with high diastolic flow (arrow).

below 35 cm/s during the maintenance phase of the erection.

The venous function of the penis is assessed by using color Doppler to detect flow in the dorsal vein and by the cavernosal arterial waveform. Scanning from the ventral side of the penis, color or pulsed Doppler is applied to the dorsal vein.[1,4,20–22,24,25] With normal venous competence, there should be no or minimal flow in the dorsal vein during the development and maintenance of an erection. A high resistance cavernosal arterial waveform is also indicative of venous competence.

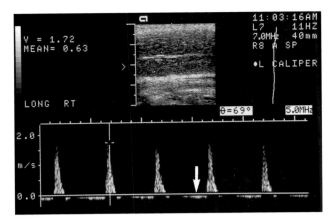

Figure 12.7 Normal cavernosal arterial waveform after erection is obtained. Longitudinal sonogram with Doppler waveform below demonstrates high resistance pattern with normal peak systolic velocity (caliper) of 172 cm/s and sharp systolic peaks and with absent, sometimes reversed, diastolic flow (arrow).

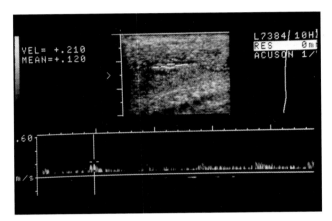

Figure 12.8 Arterial insufficiency. Longitudinal sonogram with Doppler waveform below demonstrates abnormally low peak systolic velocity (caliper) of 21 cm/s, consistent with arterial insufficiency.

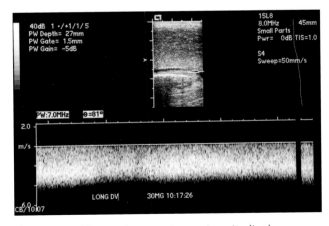

Figure 12.9 Venous incompetence. Longitudinal sonogram of penis scanned from the ventral side with Doppler gate on the dorsal vein, demonstrates a large amount of flow in the dorsal vein.

Arterial insufficiency

The cavernosal arterial peak systolic velocity, measured on the spectral waveform, is the best indicator of arterial function. The lower the peak systolic velocity, the greater the severity of arterial insufficiency. Patients with maximum peak systolic velocities of < 25 cm/s (*Fig. 12.8*) have severe arterial insufficiency that usually cannot be treated with medication. Maximum peak systolic velocities in the range 25–35 cm/s indicate mild to moderate arterial insufficiency, which can often be treated with pharmacologic agents that promote peripheral arterial flow. In addition, discrepancies of > 10 cm/s between the two cavernosal arteries are often indicative of some degree of arterial insufficiency.

Doppler studies of penile arterial function may be limited by patient anxiety. In particular, significant anxiety can lower the cavernosal arterial peak systolic velocity such that maximum flow is below the normal range despite normal arterial function. Similarly, some patients with psychogenic impotence have lower than normal peak systolic velocities, despite normal penile and cavernosal arteries.[26]

Venous incompetence

The diagnosis of venous incompetence should be suspected in any patient who does not generate an adequate erection despite normal arterial function.[1,4] With venous incompetence, the end-diastolic velocity in the cavernosal arteries remains above 5 cm/s and flow can be found in the dorsal vein with pulsed or color Doppler (*Fig. 12.9*).

While color and pulsed Doppler can suggest the diagnosis of venous incompetence, definitive diagnosis can only be made by cavernosometry. This study is usually performed in conjunction with cavernosography and not only permits diagnosis of venous incompetence, but also provides a map of the leaking cavernosal veins. This is useful if surgical repair is being considered.

Combined arterial and venous disease

In patients who are impotent as a result of both arterial insufficiency and venous incompetence, Doppler studies can only be used to assess arterial function. If arterial insufficiency is present, the penile veins cannot be assessed because the arterial inflow is not adequate to fill the cavernosal sinusoids and to occlude the draining veins. Venous flow will persist and will be visible by color Doppler, whether or not the veins would be competent if arterial flow were normal. In addition, cavernosal arterial waveforms will be low resistance because the sinusoids do not fill to the point of increasing vascular resistance.

Despite this drawback, Doppler assessment is a useful first step in evaluating patients with suspected organic impotence. If the arterial function is diminished, further studies can be performed to assess venous competence if treatment for arterial insufficiency is considered.

REFERENCES

1. Benson CB, Vickers MA, Aruny J. Evaluation of impotence. *Semin Ultrasound CT MR* 1991; **12**:176–190.

2. Krysiewicz S, Mellinger BC. The role of imaging in the diagnostic evaluation of impotence. *Am J Roentgenol* 1989; **153**:1133–1139.

3. Paushter DM. Role of duplex sonography in the evaluation of sexual impotence. *Am J Roentgenol* 1989; **153**:1161–1163.

4. Benson CB, Vickers MA. Sexual impotence caused by vascular disease: diagnosis with duplex sonography. *Am J Roentgenol* 1989; **153**:1149–1153.

5. Benson CB, Aruny JE, Vickers MA. Correlation of duplex sonography with arteriography in patients with erectile dysfunction. *Am J Roentgenol* 1993; **160**:71–73.

6. Mueller SC, Lue TF. Evaluation of vasculogenic impotence. *Urol Clin North Am* 1988; **15**:65–76.

7. Lue TF, Tanagho EA. Physiology of erection and pharmacological management of impotence. *J Urol* 1987; **137**:829–836.

8. Jarow JP, Pugh VW, Routh WD, Dyer RB. Comparison of penile duplex ultrasonography to pudendal arteriography; variant penile arterial anatomy affects interpretation of duplex ultrasound. *Invest Radiol* 1993; **28**:806–810.

9. Krane RJ, Goldstein I, De Tejada IS. Impotence. *N Engl J Med* 1989; **321**:1648–1659.

10. Doubilet PM, Benson CB, Silverman SG, Gluck C. The penis. *Semin Ultrasound CT MR* 1991; **12**:157–175.

11. Benson CB, Doubilet PM, Vickers MA. Sonography of the penis. *Ultrasound Quarterly* 1991; **9**:89–109.

12. Kadioglu A, Erdogru T, Tellaloglu S. Evaluation of penile arteries in papaverine-induced erection with color Doppler ultrasonography. *Arch Esp Urol* 1995; **48**:654–648.

13. Kaufman JM, Borges FD, Fitch WP *et al.* Evaluation of erectile dysfunction by dynamic infusion cavernosometry and cavernosography (DICC). *Urology* 1993; **41**:445–451.

14. Vickers MA, Benson CB, Richie JR. High resolution ultrasonography and pulsed-wave Doppler for detection of corporo-venous incompetence in erectile dysfunction. *J Urol* 1990; **43**:1125–1127.

15. Chou YH, Tiu CM, Pan HB *et al.* High-resolution real-time ultrasound in Peyronie's disease. *J Ultrasound Med* 1987; **6**:67–70.

16. Hamm B, Friedrich M, Kelami A. Ultrasound imaging in Peyronie's disease. *Urology* 1986; **28**:540–545.

17. Hampson SJ, Cowie AGA, Rickards D, Lees WR. Independent evaluation of impotence by colour Doppler imaging and cavernosometry. *Eur Urol* 1992; **21**:27–31.

18. Herbener TE, Seftel AD, Nehra A, Goldstein I. Penile ultrasound. *Semin Urol* 1994; **12**:320–332.

19. Iacovo F, Barra S, Lotti T. Evaluation of penile deep arteries in psychogenic impotence by means of duplex ultrasonography. *J Urol* 1993; **149**:1262–1264.

20. Govier FE, Asase D, Hefty TR, McClure RD, Pritchett TR, Weissman RM. Timing of penile color flow duplex ultrasonography using a triple drug mixture. *J Urol* 1995; **153**:1472–1475.

21. Meuleman EJH, Bemelmans BLH, Doesburg WH, van Asten WNJC, Skotnicki SH, Debruyne FMJ. Penile pharmacological duplex ultrasonography: a dose-effect study comparing papaverine, papaverine/phentolamine and prostaglandin E_1. *J Urol* 1992; **148**: 63–66.

22. Schwartz AN, Wang KY, Mack LA *et al.* Evaluation of normal erectile function with color flow Doppler sonography. *Am J Roentgenol* 1989; **153**:1155–1160.

23. Shabsigh R, Fishman IJ, Quesada ET, Seale-Hawkins CK, Dunn JK. Evaluation of vasculogenic erectile impotence using penile duplex ultrasonography. *J Urol* 1989; **142**:1469–1474.

24. Quam JP, King BF, James EM *et al.* Duplex and color Doppler sonographic evaluation of vasculogenic impotence. *Am J Roentgenol* 1989; **153**:1141–1147.

25. Broderick GA, Arger P. Duplex Doppler ultrasonography: noninvasive assessment of penile anatomy and function. *Semin Roentgenol* 1993; **28**:43–56.

26. Allen RP, Engel RME, Smolev JK, Brendler CB. Comparison of duplex ultrasonography and nocturnal penile tumescence in evaluation of impotence. *J Urol* 1994; **151**:1525–1529.

13 Ovulation induction

Antonio R Gargiulo

Current role of ovulation induction in infertility treatment

Protocols for ovulation induction (OI) are aimed at promoting follicular maturation and oocyte release in patients who lack sufficient ovulation to become pregnant on their own. The goal is to enhance ovulatory function temporarily through the use of hormonal agents, and allow precisely timed intercourse or intrauterine insemination, thereby increasing cycle fecundity.[1–3]

Spontaneous ovulation involves the development of one or two dominant follicles during the early proliferative phase of the menstrual cycle. Because several OI agents interfere with hormonal feedback between the brain and the ovary, dose-dependent supraphysiologic stimulation of follicular development can be achieved. The pharmacologic induction of three or more preovulatory follicles is referred to as 'superovulation'. This can be the unplanned (and often undesirable) result of an exuberant response to standard OI protocols, but it can also be the goal of treatment in select cases. Indeed, several prospective, randomized studies indicate that superovulation in association with intrauterine insemination is an effective empirical treatment for unexplained infertility and infertility associated with endometriosis or male factor.[4–8]

As this clinical manual is intended for radiologists and infertility specialists alike, a brief review of the pharmacologic agents currently employed for OI seems relevant.

Clomiphene citrate

The most widely prescribed fertility drug today is still clomiphene citrate, which has been approved for OI by the American Food and Drug Administration (FDA) for over 30 years.[1,2] This oral agent works at the level of the hypothalamus, modifying gonadotropin-releasing hormone (GnRH) pulsatility, which results in increased follicle-stimulating hormone (FSH) secretion by the pituitary gland. Clomiphene (Clomid, Serophene) is usually given daily for five days during the mid-follicular phase. Spontaneous ovulation occurs one to ten days after the last dose. Alternatively, an artificial ovulatory stimulus can be provided by a single injection of human chorionic gonadotropin (hCG) employed as a long-acting luteinizing hormone (LH) surrogate.

Significant concerns remain about the overall efficacy and safety of clomiphene, including its documented antiestrogenic effects on the genital tract and a suggested role in ovarian carcinogenesis with prolonged use.[10,11] Moreover, owing to the long half-life of this drug, the developing fetus may be exposed to it during organogenesis. This raises theoretical concerns regarding subtle teratogenic effects on reproductive organs, owing to clomiphene's structural affinity to diethylstilbestrol. The above nonwithstanding, this agent remains popular because it is inexpensive, user-friendly and effective. Twin pregnancies occur in fewer than 10% of clomiphene cycles, and triplet pregnancies in fewer than 1%.[1,2] Moreover, severe iatrogenic ovarian hyperstimulation syndrome, a condition characterized by ovarian enlargement and potentially life-threatening fluid and electrolyte shifts, is rarely encountered following treatment with clomiphene.

Metformin

Another class of orally administered drugs is making its way into the therapeutic armamentarium, namely oral hypoglycemic agents. Hyperinsulinemia and obesity are frequently observed in patients with hyperandrogenic chronic anovulation. Spontaneous return of ovulatory function can be achieved in some of these patients with weight reduction; however, this is difficult to attain and may take years. An alternative approach is the improvement of glucose homeostasis in these patients with oral agents, such as N1,N1-dimethyl biguanide, better known as metformin (Glucophage). This drug improves glucose tolerance, lowering both basal and postprandial plasma glucose. Unlike sulfonylureas, metformin does not produce hypoglycemia in either diabetic or non-diabetic subjects and does not cause hyperinsulinemia. Insulin secretion remains unchanged, while fasting insulin levels and day-long plasma insulin response usually decrease.

Metformin has been employed successfully to reduce hyperandrogenism and hyperinsulinemia and to induce ovulation in obese anovulatory patients, alone and in combination with low dose clomiphene or gonadotropins.[12–14] The FDA does not currently approve the use of metformin as an OI agent. As is customary for all off-label drugs, oral hypoglycemic agents should only be employed on carefully selected and thoroughly informed patients.

Gonadotropins

Human menopausal gonadotropins (hMG), isolated and characterized in Italy in 1966 by Donini and colleagues,[15,16] quickly became the mainstay of aggressive OI and superovulation. This class of drugs allows a degree of ovarian stimulation unmatched by even the highest doses of clomiphene. However, the level of response over different cycles is variable not only from patient to patient, but also, to a lesser extent, within the same individual.

Whereas monitoring of ovarian response is useful with clomiphene (mostly for timing of insemination/intercourse), this becomes essential with protocols employing gonadotropins. No matter how experienced the physician: there is a very fine line between the minimal effective dose that will induce ovulation and the dose that will trigger ovarian hyperstimulation syndrome and/or undesired superovulation. This principle has remained true for second, third and fourth generation gonadotropins, such as purified urinary FSH, highly purified urinary FSH, and recombinant FSH. Human menopausal gonadotropins (Humegon, Pergonal, Repronex) contain equal amounts (approx. 75 or 150 IU) of extracted LH and FSH, and purified urinary FSH (Metrodin) contains approx. 75 IU of FSH, plus small amounts of LH. Both of these products must be administered intramuscularly owing to their heavy protein content. Highly purified urinary FSH (Fertinex) and recombinant FSH (Follistim/Puregon, Gonal-F) contain 75 iu of FSH, and negligible or no amount of LH, respectively. Because they are free of heavy urinary protein, they can be administered safely subcutaneously.

Recombinant FSH has proven to be at least as effective as purified urinary FSH in the induction of ovulation,[3] and has now replaced extractive gonadotropins in many centers. The main advantage of recombinant, over highly purified urinary, FSH is reproducibility of dosage. Provided that storage, reconstitution and administration of the product are handled correctly, such dose consistency allows the clinician to assess with more confidence the degree of response in individual patients. Another advantage of recombinant technology (which will become more evident with the future introduction of recombinant LH) is the flexibility that it affords in treating different classes of anovulatory patients with individualized gonadotropin combinations. In addition, recombinant drugs avoid the theoretical risk of viral transmission through parenteral use of human-derived proteins, a risk that has never been confirmed by clinical observation. Fortunately, several steps in the preparation of extractive gonadotropins (including the final process of lyophilization) are incompatible with the survival of infectious viruses, including HIV.

Current indications for gonadotropin use in OI include:

- clomiphene-resistant anovulation;
- failure to achieve pregnancy despite multiple cycles of documented induction of ovulation or superovulation with clomiphene;
- low estrogen status (as demonstrated by a delayed or scarce withdrawal bleed in response to progestins);
- frank hypogonadotropic amenorrhea.

Gonadotropins exert a direct and vigorous effect on ovarian follicles and should be used exclusively by physicians specifically trained in the prevention, recognition and treatment of the potential complications associated with their use. To reinforce this point, we should point out that currently the majority of low and high-order multiple pregnancies resulting from infertility treatment are not derived from cycles of in vitro fertilization, but from OI – a fact that too many practitioners seem to ignore.[17] Moreover, the incidence of ovarian hyperstimulation syndrome and superovulation with gonadotropin OI is as high as 16%, including a 1–2% incidence of severe cases requiring hospitalization.[18] Finally, the incidences of spontaneous abortion and ectopic pregnancy are increased following OI with gonadotropins.[19,20]

Gonadotropin-releasing hormone and its analogues

Gonadotropin-releasing hormone (GnRH) and its agonistic and antagonistic analogues have a surprisingly limited role in the current practice of OI. The synthetic form of the native GnRH decapeptide, administered parenterally over an average span of 14 days by means of a portable infusion pump, has been successfully employed for OI in cases of hypogonadotropic hypogonadism. It is also used in select cases of polycystic ovary syndrome, resulting in a level of multiple conceptions comparable to that of normal, unstimulated women.[21] Owing to the physiologic nature of this treatment, ultrasound is performed mostly to synchronize insemination/intercourse with ovulation. Regrettably, owing to logistic and cost factors, this safe OI modality has never reached popularity, and is currently offered by very few centers worldwide, mostly for infertility associated with hypogonadotropic hypogonadism.

Agonistic analogues of GnRH have been in use for over two decades. These synthetic decapeptides have an exceptional affinity for the GnRH receptor and a longer half-life compared to the endogenous hormone. This results in an initial stimulation of gonadotropin secretion, followed by a profound suppression, mostly due to receptor depletion. The main clinical use of GnRH agonists in OI is to avoid untimely ovulation through prevention of the LH surge. GnRH agonists are administered parenterally. Some of them, such as goserelin, leuprolide and triptorelin, are available in injectable forms (Zoladex, Lupron Depot, Decapeptyl Depot), which allows a single administration, usually in the luteal phase preceding the induction cycle. During OI, however, more flexibility is usually allowed by preparations for daily administration, such as intranasal buserelin or nafarelin (Suprefact Nasal, Synarel) or for subcutaneous injection, such as buserelin, leuprolide and triptporelin (Suprefact, Lupron Injection, Decapeptyl).

Analogues of GnRH are currently regarded as pivotal components of controlled ovarian hyperstimulation protocols for in vitro fertilization. However, they are rarely employed in protocols of OI and superovulation. Some have proposed that the use of GnRH agonists as an adjunct to gonadotropin therapy in patients with polycystic ovarian syndrome may decrease the incidence of severe ovarian hyperstimulation syndrome and that of spontaneous abortion. However, a recent metanalysis seems to disprove both of these claims.[22]

Finally, a new class of drugs, the GnRH antagonists, has recently been introduced. Because these agents work by direct competitive inhibition of the pituitary GnRH receptor, they cause rapid inhibition of the gonadothoph without the initial stimulatory effect of GnRH agonists. This provides the clinician with the means of suppressing the midcycle LH surge without compromising endogenous FSH secretion during the early follicular phase. Moreover, because these agonists are administered during gonadotropin stimulation, the overall treatment time can be significantly shortened.

Cetrorelix (Cetrotide) has been applied in single- and multiple-dose protocols, while ganirelix (Antagon/Orgalutran) has until now only been used in the multiple-dose protocol. The incidence of a premature LH surge is below 2% for either regimen, and the incidence of severe ovarian hyperstimulation syndrome appears to be lower than that observed in long protocols employing GnRH agonists.[23]

As also observed with GnRH agonists, the GnRH antagonists may prove of limited value as an adjunct to exogenous gonadotropins for OI. Ultrasound monitoring is particularly important when using GnRH antagonists because a plateau or drop in serum estradiol is often observed after the first dose. This means that clinicians may have to rely solely on follicular dimensions to time the final hCG injection when these agents are used.

Follicular monitoring during ovulation induction

The goal of follicular monitoring during OI can be summarized in four general points:

- establish if anatomic conditions exist for safe and effective OI;
- assist in titrating the dose of medication to achieve OI or superovulation while aiming to avoid ovarian hyperstimulation syndrome and high-order multiple gestations;
- optimize synchronization of ovulation and insemination/intercourse;
- allow early recognition of complications associated with OI.

The type and extent of follicular monitoring required differs according to patient diagnosis and type of drugs employed. Transvaginal sonography (TVS) provides reliable and non-invasive biophysical indicators of follicular growth, while at the same time allowing detailed imaging of pelvic anatomy. However, although every patient will benefit from some form of surveillance, many do not need an ultrasound. Useful biochemical indicators of follicular development are available, and can be used either alone or in combination with ultrasonography. These are serum estradiol, serum progesterone and either urine or serum LH. Their role in current protocols of OI will be described later in this section.

Sonographic technique and instrumentation

Transvaginal sonography (TVS) makes OI with gonadotropins possible. It is also often useful in other protocols of OI. Use of this technique in the evaluation of ovarian follicles was first proposed as a complement to transabdominal sonography (TAS) for the minority of cases where anatomic constraints required an alternative port of access to the pelvis.[24] However, with the development of 7.5 MHz transducers, which allow superior realtime anatomic definition, it soon became clear that TVS is the technique of choice to assess follicular growth and uterine/salpingeal anatomy, including early pregnancy.[25] Currently TAS is considered complementary to TVS, and mostly useful in the evaluation of grossly abnormal pelvic anatomy, such as an enlarged uterus with multiple leiomyomata or a large ovarian or paraovarian cyst.[26] Transabdominal scanning, which employs lower-frequency transducers with higher tissue penetration, is also a practical way to visualize pelvic structures located more than 6–8 cm from the vaginal vault.

TVS has both a higher patient acceptance and the logistic advantage of not requiring a full urinary bladder. As in any endocavitary sonographic technique, antisepsis is of paramount importance. The portion of the transducer that comes in contact with the patient needs to be sterilized by prolonged immersion in a concentrated antiseptic solution. If frequent use of the transducer is expected, two transducers should be available so that one can be sterilized while the other is in use.

The practice of covering the vaginal transducer with condoms should be avoided for several reasons. There is evidence that current techniques employing condoms do not prevent transducer contamination.[27] Moreover, latex condom use may trigger allergic reactions or induce de novo allergy to latex. Finally, a case can be made that condoms are devices so deeply associated with sexual intercourse in the public imagination that their use on a vaginal probe may make some women uncomfortable. Currently, sterile non-latex transducer cover sheets are available, although they tend to be somewhat expensive. As an alternative, we employ non-sterile clear plastic bags, secured to the transducer shaft with a rubber band. A small amount of non-sterile transducer gel is placed inside the tip of the transducer cover. Gel should not be applied to the outside of the cover as it may interfere with sperm function if intercourse is timed to occur shortly after the exam. If vaginal secretions are not adequate for comfortable placement and proper transducer contact, the cover can be wet with tap water.

Once the transducer probe is in place, its contact surface in the mid-line will be the uterine cervix and the anterior or posterior vaginal fornix (depending on whether the uterus is in anteversion or retroversion, respectively). Orientation in TVS may be challenging at first, especially if the operator is used to the planes and orientation of TAS. By convention the sector field produced by TVS, usually encompassing 90° with a 10 cm depth, is imaged on the screen with the top of the sector at the top of the monitor, like TAS. This often confuses novice users.

The classic anatomical planes employed to identify images obtained with TAS, such as the sagittal, coronal and transverse planes, are inadequate to describe TVS images. The concepts of transpelvic plane and anteroposterior pelvic plane have been proposed to define imaging obtained with a sound beam directed respectively from side to side in the pelvis or anteriorly and posteriorly.[28] Currently, however, most sonographers employ targeted organ scanning, a technique that focuses on each specific organ as the main target, rather than describing the organs within anatomical planes. The exam describes longitudinal and transverse views of the pelvic organs, which resolves the issues of correct orientation and greatly simplifies the procedure.[29] For example, for a uterus in acute retroversion and with fundal deviation to the left, imaging obtained across true anatomic planes would be difficult to interpret. Targeted organ scanning should provide a written comment on the uterine retroversion and lateral displacement, and clear images obtained across uterine longitudinal and transverse planes.

The baseline scan

The baseline ultrasound examination during the early follicular phase in cycles of OI provides the clinician with fundamental information. This examination should be a complete survey of pelvic anatomy.

The uterus should be carefully evaluated in both axes for the presence of anomalies of the cervix and the corpus. In particular, size and number of all intramural and submucosal leiomyomata (*Fig. 13.1*), as well as any suspected endometrial polyps, should be described. During the early proliferative phase, the thin endometrium may limit adequate visualization of any abnormality within or immediately adjacent to the uterine cavity. For this reason, the endometrial cavity should be thoroughly re-evaluated at every subsequent examination during OI cycles. Intracavitary polyps and myomata may be

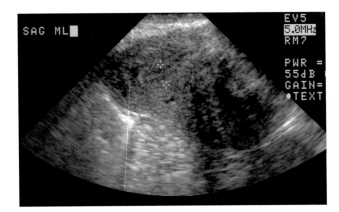

Figure 13.1 Longitudinal view of the uterus showing a large transmural myoma. These lesions usually appear as hypo- or isoechoic round structures. The extent of their relationship with the endometrium is clinically relevant but often difficult to assess at baseline ultrasound, because the early proliferative phase endometrium is isoechoic to the surrounding myometrium.

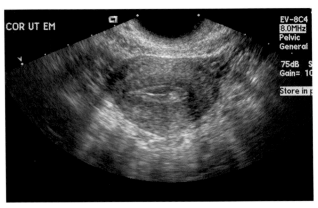

Figure 13.2 Endometrial polyp highlighted by surrounding endometrium during the late proliferative phase of the cycle. These lesions are typically hyperechoic and the differential diagnosis of an intracavitary blood clot must be considered, especially during the early proliferative phase. Small polyps such as this one are typically not detectable at baseline ultrasound.

more visible later in the cycle, when the menstrual effluvium is complete and newly formed endometrium functionalis lends itself as natural contrast (*Fig. 13.2*).

Version and flexion of the uterus should be noted as this knowledge may be useful in cases of difficult intrauterine insemination (*Fig. 13.3*). Most patients undergoing OI should be preliminarily evaluated for the presence of congenital anatomic abnormalities with techniques such as hysterosalpingography or combined laparoscopy hysteroscopy. Nevertheless TVS may sometimes provide the first indication of otherwise unsuspected Müllerian anomalies (*Fig. 13.4*).

Transvaginal sonography is a sensitive and reliable method for the detection of free peritoneal fluid in the female pelvis, as demonstrated by correlation with laparoscopic findings.[30] It is estimated that TVS can detect as little as 0.8 ml of free fluid. A small amount of free fluid is a normal finding in most women at any time during the menstrual cycle, and is most commonly demonstrated in the posterior cul-de-sac. An increase in pelvic free fluid may be suggestive of ovulation when found in association with more specific signs (see below). However, free fluid is not usually indicative of oocyte release. In fact, it is commonly observed during the late luteal phase of ovulatory women.[31] Free fluid should be

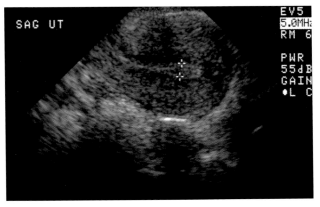

Figure 13.3 Retroverted uterus, longitudinal view. Knowledge of uterine version, of any unusual flexion between cervix and corpus, and of lateral displacement can be of assistance during OI cycles, if intrauterine insemination is planned.

routinely noted during TVS and grossly quantified (small, moderate, large amount) (*Fig. 13.5*). Knowledge of baseline amounts of free fluid may assist in the evaluation of early stages of ovarian hyperstimulation syndrome.

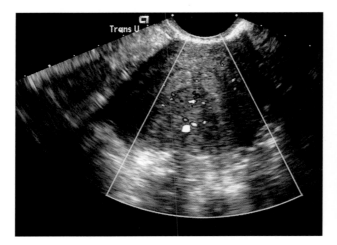

Figure 13.4 Transverse view of the upper uterine corpus during the secretory phase showing a septate versus bicornuate uterus. Two distinct round hypoechoic endometrial cavities can be identified. At baseline the diagnosis is also possible, though more challenging. Ultrasonographic diagnosis is never definitive, and clinical correlation with additional radiological or endoscopic findings is needed.

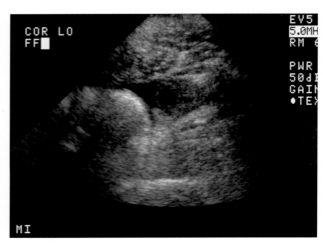

Figure 13.5 Small amount of free fluid in the adnexal region at baseline ultrasound. Peritoneal fluid is hypoechoic and highlights the contour of the surrounding pelvic structures. True quantitative assessment is impossible.

Tubal anatomy cannot be assessed by routine TVS except with sonohysterography. Identification of the tubal lumen suggests pathology almost without exception. A hypoechoic tubular structure in the adnexal region is likely due to distal tubal obstruction or frank hydrosalpinx (*Fig. 13.6*).[32] One can hardly overstate the clinical relevance of such a finding at the outset of an OI cycle. Finally, although rare, an unsuspected early tubal pregnancy may be detected at the time of baseline pelvic scan (*Fig. 13.7*).

TVS of the ovary in the early follicular phase should report the ovarian dimensions in three perpendicular planes. Ovarian volume calculated from these

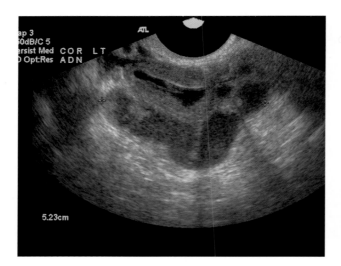

Figure 13.6 Adnexal structure with tubular shape and hypoechoic content – a picture highly suggestive of a hydrosalpinx.

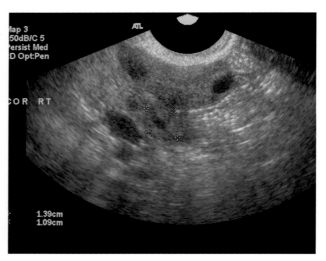

Figure 13.7 Ectopic pregnancy at 5.2 weeks' gestational age. This patient had experienced menstrual flow following a cycle of OI, and a ring-shaped adnexal structure with hypoechoic center was identified at the following baseline ultrasound. The structure was clearly separate from the ovary and was subsequently diagnosed as a tubal pregnancy.

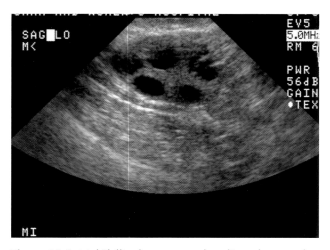

Figure 13.8 Multifollicular ovary at baseline ultrasound. This pattern is usually associated with a somewhat delayed but exuberant response to gonadotropins.

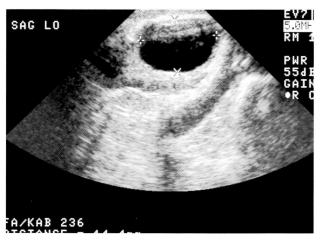

Figure 13.9 Simple ovarian cyst at baseline. Differentiation between a simple (homogeneously hypoechoic) and complex cyst is very important as the therapeutic implications are quite different.

dimensions has been proposed as a predictor of ovarian sensitivity to gonadotropins.[33,34] The normal ovary between cycle day 1 and 4 is in the recruitment phase and rare antral follicles may be seen. The lower limit of resolution of TVS for such early follicles is about 2 mm. A typical multifollicular pattern of the ovarian cortex (string of pearls) is noted in

many patients with chronic anovulation and in up to 10% of normally ovulatory women. This pattern is not consistently associated with polycystic ovarian syndrome but should be reported nonetheless, as it can predict an abnormal response to OI with gonadotropins (*Fig. 13.8*).[35–37] Even more important is the recognition of larger functional cysts (most often representing persistent unruptured follicles or cystic corpora lutea), which should be measured in three dimensions (*Fig. 13.9*). The presence of baseline ovarian cysts above 10 mm in average diameter is associated with decreased pregnancy rates in OI cycles employing gonadotropins.[38] It should also be noted that, provided no cysts above 10 mm are present on baseline scan, consecutive gonadotropin cycles can be safely offered without impairment of cycle fecundity.[39,40] Because of this, special effort should be made to correctly identify paraovarian and paratubal cysts, which can mimic simple ovarian cysts at TVS (*Fig. 13.10*). Non-simple cysts and other intraparenchymal echogenic lesions must also be measured in three dimensions. They often represent corpora lutea or albicantia, which have no impact on treatment. However, endometriomata and, more rarely, ovarian neoplasias, can also appear as non-simple cysts (*Fig. 13.11*).

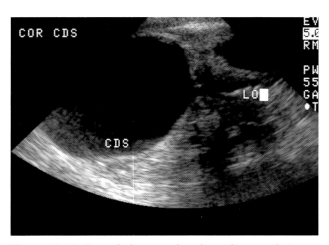

Figure 13.10 Paratubal cyst at baseline ultrasound. A two-hand scanning technique, with the nondominant hand palpating in a manner similar to that of the classic bimanual pelvic examination, may help better to define separate but adjacent pelvic structures.

Often the evaluation of the adnexa by TVS cannot be completed with a one-hand technique. Instead, the non-dominant hand of the ultrasonographer should be used as an abdominal support to help mobilize and better define pelvic structures, as well as to acquire information on focal tenderness. Most

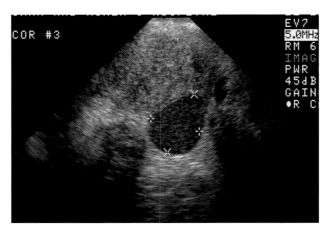

Figure 13.11 Complex ovarian cyst at baseline ultrasound. This particular cyst has a classic broken glass appearance highly suggestive of endometrioma.

of the newer ultrasound units provide a pedal remote for freeze-frame and image capture/storage, which has been designed exactly for this purpose. Such two-hand TVS techique is truly an extension of the pelvic exam for the information age. A corollary of this consideration should be that, given the current medical legal climate, a chaperon is never optional.

In conclusion, the baseline scan for cycles of OI should follow a standard protocol to provide all of the above information in a consistent way. Knowledge of the ultimate goal of the ovarian stimulation protocol (i.e. OI versus superovulation) should not change the quality of the baseline exam.

Follicular monitoring in OI cycles with intact pituitary–ovarian feedback

Certain OI protocols restore spontaneous follicular maturation and ovulation by addressing specific hormonal defects. Examples of these are the above-mentioned regimens with metformin and GnRH, but also dopamine agonists, such as bromocriptine (Parlodel) and cabergoline (Dostinex), used in anovulatory women with hyperprolactinemia.

These treatment cycles are characterized by a restoration of normal feedback mechanisms between the ovary and the hypothalamus-pituitary complex, which allows normal follicular selection and dominance to occur. Metformin and bromocriptine are given at fixed doses on a long-term basis, and the risk of ovarian hyperstimulation syndrome and

high-order multiple gestations is not different from that of spontaneous ovulatory cycles. Therefore, the role of follicular monitoring in these cases is limited to synchronizing ovulation with insemination/intercourse, and later to confirm that ovulation did actually occur. Biochemical indicators, such as urine LH self-determination by home kits, represent the first line of monitoring in these cases. The LH surge can usually be detected biochemically 16–28 hours before ovulation is shown by ultrasonography.[41] Approximately 10% of women demonstrate ultrasonographic evidence of ovulation before a urine LH surge is detected. This is due to differences in timing and duration of individual LH surges. In patients in whom the urine LH surge is not detected, despite successful OI, follicular monitoring by ultrasound is indicated.[42]

Patients receiving GnRH are monitored with ultrasound, owing to the variable individual response with respect to timing of follicular selection and dominance. Exogenous GnRH pulse frequency and amplitude can be adjusted during the OI cycle, although this is not usually necessary until after ovulation. Following baseline evaluation on cycle days 2–3, resumption of monitoring by TVS is usually begun by day 10. By that time, follicular selection (occurring between cycle days 5 and 7) is already complete, and one or two follicles have taken the lead. This period of follicular dominance usually lasts seven days, with a linear rate of follicular growth of 2–3 mm/day, and ends with a short phase of exponential growth and, finally, ovulation.

Daily ultrasound monitoring is recommended when GnRH is used. Follicles should be measured in two dimensions through a plane which provides a combination of the sharpest image and largest diameters (*Fig. 13.12*). The reporting of follicular dimensions in terms of maximum diameter, average diameter or volume is strictly a matter of preference of the infertility specialist treating the patient. Single maximum diameters are acceptable provided that dominant follicles are spherical: this is usually the case in mono or biovulatory cycles. When spherical or ellipsoid follicles are noted, their volume can be approximated by the simple formula $(\pi/6)*A*B*C$, where A, B, and C represent the diameters of the follicle in three axes.

Maximum diameters and total follicular volume are good predictors of serum estradiol levels in spontaneous as well as OI cycles.[43,44] Serum estradiol level determinations assist the clinician in determining the appropriate day for hCG administration to obtain ovulation with the minimum risk of ovarian hyperstimulation syndrome and high-order multiple pregnancies. During OI with metformin, dopamine

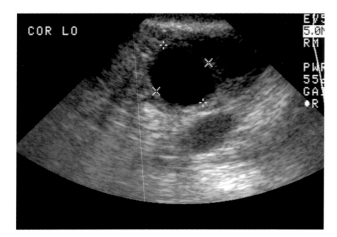

Figure 13.12 Single dominant preovulatory follicle in a previously anovulatory patient on long-term metformin treatment.

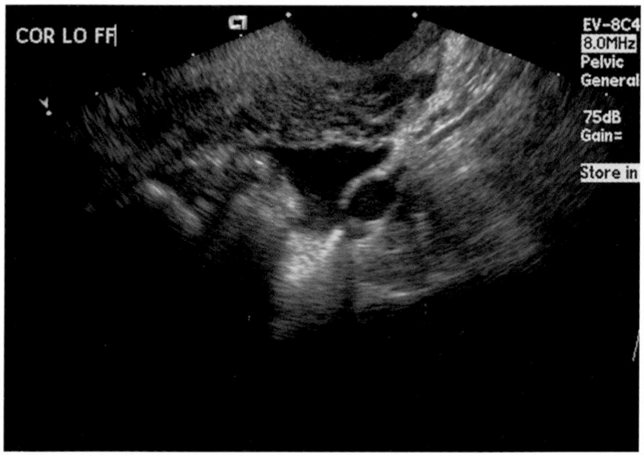

Figure 13.13 Free fluid in the periadnexal region may be a sign of recent ovulation: clearly this must be seen in the context of prior ultrasound examinations and the presence or absence of other signs of ovulation.

agonists or GnRH, the chance of either of the above happening is absolutely negligible, therefore serum estradiol determinations are not necessary. However, confident prediction of imminent ovulation by TVS alone is impossible. Modifications of the cumulus oophorus or other mural changes in the preovulatory follicle are not clinically relevant and need not be reported.[45] Rather, the combination of urine LH determinations and mean follicular diameter measured by TVS has an extremely high positive predictive value for ovulation and currently represents the preferred approach to cases where urine LH alone is insufficient.[46]

The preovulatory mean diameter in spontaneous cycles ranges between 14 and 28 mm (with an average of 20–24 mm). This is important to remember when timing insemination/intercourse in the absence of a detectable urine or serum LH surge, because conception has not been observed in spontaneous cycles when the maximum mean diameter was below 17 mm.[47]

Many physicians request daily follicular monitoring until signs of ovulation are detected to confirm that insemination/intercourse was adequately timed. This is done not only for patient reassurance, but also to rule out the occurrence of a luteinized unruptured follicle. This ovulatory abnormality is impossible to demonstrate without an ultrasound examination, because a timely LH surge, progesterone elevation and secretory transformation of the endometrium are observed with luteinized unruptured follicle.[48] The criteria for ultrasonographic diagnosis of ovulation are generally reliable, but false positives and false negatives are well known to occur.[49] Intrafollicular

echoes are sometimes observed in normal mature preovulatory follicles. After ovulation occurs, the dominant follicle may just disappear, or, more often, display a modest decrease in volume with irregularity of the follicular wall and echogenic foci due to hemorrhage. A sudden increase in the volume of free fluid in the pelvis is also seen in association with ovulation in some cases, although this sign is by no means specific (*Fig. 13.13*). Filling-in of the dehiscent follicle and increased echogenicity of its wall are signs of early luteinization (*Fig. 13.14*). The ultrasonographic diagnosis of ovulation is often difficult

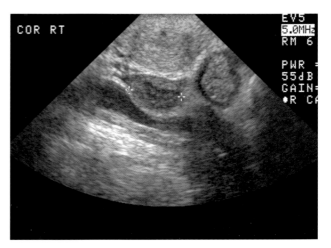

Figure 13.14 Complex ovarian cyst with features suggestive of a mature corpus luteum: echogenicity and thickness of the luteinized follicular wall and of the intracystic contents.

and frankly impossible if examinations are not done on a daily basis. Instead, correlation of clinical data with subtle morphologic modifications appreciated through frequent TVS sessions will allow the best estimate of ovulation timing.

Follicular monitoring in OI cycles induced with clomiphene

Clomiphene citrate overrides the natural process of follicular selection and dominance by interfering with the negative feedback of ovarian estradiol on the hypothalamus. Follicular stimulation is still the result of endogenous FSH, and response to medication is extremely variable. It is possible to achieve true superovulation with clomiphene, depending on the dose employed and the individual sensitivity to the drug. Secretion of LH is not usually affected by clomiphene, therefore an ovulatory trigger with hCG is not absolutely necessary.

Classically, synchronous selection of multiple co-dominant follicles is observed in cycles with clomiphene. Individual follicular growth rate thereafter is often inconsistent. It is not uncommon to observe unexpected shifts in leading follicles from one day to the next. The rate of follicular growth is overall accelerated compared to spontaneous ovulatory cycles and to OI cycles with intact pituitary–ovarian feedback. Despite this, clomiphene cycles are on average one day longer than spontaneous or OI cycles.[50] Therefore, follicular monitoring during clomiphene-stimulated cycles is safely begun on cycle day 12 rather than 10.

Follicular dimensions in clomiphene-stimulated cycles are always greater than those of natural, GnRH-stimulated, and even gonadotropin-stimulated cycles. Correlation analysis of several biophysical and biochemical variables with the day of serum LH surge demonstrates that the best predictor of oocyte maturation in clomiphene cycles is the diameter of the largest follicle (range 22–31 mm) (*Fig. 13.15*). Serum estradiol (either absolute value or normalized for the number of follicles with a diameter above 10 mm) does not improve prediction of the timing of ovulation.[50] Because estradiol levels do not assist in predicting ovulation, and in consideration of the fact that ovarian hyperstimulation syndrome and high-order multiple pregnancies are exceedingly rare following OI with clomiphene, this biochemical marker is not useful in this setting.

Controversy remains as to whether it is advantageous to induce ovulation by administration of hCG in clomiphene-stimulated cycles. A prospective, randomized, cross-over study reported a comparable

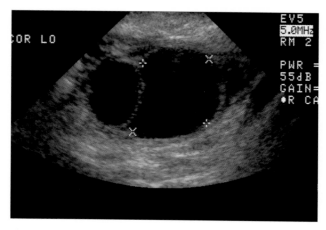

Figure 13.15 Preovulatory follicle during OI with clomiphene citrate. Diameters are typically larger than those observed in spontaneous or gonadotropin-induced cycles.

pregnancy rate in cycles where TVS was used to time hCG administration and inseminations, and cycles where inseminations were performed after urine LH detection.[51] Despite its low statistical power, this study suggests that in cycles where clomiphene is used for OI or superovulation, use of TVS as a first-line monitoring approach may not provide a significant advantage.

Follicular monitoring in OI cycles induced with gonadotropins

Owing to the significant risk of severe complications, OI and superovulation with gonadotropins require intense biochemical and biophysical monitoring with parallel determinations of serum estradiol and follicular size by TVS.

The goal is to achieve an acceptably high pregnancy rate while maintaining an acceptably low risk of severe ovarian hyperstimulation syndrome and high-order multiple pregnancies. Depending on what one defines as acceptable, this goal may or may not ever be achievable. A retrospective analysis of 3347 cycles of gonadotropin OI and superovulation in association with intrauterine insemination identified three independent risk factors for high-order multiple pregnancies:

- large number of follicles;
- elevated peak serum estradiol concentrations;
- young patient age.[52]

The authors provide an ordinal logistic-regression model of increasing incidence of high-order multiple pregnancies according to these three parameters. Threshold values for an increased risk of high-order multiple pregnancies are a peak estradiol concentration of 1385 pg/ml or higher and the presence of seven or more follicles. The risk increases further with increasing estradiol concentrations, total follicle number and younger age, where each is an independent predictor. One of the most striking findings of this study is the fact that the number of follicles with a maximum diameter of 16 mm or more is not a predictor of high-order multiple pregnancies. This means that unless a precise assessment of the total number of follicles (regardless of size) is provided, ultrasound may not be a valuable tool in reducing the risk of high-order multiple pregnancies. The authors conclude that the current criteria guiding OI and superovulation with gonadotropins may not be improved without negatively affecting pregnancy rates.

As for ovarian hyperstimulation syndrome, its incidence increases with increasing numbers of small and intermediate follicles.[53,54] Most centers would not proceed with hCG administration if the total number of follicles exceeds ten. A more aggressive approach is made possible by the knowledge of the serum estradiol level. A 5% risk of severe ovarian hyperstimulation syndrome is reported in anovulatory women and in women with hypothalamic amenorrhea with serum estradiol values of 3800 pg/ml and 2400 pg/ml, respectively.[55] These values are well above the safe threshold for high-order multiple pregnancies and should never be reached unless the cycle is converted to in vitro fertilization.

Parallel biochemical and biophysical follicular monitoring is not only important to avoid complications in cycles with an exuberant response, but also to assess optimal timing of hCG administration.[56] Superovulation with gonadotropins does not inhibit the endogenous LH surge at mid-cycle, which is always present, although blunted.[57] Analyses of OI cycles employing gonadotropins indicate that both serum estradiol and maximum follicular diameter should be used to predict the spontaneous LH surge.[50] Monitoring of serum progesterone may also be of some value in anticipating an LH surge (which will impair timing of insemination).[58] However, in most cases, this additional test is not needed. The overall duration of OI cycles is shorter and the maximum follicular diameter (15–18 mm) is smaller than that seen with spontaneous cycles and clomiphene-stimulated cycles.[41] Follicular monitoring is therefore started, at the latest, by cycle day 8 (which usually corresponds to day 6 of medication) and is continued at daily intervals unless estradiol values and follicular number and sizes are low. Owing to the variable rate of follicular growth and estradiol secretion, it is recommended that daily monitoring is systematically adopted until the physician becomes very familiar with the expected patient response to various doses of different gonadotropins.

Three patterns of folliculogenesis can be observed in response to exogenous gonadotropins. One should become familiar with all, understanding, however, that the great majority of patients fit somewhere in between. In women with hypogonadotropic hypogonadism [World Health Organization (WHO) group I] a prompt response to the drug is observed. Usually, a small number of follicles are recruited from the otherwise inactive gonads and they enlarge uniformly during the preovulatory stage. The growth rate is linear and correlates well with serum estradiol levels. Owing to such predictable growth, the risks of ovarian hyperstimulation syndrome and high-order multiple pregnancies are low in this group of patients. In contrast, the ovaries of normogonadotropic chronic anovulatory women (WHO group II) already harbor follicles at several stages of development, all invariably destined to atresia in a hyperandrogenic microenvironment. Gonadotropin administration initially reduces the rate of follicular atresia, thereby leading to accumulation of multiple small antral follicles. These follicles do not possess high numbers of FSH receptors owing to local androgen inhibition and, therefore, a surprisingly low and often stationary estradiol level is seen over several days. Eventually, and quite abruptly, exogenous FSH induces its own receptors in this non-homogeneous follicular cohort and an exponential rate of follicular growth and rise of estradiol levels begin (*Figs. 13.16 and 13.17*). This cascade of events should be anticipated rather than controlled, but often neither option is possible and the cycle must be canceled due to the high risk of ovarian hyperstimulation syndrome and/or high-order multiple pregnancies. Finally, patients with hypergonadotropic hypogonadism (WHO group III) display a weak or absent response to high doses of gonadotropins. Both the clinical and the ultrasonographic pictures (lack of multiple antral follicles) reassure the physician that the likelihood of unpredictable accelerations of follicular growth and development of ovarian hyperstimulation syndrome/ high-order multiple pregnancies is quite low.

Physicians treating patients with gonadotropins are often faced with difficult decisions as to whether to allow hCG administration and risk uncontrolled

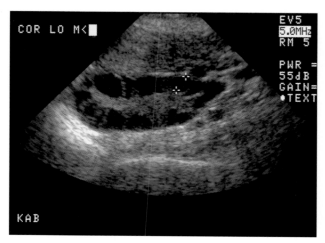

Figure 13.16 Typical follicular pattern in a woman with normogonadotropic chronic anovulation undergoing ovulation induction with low-dose gonadotropins. Note the crowded appearance of the ovary, with multiple follicles below 10–12 mm in maximum diameter. This pattern calls for a swift reassessment of the ovulation induction strategy in order to salvage the cycle.

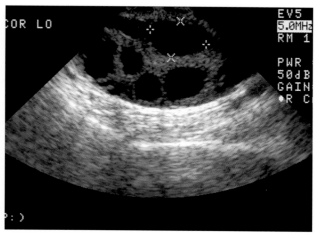

Figure 13.17 The same patient as in Figure 13.16, 48 hours later. An abrupt increase in size of multiple follicles has resulted in an undesired superovulation pattern. Owing to the unacceptably elevated risk of high order multiple gestation, the only options at this point are cycle cancellation or conversion to in vitro fertilization.

multiple ovulation and the related consequences, or to cancel the cycle at the last minute.[52] When faced with a non-homogeneous cohort of follicles on the day of potential hCG administration, knowledge of how many of these are likely to ovulate may be of assistance in borderline situations. In a prospective observational study of OI employing clomiphene/gonadotropins, the authors performed individual TVS follow-up of individual follicles in multifollicular cycles (mean follicle number per ovary 3.5). All follicles with maximum diameter over 10 mm were measured 12 hours before and 35 and 45 hours after hCG. The authors arbitrarily defined ovulation as a decrease in follicular diameter of at least 3 mm. They reported an overall incidence of luteinized unruptured follicles of over 50%. Only 20% of cycles showed complete luteinized unruptured follicles, whereas 70% of cycles had partial luteinized unruptured follicles, and 10% had no luteinized unruptured follicles. More than 80% of follicles ruptured between 35 and 45 hours after hCG. As expected, the chance of a follicle rupturing after hCG was noted to be proportional to its size (*Fig. 13.18*). The authors also performed a TVS on day 7 after hCG, which showed that functional cysts and cystic corpora lutea derive from both ruptured and unruptured follicles. Therefore, based on a luteal phase ultrasound only, one cannot assume anything about the incidence of luteinized unruptured follicle in a given cycle.[59]

Endometrial monitoring during ovulation induction

Endometrial thickness is the distance between the anterior and posterior endometrial–myometrial junctions at the point of maximum thickness. This is occasionally called double endometrial thickness. This highly reproducible measurement represents two apposing layers of endometrium and has been validated with a classic anatomical study (*Fig. 13.19*).[60,61]

The importance of endometrial evaluation during OI cycles cannot be overstated. As mentioned above, some significant intracavitary lesions, such as polyps, may only be evident during the mid-to-late proliferative phase. Moreover, there have been a number of studies to suggest that the overall thickness of the endometrium at mid-cycle can predict implantation potential. The chance of implantation is greatest with endometrial thickness above 9–10 mm regardless of the OI protocol used.[62,63] Clomiphene citrate has a well demonstrated inhibitory effect on endometrial growth,[64] and no pregnancies have been observed in clomiphene or gonadotropin OI when the endometrial thickness is less than 6 mm.[65]

Besides its thickness, the structural pattern of the endometrium has also been evaluated as a predictor of OI cycle success. TVS can consistently allow an

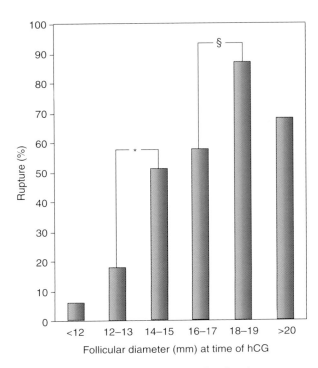

Figure 13.18 Correlation between follicular diameter measured 12 hours before hCG administration and probability of follicular rupture (defined as a decrease in mean follicular diameter of ≥ 3 mm) by 45 hours after hCG administration. * and § indicate statistically significant differences. *Source:* Redrawn from reference 59.

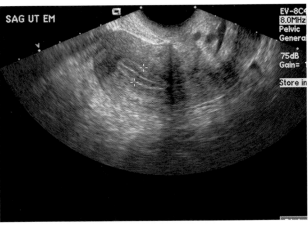

Figure 13.19 Conventionally, measurement of the endometrial stripe's thickness is performed by placing the calipers at the outer margin of the echogenic rim indicating the interface between endometrium basalis and myometrium. This measurement is always done at the point of maximum thickness in the longitudinal view. If intracavitary fluid is noted, then the two apposing endometrial surfaces are measured separately and their values added.

impressive level of endometrial detail: a multilayered appearance (trilaminar endometrium) is noted at mid-cycle in most women (*Fig. 13.20*). This multilayered pattern is associated with a higher pregnancy rate when compared to women who do not display this pattern (*Fig. 13.21*).[66,67]

Monitoring of complications of ovulation induction

Strategies should be systematically applied to avoid the occurrence of ovarian hyperstimulation syndrome in women undergoing OI with gonadotropins, including careful choice of the initial dose of medication and aggressive monitoring of serum estradiol levels and TVS for follicular growth. Nonetheless, cases of ovarian hyperstimulation syndrome will occur in every infertility practice. Ultrasonagraphy is used to establish the diagnosis in a prompt and relatively non-invasive fashion. It also has a role in the follow-up of these patients, in whom symptomatic ovarian enlargement can persist for up to six weeks after hCG injection.

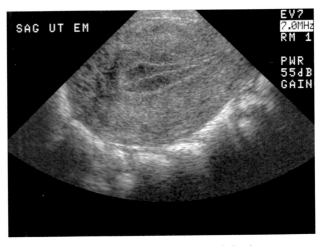

Figure 13.20 Trilaminar endometrium of the late proliferative phase; note the hypoechoic area of the inner endometrium, likely due to periovulatory edema of the compactum layer.

When ovarian hyperstimulation syndrome is suspected by history and physical examination, a gynecologic ultrasound is performed to assist in determining the degree of severity of the

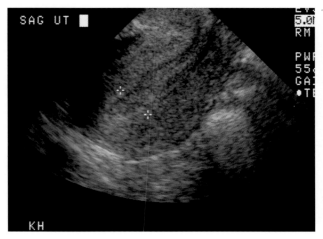

Figure 13.21 Homogeneously echogenic endometrium during the proliferative phase of an OI cycle. This finding should always be documented owing to its potential prognostic implications.

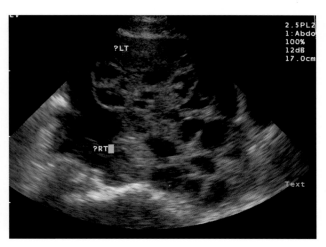

Figure 13.22 Severe ovarian hyperstimulation syndrome. TAS showing enlarged ovaries with massive stromal edema and hypoechoic areas (hemorrhagic and atretic follicles).

syndrome. An examination done in this setting often demonstrates enlarged cystic ovaries that are at risk for rupture, bleeding, and torsion. A bimanual examination is discouraged, as is a TVS with the two-hand technique. Instead, TAS is performed, because it has a low potential of causing trauma to the ovaries, provides a better assessment of extreme ovarian enlargement, and can quantify the amount of ascites (*Figs. 13.22 and 13.23*).

The ovarian hyperstimulation syndrome survey should provide a detailed description of the ovaries including size and structure. Typically the ovary is edematous and contains multiple immature follicles and some larger hypoechoic cysts (measurements of all cysts are not clinically helpful here). Ovarian enlargement is almost always bilateral and can be massive, sometimes over 10 cm in maximal dimension. Detailed documentation is useful if the same patient should present shortly thereafter with symptoms suggestive of adnexal torsion or cyst rupture. Gentle TVS can be performed if the adnexa are difficult to identify through TAS, or if early obstetrical ultrasound is part of the examination, as is often the case with late-onset ovarian hyperstimulation syndrome. If paracentesis is needed, this is more safely performed with TAS guidance, to avoid unintentional injury to the enlarged ovaries.

Finally, an evaluation of the lower pleural spaces to rule out the presence of effusion should be performed routinely on patients with suspected ovarian hyperstimulation syndrome (*Fig. 13.24*).

Adnexal torsion can occur with or without the presence of ovarian hyperstimulation syndrome. It is a rare event and in many cases appears to be incomplete and self-limited. Catastrophic torsion requiring immediate surgical intervention and possible oophorectomy is rare, even in programs that employ aggressive superovulation protocols. Unless peritoneal signs or other clinical indications of immediate danger to the patient are present, the surgeon usually relies on TVS imaging to decide whether exploration is needed. Unfortunately there is no pathognomonic ultrasonographic finding associated with adnexal torsion. Torsion causes venous compromise, and arterial flow is rarely altered enough to allow diagnosis of torsion with Doppler. Moreover, vascular supply to the ovary is provided not only by the ovarian artery and vein, but also by the utero-ovarian vessels. Because of this, color Doppler flow assessment will rarely detect significantly impaired arterial flow, therefore the test lacks sufficient sensitivity to be clinically helpful. The most useful radiologic study in the workup of a possible adnexal torsion is a classic gray-scale. Findings of marked ovarian enlargement, an edematous fallopian tube, and periadnexal free fluid should raise the suspicion of torsion (*Fig. 13.25*).

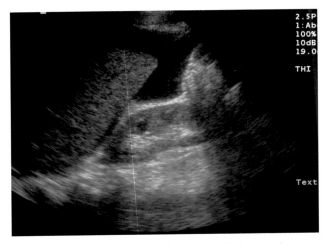

Figure 13.23 Severe ovarian hyperstimulation syndrome. TAS showing large ascites highlighting the contour of the upper abdominal organs.

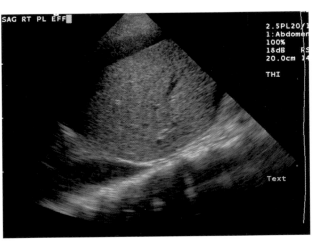

Figure 13.24 Severe ovarian hyperstimulation syndrome. TAS showing a large pleural effusion (seen posteriorly to the right hepatic lobe).

Pregnancy-related complications of OI and superovulation such as ectopic pregnancy, are discussed in detail in other chapters of this book.

Conclusions

Ovulation induction and superovulation remain fundamental tools in modern infertility treatment. The role of ultrasonography is to make ovulation induction effective and safe. Given the availability of alternative non-invasive markers of impending ovulation, ultrasonography is not recommended in all ovulation induction protocols. However, ovulation induction and superovulation with gonadotropins mandate ultrasound monitoring. Transvaginal sonography is undoubtedly the modality of choice; transabdominal sonography is a complementary technique that may be useful in select cases. Doppler flow analysis and tridimensional ultrasound have not yet entered general infertility practice and were therefore not discussed here. The importance of a formal baseline ultrasound during OI cycles cannot be overestimated. Indeed, because of today's preoccupation with cost-containment the baseline scan may represent the first pelvic ultrasound ever for some patients. A two-hand technique, using the abdominal hand to increase discrimination between adnexal structures, is often helpful. A polycystic or multifollicular pattern of the

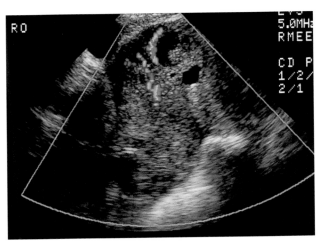

Figure 13.25 TVS with color Doppler of an ovary subsequently shown by laparoscopy to have undergone a complete torsion around the utero-ovarian ligament. Normal flow is demonstrated through the infundibulo-pelvic vessels. Ovarian edema and a moderate amount of free fluid are noted, suggesting the possibility of torsion (especially in a case such as this, where there was no evidence of ovarian hyperstimulation syndrome).

ovarian cortex may have clinical implications in predicting the type of response to OI and should be recognized. During OI, follicular number and size must be documented carefully because the number of ovarian follicles is a predictor of high-order multiple pregnancies. Likewise, endometrial structure and thickness have important prognostic implications for successful pregnancy and should be accurately described. Finally, ultrasonography can assist in the prevention, recognition and management of complications of ovulation induction, such as ovarian hyperstimulation syndrome and adnexal torsion.

References

1. Hammond MG, Halme JK, Talbert LM. Factors affecting the pregnancy rate in clomiphene citrate induction of ovulation. *Obstet Gynecol* 1983; **62**:196–202.

2. Hull MG, Savage PE, Jacobs HS. Investigation and treatment of amenorrhoea resulting in normal fertility. *Br Med J* 1979; **1**:1257–61.

3. Coelingh Bennink HJ, Fauser BC, Out HJ. Recombinant follicle-stimulating hormone (FSH; Puregon) is more efficient than urinary FSH (Metrodin) in women with clomiphene citrate-resistant, normogonadotropic, chronic anovulation: a prospective, multicenter, assessor-blind, randomized, clinical trial. European Puregon Collaborative Anovulation Study Group. *Fertil Steril* 1998; **69**:19–25.

4. Deaton JL, Gibson M, Blackmer KM, Nakajima ST, Badger GJ, Brumsted JR. A randomized, controlled trial of clomiphene citrate and intrauterine insemination in couples with unexplained infertility or surgically corrected endometriosis. *Fertil Steril* 1990; **54**:1083–8.

5. Chung CC, Fleming R, Jamieson ME, Yates RW, Coutts JR. Randomized comparison of ovulation induction with and without intrauterine insemination in the treatment of unexplained infertility. *Hum Reprod* 1995; **10**:3139–41.

6. Tummon IS, Asher LJ, Martin JS, Tulandi T. Randomized controlled trial of superovulation and insemination for infertility associated with minimal or mild endometriosis [see comments]. *Fertil Steril* 1997; **68**:8–12.

7. Zeyneloglu HB, Arici A, Olive DL, Duleba AJ. Comparison of intrauterine insemination with timed intercourse in superovulated cycles with gonadotropins: a meta-analysis. *Fertil Steril* 1998; **69**:486–91.

8. Guzick DS, Carson SA, Coutifaris C, *et al.* Efficacy of superovulation and intrauterine insemination in the treatment of infertility. National Cooperative Reproductive Medicine Network [see comments]. *N Engl J Med* 1999; **340**:177–83.

9. Dickey RP, Holtkamp DE. Development, pharmacology and clinical experience with clomiphene citrate. *Hum Reprod Update* 1996; **2**:483–506.

10. Rossing MA, Daling JR, Weiss NS, Moore DE, Self SG. Ovarian tumors in a cohort of infertile women [see comments]. *N Engl J Med* 1994; **331**:771–6.

11. Birkenfeld A, Beier HM, Schenker JG. The effect of clomiphene citrate on early embryonic development, endometrium and implantation. *Hum Reprod* 1986; **1**:387–95.

12. Velazquez EM, Mendoza S, Hamer T, Sosa F, Glueck CJ. Metformin therapy in polycystic ovary syndrome reduces hyperinsulinemia, insulin resistance, hyperandrogenemia, and systolic blood pressure, while facilitating normal menses and pregnancy. *Metab Clin Exper* 1994; **43**:647–54.

13. Nestler JE, Jakubowicz DJ, Evans WS, Pasquali R. Effects of metformin on spontaneous and clomiphene-induced ovulation in the polycystic ovary syndrome. *N Engl J Med* 1998; **338**:1876–80.

14. De Leo V, la Marca A, Ditto A, Morgante G, Cianci A. Effects of metformin on gonadotropin-induced ovulation in women with polycystic ovary syndrome. *Fertil Steril* 1999; **72**:282–5.

15. Donini P, Puzzuoli D, D'Alessio I, Lunenfeld B, Eshkol A, Parlow AF. Purification and separation of follicle stimulating hormone (FSH) and luteinizing hormone (LH) from human postmenopausal gonadotrophin (HMG). II. Preparation of biological apparently pure FSH by selective binding of the LH with an anti-HGG serum and subsequent chromatography. *Acta Endocrinol* 1966; **52**:186–98.

16. Donini P, Puzzuoli D, D'Alessio I, Lunenfeld B, Eshkol A, Parlow AF. Purification and separation of follicle stimulating hormone (FSH) and luteinizing hormone (LH) from human postmenopausal gonadotrophin (HMG). I. Separation of FSH and LH by electrophoresis, chromatography and gel filtration procedures. *Acta Endocrinol* 1966; **52**:169–85.

17. Evans MI, Littmann L, St. Louis L, *et al.* Evolving patterns of iatrogenic multifetal pregnancy generation: implications for aggressiveness of infertility treatments. *Am J Obstet Gynecol* 1995; **172**:1750–3; discussion 1753–5.

18. Navot D, Relou A, Birkenfeld A, Rabinowitz R, Brzezinski A, Margalioth EJ. Risk factors and prognostic variables in the ovarian hyperstimulation syndrome. *Am J Obstet Gynecol* 1988; **159**:210–5.

19. Fernandez H, Coste J, Job-Spira N. Controlled ovarian hyperstimulation as a risk factor for ectopic pregnancy [see comments]. *Obstet Gynecol* 1991; **78**:656–9.

20. Ben-Rafael Z, Dor J, Mashiach S, Blankstein J, Lunenfeld B, Serr DM. Abortion rate in pregnancies following ovulation induced by human menopausal gonadotropin/human chorionic gonadotropin. *Fertil Steril* 1983; **39**:157–61.

21. Filicori M, Cognigni GE, Arnone R, *et al.* Is multiple pregnancy an unavoidable complication of ovulation induction? The case for pulsatile GnRH. *Eur J Obstet Gynecol Reprod Biol* 1996; **65**(suppl):S19–21.

22. Hughes E, Collins J, Vandekerckhove P. Gonadotrophin-releasing hormone analogue as an adjunct to gonadotropin therapy for clomiphene-resistant polycystic ovarian syndrome. *Cochrane Database of Systematic Reviews* [computer file] 2000:CD000097.

23. Devroey P. GnRH antagonists [editorial]. *Fertil Steril* 2000; **73**:15–7.

24. Meldrum DR, Chetkowski RJ, Steingold KA, Randle D. Transvaginal ultrasound scanning of ovarian follicles. *Fertil Steril* 1984; **42**:803–5.

25. Guy RL, King E, Ayers AB. The role of transvaginal ultrasound in the assessment of the female pelvis. *Clin Radiol* 1988; **39**:669–72.

26. Andolf E, Jorgensen C. A prospective comparison of transabdominal and transvaginal ultrasound with surgical findings in gynecologic disease. *J Ultrasound Med* 1990; **9**:71–5.

27. Storment JM, Monga M, Blanco JD. Ineffectiveness of latex condoms in preventing contamination of the transvaginal ultrasound transducer head. *South Med J* 1997; **90**:206–8.

28. Dodson MG, Deter RL. Definition of anatomical planes for use in transvaginal sonography. *J Clin Ultrasound* 1990; **18**:239–42.

29. Rottem S, Thaler I, Goldstein SR, Timor-Tritsch IE, Brandes JM. Transvaginal sonographic technique: targeted organ scanning without resorting to 'planes'. *J Clin Ultrasound* 1990; **18**:243–7.

30. Nichols JE, Steinkampf MP. Detection of free peritoneal fluid by transvaginal sonography. *J Clin Ultrasound* 1993; **21**:171–4.

31. Davis JA, Gosink BB. Fluid in the female pelvis: cyclic patterns. *J Ultrasound Med* 1986; **5**:75–9.

32. Tessler FN, Perrella RR, Fleischer AC, Grant EG. Endovaginal sonographic diagnosis of dilated fallopian tubes. AJR. *Am J Roentgenol* 1989; **153**:523–5.

33. Oyesanya OA, Parsons JH, Collins WP, Campbell S. Total ovarian volume before human chorionic gonadotrophin administration for ovulation induction may predict the hyperstimulation syndrome. *Hum Reprod* 1995; **10**:3211–12.

34. Danninger B, Brunner M, Obruca A, Feichtinger W. Prediction of ovarian hyperstimulation syndrome by ultrasound volumetric assessment [corrected] of baseline ovarian volume prior to stimulation [see comments] [published erratum appears in *Hum Reprod* 1997 Feb;12(2):401]. *Hum Reprod* 1996; **11**:1597–9.

35. Shoham Z, Conway GS, Patel A, Jacobs HS. Polycystic ovaries in patients with hypogonadotropic hypogonadism: similarity of ovarian response to gonadotropin stimulation in patients with polycystic ovarian syndrome [see comments]. *Fertil Steril* 1992; **58**:37–45.

36. MacDougall MJ, Tan SL, Balen A, Jacobs HS. A controlled study comparing patients with and without polycystic ovaries undergoing in-vitro fertilization. *Hum Reprod* 1993; **8**:233–7.

37. Wong IL, Morris RS, Lobo RA, Paulson RJ, Sauer MV. Isolated polycystic morphology in ovum donors predicts response to ovarian stimulation. *Hum Reprod* 1995; **10**:524–8.

38. Akin JW, Shepard MK. The effects of baseline ovarian cysts on cycle fecundity in controlled ovarian hyperstimulation. *Fertil Steril* 1993; **59**:453–5.

39. Diamond MP, DeCherney AH, Baretto P, Lunenfeld B. Multiple consecutive cycles of ovulation induction with human menopausal gonadotropins. *Gynecol Endocrinol* 1989; **3**:237–40.

40. Silverberg KM, Klein NA, Burns WN, Schenken RS, Olive DL. Consecutive versus alternating cycles of ovarian stimulation using human menopausal gonadotrophin. *Hum Reprod* 1992; **7**:940–4.

41. Martinez AR, Bernardus RE, Kucharska D, Schoemaker J. Urinary luteinizing hormone testing and prediction of ovulation in spontaneous, clomiphene citrate and human menopausal gonadotropin-stimulated cycles. A clinical evaluation. *Acta Endocrinol* 1991; **124**:357–63.

42. Lloyd R, Coulam CB. The accuracy of urinary luteinizing hormone testing in predicting ovulation. *Am J Obstet Gynecol* 1989; **160**:1370–2; discussion 1373–5.

43. Fleischer AC, Pittaway DE, Beard LA, et al. Sonographic depiction of endometrial changes occurring with ovulation induction. *J Ultrasound Med* 1984; **3**:341–6.

44. Hoffman DI, Lobo RA, Campeau JD, et al. Ovulation induction in clomiphene-resistant anovulatory women: differential follicular response to purified urinary follicle-stimulating hormone (FSH) versus purified urinary FSH and luteinizing hormone. *J Clin Endocrinol Metab* 1985; **60**:922–7.

45. Zandt-Stastny D, Thorsen MK, Middleton WD, et al. Inability of sonography to detect imminent ovulation. AJR. *Am J Roentgenol* 1989; **152**:91–5.

46. Fedele L, Brioschi D, Dorta M, Parazzini F, Bocciolone L. Timing of ovulation in spontaneous and induced cycles. *Int J Gynaecol Obstet* 1990; **32**:369–75.

47. Ritchie WG. Sonographic evaluation of normal and induced ovulation. *Radiology* 1986; **161**:1–10.

48. Check JH, Dietterich C, Nowroozi K, Wu CH. Comparison of various therapies for the luteinized unruptured follicle syndrome. *Int J Fertil* 1992; **37**:33–40.

49. Elkind-Hirsch K, Goldzieher JW, Gibbons WE, Besch PK. Evaluation of the OvuSTICK urinary luteinizing hormone kit in normal and stimulated menstrual cycles. *Obstet Gynecol* 1986; **67**:450–3.

50. Fossum GT, Vermesh M, Kletzky OA. Biochemical and biophysical indices of follicular development in spontaneous and stimulated ovulatory cycles. *Obstet Gynecol* 1990; **75**:407–11.

51. Zreik TG, Garcia-Velasco JA, Habboosh MS, Olive DL, Arici A. Prospective, randomized, crossover study to evaluate the benefit of human chorionic gonadotropin-timed versus urinary luteinizing hormone-timed intrauterine inseminations in clomiphene citrate-stimulated treatment cycles. *Fertil Steril* 1999; **71**:1070–4.

52. Gleicher N, Oleske DM, Tur-Kaspa I, Vidali A, Karande V. Reducing the risk of high-order multiple pregnancy after ovarian stimulation with gonadotropins [see comments]. *New Engl J Med* 2000; **343**:2–7.

53. Tal J, Paz B, Samberg I, Lazarov N, Sharf M. Ultrasonographic and clinical correlates of menotropin versus sequential clomiphene citrate: menotropin therapy for induction of ovulation. *Fertil Steril* 1985; **44**:342–9.

54. Blankstein J, Shalev J, Saadon T, *et al.* Ovarian hyperstimulation syndrome: prediction by number and size of preovulatory ovarian follicles. *Fertil Steril* 1987; **47**:597–602.

55. Haning RV, Jr., Boehnlein LM, Carlson IH, Kuzma DL, Zweibel WJ. Diagnosis-specific serum 17 beta-estradiol (E2) upper limits for treatment with menotropins using a 125I direct E2 assay. *Fertil Steril* 1984; **42**:882–9.

56. Tulandi T, Hamilton EF, Arronet GH, Coleman PW, McInnes RA. Ovulation induction by human menopausal gonadotropin with ultrasonic monitoring of the ovarian follicles. *Int J Fert* 1987; **32**:312–5.

57. Glasier A, Thatcher SS, Wickings EJ, Hillier SG, Baird DT. Superovulation with exogenous gonadotropins does not inhibit the luteinizing hormone surge. *Fertil Steril* 1988; **49**:81–5.

58. Serafini P, Stone B, Kerin J, Batzofin J, Quinn P, Marrs RP. Occurrence of a spontaneous luteinizing hormone surge in superovulated cycles-predictive value of serum progesterone. *Fertil Steril* 1988; **49**:86–9.

59. Coetsier T, Dhont M. Complete and partial luteinized unruptured follicle syndrome after ovarian stimulation with clomiphene citrate/human menopausal gonadotrophin/human chorionic gonadotrophin. *Hum Reprod* 1996; **11**:583–7.

60. Fleischer AC, Kalemeris GC, Entman SS. Sonographic depiction of the endometrium during normal cycles. *Ultrasound Med Biol* 1986; **12**:271–7.

61. Delisle MF, Villeneuve M, Boulvain M. Measurement of endometrial thickness with transvaginal ultrasonography: is it reproducible? *J Ultrasound Med* 1998; **17**:481–4; quiz 485–6.

62. Shapiro H, Cowell C, Casper RF. The use of vaginal ultrasound for monitoring endometrial preparation in a donor oocyte program. *Fertil Steril* 1993; **59**:1055–8.

63. Isaacs JD, Jr., Wells CS, Williams DB, Odem RR, Gast MJ, Strickler RC. Endometrial thickness is a valid monitoring parameter in cycles of ovulation induction with menotropins alone. *Fertil Steril* 1996; **65**:262–6.

64. Randall JM, Templeton A. Transvaginal sonographic assessment of follicular and endometrial growth in spontaneous and clomiphene citrate cycles. *Fertil Steril* 1991; **56**:208–12.

65. Dickey RP, Olar TT, Taylor SN, Curole DN, Matulich EM. Relationship of endometrial thickness and pattern to fecundity in ovulation induction cycles: effect of clomiphene citrate alone and with human menopausal gonadotropin. *Fertil Steril* 1993; **59**:756–60.

66. Fleischer AC, Gordon AN, Entman SS, Kepple DM. Transvaginal scanning of the endometrium. *J Clin Ultrasound* 1990; **18**:337–49.

67. Gonen Y, Casper RF. Prediction of implantation by the sonographic appearance of the endometrium during controlled ovarian stimulation for in vitro fertilization (IVF) [see comments]. *J in Vitro Fertil Embryo Transfer* 1990; **7**:146–52.

14 Assisted reproductive technology (ART)

Lawrence Grunfeld

Ultrasonographic assessment of follicle growth was first introduced in the 1970s when Hackeloer described a linear relationship between follicle size and estradiol levels[1] (*Fig. 14.1*). This fortuitous relationship has allowed ultrasound to become a standard tool in reproductive medicine for the assessment of oocyte maturity. Later that decade, in 1978, Steptoe and Edwards introduced to the world the birth of the first human conceived through in vitro fertilization (IVF).[2] The disappointing results that were achieved with tubal surgery were replaced by excitement about this innovation. Unfortunately, many patients who most needed IVF could not safely undergo this procedure because their ovaries were not accessible to abdominal retrieval techniques. The introduction of endovaginal ultrasonography in the late 1980s enabled oocyte harvesting to be performed for patients who could benefit from IVF but whose ovaries were inaccessible. The combination of a rapid non-invasive technique for the detection of follicle maturity with the easy harvesting of oocytes led to the rapid proliferation of endovaginal ultrasonography in reproductive medicine.

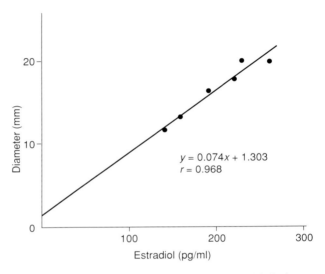

$$y = 0.074x + 1.303$$
$$r = 0.968$$

Figure 14.1 Ultrasonographic measurement of follicle maturity is possible because of a linear relationship between E2 and follicle size. (From Hackeloer *et al.*[1])

Assisted reproductive technology (ART)

Assisted reproduction consists of several medical procedures used to enhance fertilization through either natural ovulation or controlled ovarian hyperstimulation (COH). Ovulation is precisely timed and spermatozoa are introduced through either timed intercourse or some form of insemination. In advanced reproductive techniques oocytes are extracted and insemination is performed in vitro either by adding prepared spermatozoa or by directly injecting spermatozoa into the egg (intracytoplasmic insemination—ICSI).

The first successful in vitro fertilization, in 1978, was achieved with an egg that was harvested in a natural menstrual cycle.[2] Steptoe and Edwards observed their patient for 24 hours until the spontaneous luteinizing hormone (LH) surge was detected. Some time in the middle of the night a laparoscopic egg retrieval yielded an egg that developed into the first human birth conceived in vitro. Their monumental feat was achieved through an intimate knowledge of the events of the natural menstrual cycle.

During the normal menstrual cycle, endovaginal ultrasound is able to discern ovarian as well as endometrial changes. The initiation of follicular growth is a continuous process, which is independent of gonadotropin stimulation and proceeds until the follicle reaches 5 mm.[3] Ultrasonography of the ovary, in women of reproductive age, will always demonstrate follicles at this stage of development, even if ovulation is suppressed by oral contraceptives. However, further growth of the follicle is impossible in the absence of an appropriate gonadotropin stimulation. Later in the follicle phase, the most dominant follicle contains enough receptors to follicle stimulating hormone (FSH) to continue growth despite declining serum FSH. Follicles with fewer FSH receptors on their surface will become atretic with the withdrawal of gonadotropin support (*Fig. 14.2*). Once the leading follicle reaches a diameter of 14 mm, the daily growth rate is approximately 1.5–2 mm until ovulation, which occurs at a diameter of 20–24 mm. In the natural cycle, a follicle diameter of 20 mm indicates follicle maturity and ovulation can be triggered through the administration of human chorionic gonadotropin (hCG). This hormone has a similar action to pituitary LH, but is longer in duration.

Characteristic sonographic events at the time of ovulation include diminution in follicle size, blurring of the follicle borders, appearance of intrafollicular echoes, and the demonstration of free fluid in the cul-de-sac. Thereafter, an irregular, mildly cystic structure representing the corpus luteum diminishes in size throughout the luteal phase of the cycle until luteolysis, which precedes menses. The corpus luteum can assume many forms and there is no characteristic appearance to the ovary in the luteal phase (*Fig. 14.3*). Cystic corpora lutea can be quite sonolucent, although increasing the gain settings can usually detect more echogenicity than in the preovulatory follicle. The walls of the corpus luteum tend to be thicker and less regularly shaped than the preovulatory follicle. Many corpora lutea are echogenic and have the typical speckled appearance associated with blood. Some corpora lutea can layer out serum and solid clots.

The endometrium also demonstrates marked changes throughout the menstrual cycle (*Fig. 14.4*). Beginning with a thin echo during menses the endometrium gradually thickens throughout the proliferative phase. Prior to ovulation when estrogen levels peak and progesterone is not detectable, the endometrium is represented by three lines.[4] An inner luminal interface is surrounded by the functional hypoechoic endometrium and the echogenic myometrial–endometrial interface. A sonolucent halo, the origin of which is subject to debate, most likely represents the inner compact myometrium. The rise in progesterone that occurs following ovulation causes an increase in stromal edema and the growth of spiral arterioles, which is depicted sonographically as an increase in echogenicity.[5] The luteal phase begins with an

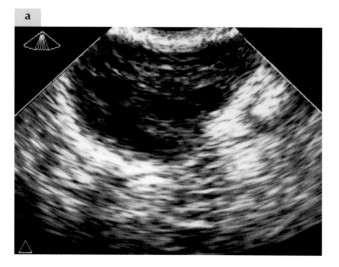

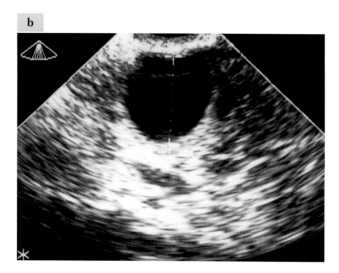

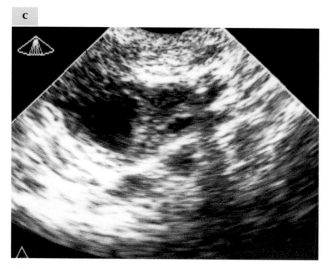

Figure 14.2 Follicle maturation. (a) Early follicle phase ovaries demonstrate follicles smaller than 10 mm. (b) Late follicle phase ovaries demonstrate a single Graafian follicle and several atretic follicles. (c) Luteal phase demonstrates follicle rupture and the development of the corpus luteum.

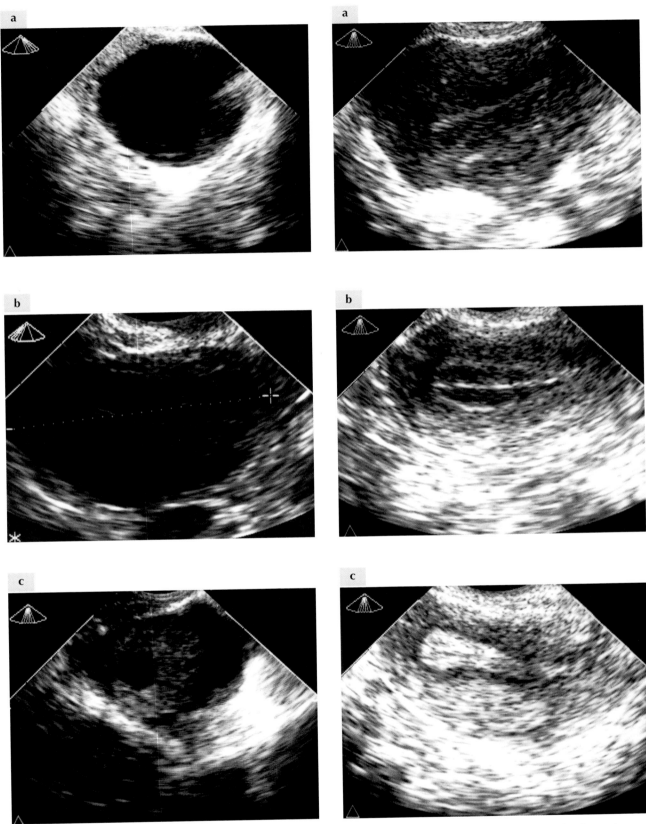

Figure 14.3 The corpus luteum is typically cystic (a), but can be hemorrhagic with layering of clots (b). In some cases, the corpus luteum may not be visible on ultrasonography and the only finding is a disappearance of a previously visible follicle and free fluid around the ovary (c).

Figure 14.4 The endometrium is thin and echogenic during menses (a) and progressively thickens up to the late follicular phase (b) when it is characterized by the three-layered pattern. In the luteal phase, the endometrium is hyperechoic (c).

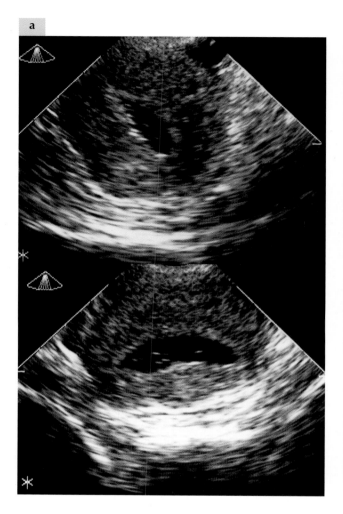

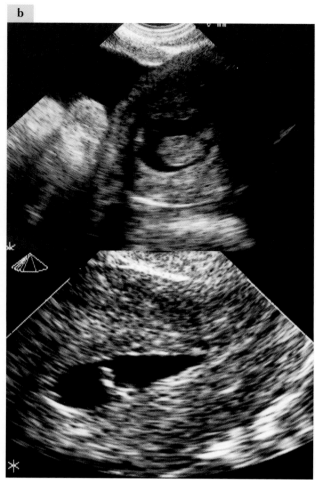

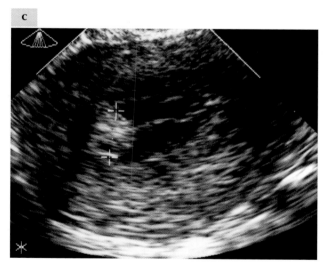

Figure 14.5 (a) Sonohysterogram of normal endometrial cavity in longitudinal (top) and transverse (bottom) section. (b) Large endometrial polyp and endometrial adhesion. (c) Polyps can be visible in the late follicular phase, even without saline instillation.

increase in peripheral echogenicity, which gradually progresses to the lumen and eventually causes its obliteration. The pattern of echogenicity follows the direction of growth of the spiral arterioles that form in the basalis and grow into the endometrium (peripheral to central). Echogenicity in the luteal phase is maintained until menses when there is breakdown of the endometrium.

Pretreatment assessment

Although IVF can overcome many causes of infertility it is important to ensure that the patient has a normal endometrial cavity, healthy oocytes, and at least a minimal number of spermatozoa before beginning therapy. A healthy endometrial cavity can usually be reliably determined through sonohysterography, as

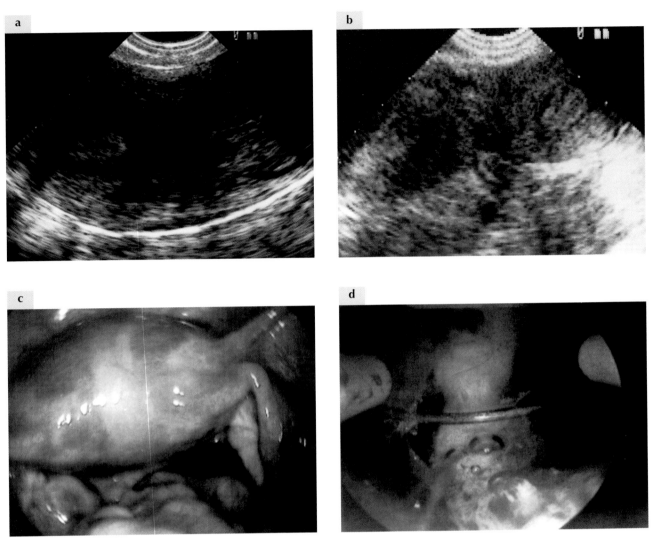

Figure 14.6 (a) Uterine septum on transverse view demonstrates the presence of myometrium between two separate endometrial cavities. (b) Didelphic uteri demonstrate two completely separate uteri with separate cavities and separate serosal contours. (c) Serosa of uterine septum demonstrates a ridge, but only a single contour. (d) Hysteroscopic view of a septum demonstrates a thick muscular ridge between two endometrial cavities.

described elsewhere in this book. Saline infusion sonohysterography has the advantage of being relatively painless and can usually detect fibroids, polyps, adhesions, and endometrial deformities. Parsons and colleagues[6,7] demonstrated good correlation between X-ray hysterosalpingography (HSG) and sonohysterography (*Fig. 14.5*). Ayida et al utilized sonohysterography prior to IVF and demonstrated a sensitivity of 87% and a specificity of 91%.[8] When sonography is performed in the follicular phase, saline instillation is not necessary to see most filling defects.[9] In the follicular phase the endometrium is hypoechoic, while echogenic fibroids and polyps are readily apparent. Uterine septum can also be visualized by observing the endometrial cavity in transverse section

through the fundus. Uterine septum appears as a single serosal contour, but with two separate endometrial cavities (*Fig. 14.6*). In contrast, the didelphic uterus has two separate endometrial contours with two separate serosal contours (*Fig. 14.6*). A formal assessment of the endometrial cavity is mandatory prior to IVF to eliminate correctable causes of implantation failure.

Ovaries deformed by endometriosis can still yield healthy eggs, but ovarian tumors need to be assessed prior to IVF (*Fig. 14.7*). Oocyte harvesting in the presence of a dermoid tumor can lead to peritonitis, if the dermoid is inadvertently punctured.[10] It is also important to keep in mind that ovarian neoplasms are a cause of infertility, and suspicious masses need

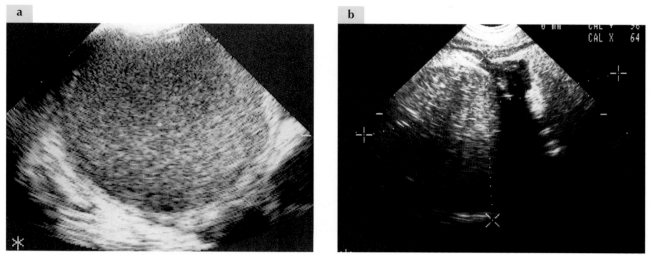

Figure 14.7 (a) Large endometrioma. Typical speckled sonographic appearance of endometriotic fluid. (b) Dermoid cyst containing fat.

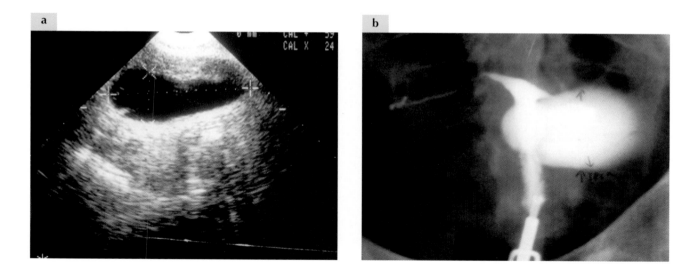

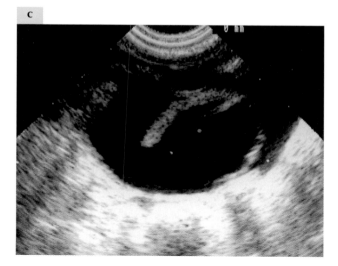

Figure 14.8 Hydrosalpinx on sonogram (a) and HSG (b). Hydrosalpinges are tubular. Rotating the transducer demonstrates the tubular nature of this structure. Many hydrosalpinges have a serpentine course (c).

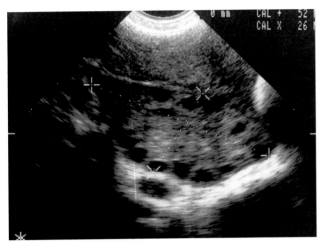

Figure 14.9 Ovary demonstrating typical signs of polycystic ovary syndrome. Note the dense stroma and peripheral distribution of oocytes.

to be investigated prior to initiating ovarian stimulation. However, functional ovarian cysts do not interfere with ovarian stimulation and small cysts can safely be ignored once the possibility of neoplasm has been reliably eliminated.[11]

In vitro fertilization usually demonstrates good success in patients with tubal blockage, but patients with severe tubal obstruction and hydrosalpinges do not achieve ideal rates of success (*Fig. 14.8*). This is thought to be caused by the secretion of hydrosalpinx fluid into the endometrial cavity. Hydrosalpinx fluid has been demonstrated to be toxic to

the developing embryo in a dose-dependent fashion.[12] The presence of a hydrosalpinx large enough to be visible on transvaginal ultrasonography is considered to be the criterion for either salpingectomy or transection of the tube prior to IVF.[13]

Observation of ovarian volume prior to selecting an ovarian stimulation protocol is important. Ovaries with more than 10 follicles per section will likely overstimulate, particularly if a thickened stroma is observed[14] (*Fig. 14.9*). Ovarian hyperstimulation syndrome (OHSS), a life-threatening complication of ovulation induction where fluid transudates into the peritoneal and pleural spaces, is most reliably predicted by ultrasonography (*Fig. 14.10*). Many patients who over-respond to gonadotropins have regular menses and no stigmata of polycystic ovary syndrome, other than the appearance of their ovaries on ultrasonography. Normal ovaries have a volume of approximately 6.3 cm^3, while patients with small ovaries (< 3 cm^3) will probably need more aggressive stimulation protocols[15] (*Fig. 14.11*). It is important to recognize poorly responding patients since this group carries a very poor prognosis for successful outcome with IVF.

Superovulation

Early in the course of the development of IVF it became apparent that the process of fertilizing an embryo and transferring it into the endometrial cavity is very inefficient. Steptoe and Edward's efforts utilized single embryo transfers and achieved only a 5% pregnancy rate.[2] Although this was

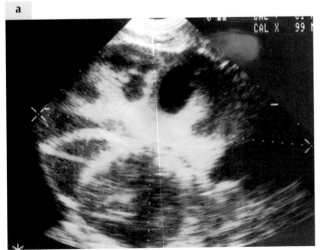

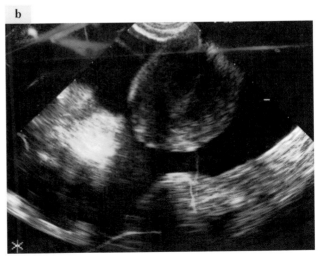

Figure 14.10 Case of severe ovarian hyperstimulation syndrome. (a) Enlarged ovary. (b) The 'floating uterus' is due to ascites.

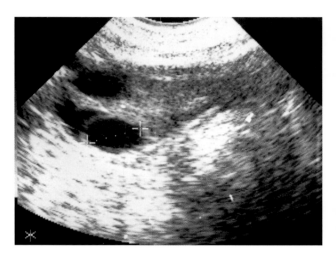

Figure 14.11 Small ovaries are associated with poor response to gonadotropins.

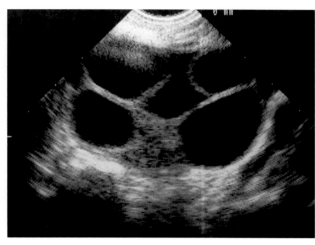

Figure 14.12 A favorable response to gonadotropins is associated with the production of four to eight follicles of mature size.

clearly a milestone in the advancement of therapy for infertility, early success rates would not be acceptable today. The major advancement resulting in an enhanced success rate was the use of controlled ovarian hyperstimulation (COH) for the recruitment of several oocytes.[16] Today, superovulation with a combination of human menopausal gonadotropins (hMG), and gonadotropin releasing hormone (GnRH) analogs, is standard. COH permits the retrieval of many oocytes, while in natural cycles only one oocyte matures. This increase in the pool of fertilizable oocytes will increase the number of embryos transferred into the endometrial cavity with a resultant increase in the chance of at least one embryo implanting (*Fig. 14.12*).

Oocytes can be aspirated in natural cycles as an alternative to COH.[17] Natural ovulatory cycles, such as that utilized by Steptoe and Edwards, result in the production of only a single mature oocyte and several immature oocytes. Unlike the earliest efforts where a completely natural ovulation was detected before follicle aspiration, today's natural cycles are triggered with a chemical surge of human chorionic gonadotropin (hCG) at follicle maturity. This allows oocyte retrieval to be performed during regular clinic hours. Although the yield of oocytes is poor, there is an advantage to the patient in the omission of superovulatory drugs. This procedure may have cost benefit to the patient, but is not as efficient as COH in the production of implantable oocytes. The immature oocytes that are retrieved can be matured in vitro, but to date the implantation rates of these oocytes are poor.[18]

In natural cycles ovulation occurs at follicular diameters of 2.0–2.5 cm. However, menotropin treatment is associated with more rapid increases in oocyte maturity as reflected by follicle diameters. Correlation between follicle diameter as measured on ultrasound demonstrates that mature eggs are almost never retrieved from follicles smaller than 15 mm, while follicles larger than 18 mm typically contain fertilizable oocytes.[19] GnRH analogs offer the advantage of prolonging stimulation until follicle maturity is achieved without the concern of premature ovulation.

Endometrial assessment

Ultrasonic measurement of the endometrium has received a great deal of attention in the analysis of factors that affect implantation. Gonen et al demonstrated that pregnancy was not associated with significantly thicker endometrium when patients were treated with a combination of clomiphene and pergonal.[20] Using the classification introduced by Welker et al, Gonen et al demonstrated improved implantation rates when a pattern associated with the late follicular phase was present on the day of hCG administration (pattern C).[21] There is no uniformity in endometrial pattern classification and this pattern has been described by various authors as either multilayered pattern I,[5] or pattern IIB,[22] or triple line. The follicular phase pattern consists of a luminal echo surrounded by a hypoechoic endometrium and an echogenic endometrium–myometrium interface (*Fig. 14.13*). An endometrium that is echogenic and characteristic of the luteal phase rarely results in pregnancy when present on the day of hCG administration. Sher et al demonstrated a reduction in pregnancy rates from 29% to 6% in over 1300 cycles with advanced patterns.[22]

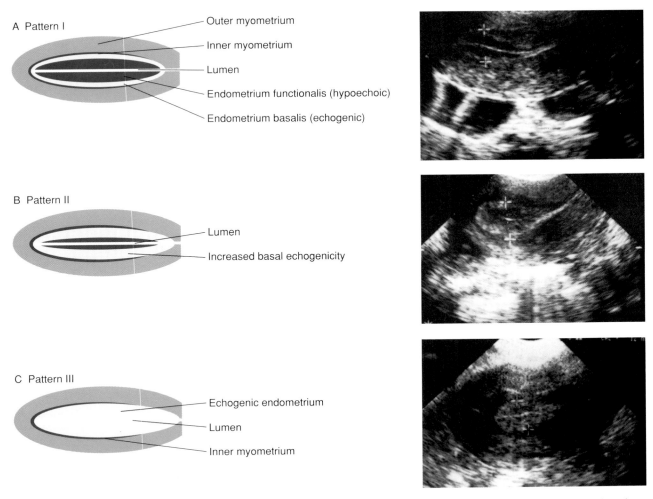

A Pattern I

- Outer myometrium
- Inner myometrium
- Lumen
- Endometrium functionalis (hypoechoic)
- Endometrium basalis (echogenic)

B Pattern II

- Lumen
- Increased basal echogenicity

C Pattern III

- Echogenic endometrium
- Lumen
- Inner myometrium

Figure 14.13 There is a transitional endometrium in the early luteal phase where echogenicity progresses from basalis to the lumen. (From Grunfeld et al.[5])

The likely explanation for this finding is that the endometrium and embryo must be synchronized and if the endometrium is advanced or retarded in its development implantation will not occur.

Authors who have studied endometrial patterns in patients treated with the addition of GnRH analogs to suppress premature ovulation have failed to demonstrate a strong dependence on the multilayered endometrium with implantation.[23] The absence of premature luteinization with the administration of GnRH analogs diminishes the predictive value of endometrial patterns. This is probably because very few patients demonstrate advanced endometrial patterns when progesterone levels are inhibited in the late follicular phase by GnRH analogs.

The endometrial pattern does provide useful information in cycles supplemented with estrogen and progesterone. Supplemented cycles are used to permit transfer of embryos from third parties in oocyte donation. Patients who require oocyte donation do not develop eggs that can sustain pregnancy, although the endometrium is normal in these patients and can support pregnancy if healthy embryos are transferred. Shapiro et al found a 60% pregnancy rate in oocyte recipients who demonstrated a favorable pattern and no pregnancies when < 6 mm of endometrium growth was achieved.[24] Increasing the dosage of estrogen was shown by Sher et al to convert unfavorable to favorable endometrial patterns.[25] Patients exposed to DES in utero have endometria that do not implant embryos well. Ultrasonography in the mid-cycle demonstrates a thin irregularly developed endometrium[26] (Fig. 14.14).

Doppler measurements of vascular resistance

Implantation is dependent upon the interplay of embryonic factors and uterine receptivity. While

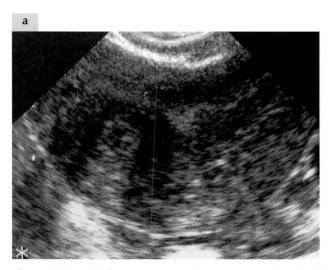

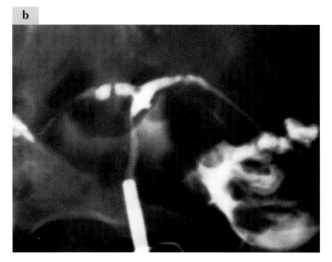

Figure 14.14 (a) The DES-exposed uterus is associated with a thin irregular endometrium. (b) On HSG the uterus demonstrates a 'T' shape.

embryo quality is critical for successful implantation, endometrial receptivity has a major role. Pulsed Doppler has been used to obtain flow waveforms from the uterine arteries during various phases of the menstrual cycle (*Fig. 14.15*). Preliminary data have suggested that decreased uterine perfusion may be responsible for some forms of infertility. Steer et al have analysed 82 cycles of assisted reproduction in which the flow through the uterine arteries was measured by transvaginal color flow Doppler.[27] The mean pulsatility index of the two uterine arteries was calculated and was used as a quantitative index of endometrial receptivity. Women whose pulsatility indices were > 3.0 demonstrated decreased implantation rates. It has been suggested that this new technique could lead to improved pregnancy rates in cycles of assisted reproduction by demonstrating suboptimal conditions for embryo transfer. Embryo transfer can be postponed through cryopreservation to subsequent cycles where endometrial receptivity can be manipulated through estrogen administration.

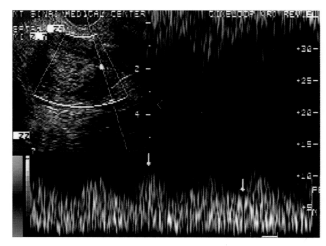

Figure 14.15 Uterine artery Doppler flow measurements on patients with a low (favorable) pulsatility index.

Oocyte retrieval

Once follicle maturity has been detected by ultrasonography, as described above, a triggering dose of human chorionic gonadotropins (hCG) is administered. This results in resumption of meiosis by the oocyte and follicular maturation that allows the oocyte to be fertilized. With resumption of meiosis there is a loss of the germinal vesicle and expulsion of the polar body. Only oocytes that have achieved this level of maturity are fertilizable. These events

require 34–38 hours in humans and oocyte aspiration is scheduled for 36 hours after injection of hCG.

The first oocyte retrieval in humans was performed in 1966 through a laparotomy. With further refinements of techniques, Edwards and Steptoe successfully fertilized human oocytes recovered laparoscopically in 1977. The first ultrasound-guided aspiration of oocytes was performed transabdominally by Lenz et al in Denmark.[28] The approach used by the Danish team was a transabdominal ultrasound with a transvesicle puncture (*Fig. 14.16*). Initially the needle was not coupled to

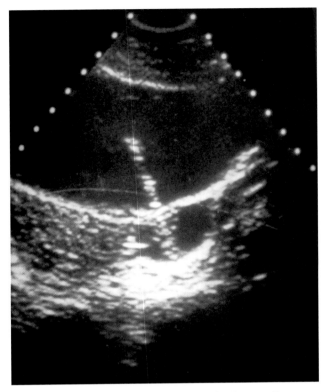

Figure 14.16 Transvesicle egg retrieval. The needle traverses the bladder into a follicle.

the transducer, but a needle guide improved the rate of oocyte recovery. Recovery rates in this series were 53%, which compares favorably with laparoscopically performed procedures. Gleicher was credited with the first oocyte retrieval through culdocentesis, although the technology of the time required transabdominal sonography.[29]

A major improvement in ultrasound retrieval occurred with the development of the transvaginal transducer.[30] Ovaries that are surrounded by dense adhesions tend to be fixed to the cul-de-sac, a location that is most easily reached transvaginally. Prior to the development of transvaginal ultrasound a surgical procedure was often necessary to fix the ovaries to the fundus of the uterus to allow access to the ovaries by laparoscopy. This is no longer performed, since the most appropriate place for the ovary after laparotomy is its usual location, in the cul-de-sac. The absence of bowel gas between the vaginal fornix and the ovaries allows the direct visualization of the ovaries without the need for a sonic window to enhance ultrasound transmission. In addition to the easier access to the ovaries in vaginal aspiration, the risks of bladder injury, hematuria, and infection which are associated with transvesical puncture are reduced. Transvaginal ultrasound-guided follicular puncture has resulted

in oocyte retrieval rates of 75%, which are comparable to those obtained by laparoscopy (*Fig. 14.17*).

It is important for ultrasound visualization of the needle that the tip be echogenic to enhance reflection of the ultrasound beam (*Fig. 14.18*). Precise placement of the needle is particularly important when the relationships of the major vessels of the pelvis are considered. The stimulated ovary lies immediately adjacent to the hypogastric artery and vein. In order to prevent injury to the vessels the tip of the needle must be visualized at all times. Another problem that can occur is misalignment of the needle with the ultrasound beam. It is important that the needle guide be secured to the transducer to prevent rotation from the proper axis (*Fig. 14.19*). Misalignment of the needle guide will result in loss of visibility of the needle with a loss of precision.

Transvaginal approaches to the ovary are less painful and this procedure can be performed on an ambulatory basis with only intravenous sedation. Patients who have a transvaginal ultrasound aspiration under local anesthesia tolerate the procedure well. Hammarberg et al found that 90% of patients experienced some pain or no pain while none described the retrieval as very painful.[31] Premedication with a sedative and paracervical block was sufficient anesthesia for 70% of patients, additional sedation was necessary for 20% of patients, and 10% of patients felt the procedure to be painful enough to require heavier anesthesia. When only a single oocyte is retrieved, such as in the natural cycle, only local anesthetic is necessary.

Dellenbach et al reported no major complications in over 800 transvaginal oocyte recoveries.[30] In a series of over 2500 retrievals, Bennett et al reported vaginal hemorrhage in 8% of cases, but most of these had insignificant blood loss.[32] Pelvic infections occurred in 0.6% of cases. Two cases resulted in hemoperitoneum requiring laparotomy. Dicker et al found nine pelvic abscesses in 3600 retrievals.[33] Most of these cases were patients with pre-existing pelvic infections. Care should be taken to avoid entering hydrosalpinges or endometriomas when performing follicle puncture, since this can predispose to pelvic infection. Furthermore, endometrioma fluid is toxic to the oocytes and inadvertent entry requires copious flushing of equipment. The hypogastric vessels are easily identified by turning the transducer 90° to see the long axis of the structure.

Embryo transfer

A major drop in the success of IVF occurs after the transfer of the embryos. While 70–80% of oocytes

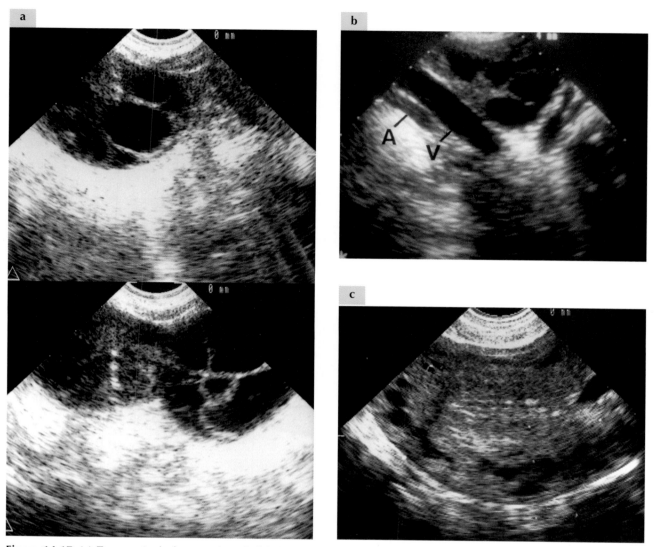

Figure 14.17 (a) Transvaginal ultrasound-guided follicular aspiration. (b) The needle punctures the lateral vaginal fornices and is introduced into the follicles. Note the position of the ovary in the cul-de-sac adjacent to the fornix. The iliac artery (A) and vein (V) are situated lateral to the ovary and care must be exercised to avoid injury. (c) The periphery of the uterus has large venous sinuses that should be avoided in oocyte aspiration.

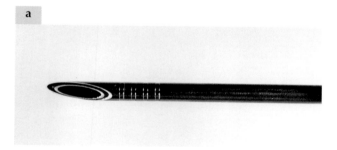

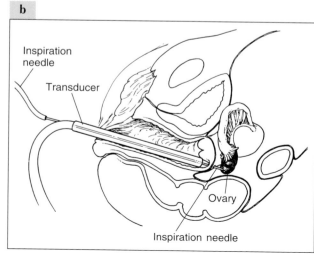

Figure 14.18 (a) Ultrasound-guided aspiration needles have an echogenic tip to aid visualization. (b) The needle is secured to the transducer to avoid rotation out of the plane of visualization.

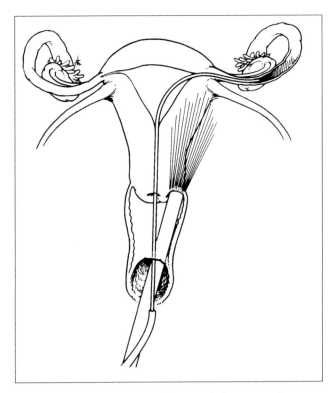

Figure 14.19 Transvaginal ultrasound depiction of transcervical fallopian tube catheterization.

aspirated will fertilize and cleave, only 20% of transferred embryos will implant.[34] Although the process of embryo placement is vital to the success of IVF, it is often performed as a blind procedure. Retention of the embryos in the cervical canal is a problem encountered with embryo transfer. As the catheter passes through the cervix, cervical mucous sticks to the catheter and embryos can become stuck to the mucous. As a result of these observations transfers have been attempted under ultrasound guidance.

Transabdominal ultrasound has been used to observe that the transfer catheter has passed into the endometrial cavity.[35] As the catheter is guided through the cervix a transabdominal ultrasound can identify the catheter tip to insure proper fundal placement of the embryos. Even when the embryos do reach the uterine cavity, bleeding into the catheter from trauma to the cervix can significantly compromise embryo viability.[36] In cases where cervical stenosis exists, passage of the embryo transfer catheter can be complicated by coiling in the cervical canal. This unfortunate complication could result in the expulsion of embryos into the cervical canal. In these cases ultrasound can be very helpful for confirming proper endometrial placement.

Transmyometrial embryo transfer has been attempted when the cervix cannot be easily traversed.[37,38]

Considerable expertise is needed and currently pregnancy rates do not approach those achieved with standard IVF. This technique is used primarily when all other techniques are destined to fail.

Tubal transfer

Embryo culturing varies in quality from laboratory to laboratory. While some laboratories can grow embryos that result in pregnancy rates of 60% per cycle in women younger than 40, other laboratories have lower success rates. It is felt that improving culturing conditions and embryo selection will optimize success rates. In less advanced laboratories, tubal transfer procedures yield better pregnancy rates for patients with normal tubes.[39] This technology is also being utilized for multiple failed cycles in patients with normal tubes. Fallopian tube transfers are typically performed laparoscopically, but less intrusive transcervical techniques have been described. Jansen and Anderson developed a technique for guiding embryos through the cervical canal and into the fallopian tube under endovaginal sonographic guidance[40] (*Fig. 14.20*). The transfer of zygotes or embryos into the fallopian tube, or ZIFT (zygote intrafallopian tube transfer), is only appropriate for patients who have normal fallopian tubes. The embryos can progress to the blastocyst stage before passage into the uterus, resulting in synchrony of endometrial and embryo development. This is in contrast to standard IVF embryo transfer where premature replacement of embryos occurs.

Transcervical ZIFT is performed by passing a coaxial catheter into the endometrial cavity by palpation. Once the catheter has successfully passed into the uterus the speculum is removed and an endovaginal

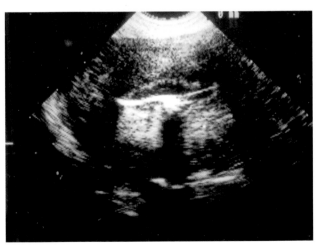

Figure 14.20 Echogenic catheter seen in the endometrial cavity prior to advancing into the cornua.

transducer is placed into the isthmic fallopian tube. The operator can feel the loss of resistance as the catheter passes up into the isthmic tube. The endovaginal transducer can confirm catheter placement in most cases. In early series fallopian tube catheterization was successful 92% of the time, and pregnancy occurred in 13% of cases. A randomized study of transcervical ZIFT as compared to traditional IVF by Scholtes did not confirm improved pregnancy rates with this technique.[41,42] It seems that the additional technology required for transcervical transfer of gametes or zygotes into the fallopian tube is not rewarded by greater success. Currently, traditional IVF with embryo replacement into the endometrial cavity is still standard and fallopian tube replacements await further studies.

GIFT

Asch et al have demonstrated in women with at least one normal fallopian tube that transferring gametes into the ampullary portion of the tube (gamete intrafallopian transfer or GIFT) achieved higher pregnancy rates than those of IVF.[43] Currently, this technique is unpopular because improved laboratory conditions have increased the success of transcervical embryo transfer while GIFT is usually performed under general anesthesia via laparoscopy. Transcervical GIFT procedures have also been developed.[40] Oocyte retrieval is performed routinely via transvaginal retrieval. Once the oocytes have been identified they are mixed with sperm in the transfer catheter. Under ultrasound guidance the catheter is passed into the tubal ostia and into the ampullary tube where the gametes are expelled, as described above for transcervical ZIFT. The same limitations in pregnancy rates seen in ZIFT are present in transcervical GIFT. In fact, it is technically more difficult to load the larger oocyte with its surrounding cumulus complex into a small enough volume so that expulsion out of the ampullary fallopian tube does not occur. Volumes >70 μl cannot be accommodated by the fallopian tube. The initial excitement reported by Jansen and Andersen has not been confirmed by later studies.

Recently, alternatives to traditional IVF have been described in an attempt to decrease complexity and expense. One such technique is ultrasound-guided follicle puncture and cul-de-sac transfer of eggs and sperm.[44] None of these techniques achieve the pregnancy rates or the ability to diagnose embryo developmental problems that can be obtained by advanced in vitro fertilization. It is important to await clinical trials that compare these techniques to intrauterine insemination before adopting them into the clinical armamentarium. Under ideal laboratory conditions, only in vitro culturing and uterine transfer of embryos have been shown to significantly enhance pregnancy rates over controlled ovarian hyperstimulation and intrauterine insemination.

REFERENCES

1. Hackeloer BJ, Fleming R, Robinson HP et al. Correlation of ultrasonic and endocrinologic assessment of human follicular development. Am J Obstet Gynecol 1979: 135:122–128.
2. Steptoe PC, Edwards RG. Birth after the reimplantation of a human embryo. Lancet 1978; 2:366.
3. Adashi E. The ovarian follicular apparatus. In: Adashi E, Rock J, Roslenwaks Z, eds. Reproductive Endocrinology, Surgery, and Technology. Philadelphia: Lippincot-Raven, 1996:17–40.
4. Yoshimitsu K, Nakamura G, Nakano H. Dating sonographic endometrial images in the normal ovulatory cycle. Int J Gynecol Obstet 1989; 28:33–39.
5. Grunfeld L, Walker B, Bergh PA et al. High resolution endovaginal ultrasonography of the endometrium: a non-invasive test for endometrial adequacy. Obstet Gynecol 1991; 78:200–204.
6. Parsons AAD, Lense JJ. Sonohysterography for endometrial abnormalities: preliminary results. J Clin Ultrasound 1993; 21:87–95.
7. Maroulis GB, Parsons AK, Yeko TR. Hydrogynecography: a new technique enables vaginal sonography to visualize pelvic adhesions and other pelvic structures. Fertil Steril 1992; 58:1073–1975.
8. Ayida G, Kennedy S, Barlow D, Chamberlain P. Uterine cavity assessment prior to in vitro fertilization; comparison of transvaginal sonography, saline contrast hysterosonography and hysteroscopy. Ultrasound Obstet Gynecol 1997; 10:59–62.
9. Grunfeld L, Stadtmauer L. Significance of endometrial filling defects detected on routine transvaginal ultrasound. J Ultrasound Med 1995; 14:169–172.
10. Coccia ME, Becattini C, Bracco GL, Scarselli G. Acute abdomen following dermoid cyst rupture during transvaginal ultrasonographically guided retrieval of oocytes. Human Reprod 1996; 11:1897–1899.
11. Penzias AS, Jones EE, Seifer DB, Grifo JA, Thatcher SS, DeCherney AA. Baseline ovarian cysts do not affect clinical response to controlled ovarian hyperstimulation for in vitro fertilization. Fertil Steril 1992; 57:1017–1021.

12. Mukherjee T, Copperman AB, McCaffrey C, Cook CA, Bustillo M, Obasaju MF. Hydrosalpinx fluid has embryotoxic effects on murine embryogenesis: a case for prophylactic salpingectomy. *Fertil Steril* 1996; **66**:851–853.

13. Nackley A, Muasher S. The significance of hydrosalpinx in in vitro fertilization. *Fertil Steril* 1998; **69**:373–384.

14. Suikkari AM, MacLachlan V, Montalto J, Calderon I, Healy DL, McLachlan RI. Ultrasonographic appearance of polycystic ovaries is associated with exaggerated ovarian androgen and oestradiol responses to gonadotrophin-releasing hormone agonist in women undergoing assisted reproduction treatment. *Human Reprod* 1995; **10**:513–519.

15. Lass A, Winston RM, Margara R, McVeigh E, Skull J. Measurement of ovarian volume by transvaginal sonography before ovulation induction with human menopausal gonadotropin for in-vitro fertilization can predict poor response. *Human Reprod* 1997; **12**:294–297.

16. Trounson AO, Leeton JF, Wood C. Pregnancies in humans by fertilization in vitro and embryo transfer in the controlled ovulatory cycle. *Science* 1981; **212**:681–682.

17. Paulson RJ, Sauer MV, Francis MM *et al*. In vitro fertilization in unstimulated cycles: the University of Southern California experience. *Fertil Steril* 1992; **57**:290–293.

18. Russell JB, Knezevich KM, Fabian KF, Dickson JA. Unstimulated immature oocyte retrieval: early versus midfollicular endometrial priming. *Fertil Steril* 1997; **67**:616–620.

19. Scott RT, Hofmann GE, Muasher SJ, Acosta AA, Kreiner DK, Rosenwaks Z. Correlation of follicular diameter with oocyte recovery and maturity at the time of transvaginal follicular aspiration. *J In Vitro Fert Embryo Transf* 1989; **6**:73–75.

20. Gonen Y, Casper RF, Jacobson W *et al*. Endometrial thickness and growth during ovarian hyperstimulation: a possible predictor of implantation in in vitro fertilization. *Fertil Steril* 1989; **52**:446–450.

21. Welker BG, Gembruch U, Diedrich K, al Hasani S, Krebs D. Transvaginal sonography of the endometrium during ovum pickup in stimulated cycles for in vitro fertilization. *J Ultrasound Med* 1989; **8**:549–553.

22. Sher G, Dodge S, Maassarani G *et al*. Management of suboptimal endometrial patterns in patients undergoing in vitro fertilization and ET. *Human Reprod* 1993; **8**:347–349.

23. Oliveira JB, Baruffi RL, Mauri AL, Petersen CG, Borges MC, Franco JG Jr. Endometrial ultrasonography as a predictor of pregnancy in an in-vitro fertilization programme after ovarian stimulation and gonadotrophin-releasing hormone and gonadotrophins. *Human Reprod* 1997; **12**:2515–2518.

24. Shapiro H, Cowell Casper RF. Use of vaginal ultrasound for monitoring endometrial preparation in a donor oocyte program. *Fertil Steril* 1993; **59**:1055–1058.

25. Sher G, Herbert C, Maassarani G, Jacobs MH. Assessment of the late proliferative phase endometrium by ultrasonography in patients undergoing in vitro fertilization and embryo transfer (IVF/ET). *Human Reprod* 1991; **6**:232–237.

26. Noyes N, Liu HC, Sultan K, Rosenwaks Z. Endometrial pattern in diethylstilboestrol-exposed women undergoing in-vitro fertilization may be the most significant predictor of pregnancy outcome. *Human Reprod* 1996; **11**:2719–2723.

27. Steer CV, Campbell S, Tan S *et al*. The use of transvaginal color flow imaging after in vitro fertilization to identify optimum uterine conditions before embryo transfer. *Fertil Steril* 1992; **57**:372–376.

28. Lenz S, Lauritsen J, Kjellow M. Collection of human oocytes for in vitro fertilization by ultrasonically guided follicular puncture. *Lancet* 1981; **i**:1163–1164.

29. Gleicher N, Friberg J, Fullan N *et al*. Egg retrieval for in vitro fertilization by sonographically controlled vaginal culdocentesis. *Lancet* 1983; **i**:508–509.

30. Dellenbach P, Nisand I, Moreau L *et al*. The transvaginal method for oocyte retrieval. An update on our experience (1948–87). *Ann NY Acad Sci* 1988; **541**:111–124.

31. Hammarberg K, Enk L, Nilsson L, Wikland M. Oocyte retrieval under the guidance of a vaginal transducer: evaluation of patient acceptance. *Human Reprod* 1987; **2**:487–490.

32. Bennett SJ, Waterstone JJ, Cheng WL, Parsons J. Complications of transvaginal ultrasound directed follicle aspiration in a review of 2670 consecutive procedures. *J Assist Reprod Genet* 1993; **10**:72–77.

33. Dicker D, Ashkenaji J, Feldberg D, Levy T, Dekel A, Ben Rafael Z. Severe abdominal complication after transvaginal ultrasonographically guided retrieval of oocytes in vitro fertilization and embryo transfer. *Fertil Steril* 1993; **59**:1313–1315.

34. Assisted reproductive technology in the United States and Canada: 1995 results generated from the American Society for Reproductive Medicine/Society for Assisted Reproductive Technology Registry. *Fertil Steril* 1998; **69**:389–396.

35. Prapas Y, Jones EE, Vlassis B *et al*. The echoguide embryo transfer maximizes IVF results. *Acta Eur Fertil* 1995; **261**: 113–115.

36. Al Shawaf T, Dave R, Harper J, Linehan D, Riley P, Craft I. Transfer of embryos into the uterus: how much do technical factors affect pregnancy rates? *J Assist Reprod Genet* 1993; **10**:31–36

37. Groutz A, Amit A, Yovel I, Azem F, Wolf Y, Lessing JB. Comparison of transmyometrial and transcervical embryo transfer in patients with previously failed in vitro fertilization–embryo transfer cycles and/or cervical stenosis. *Fertil Steril* 1997; **67**:1073–1076.

38. Sharif K, Khalaf Y, Hunjam M, Bilalis D, Lenton W, Afnan M. Transmyometrial embryo transfer after difficult immediate mock transcervical transfer. *Fertil Steril* 1996; **65**:1071–1074.

39. Levran D, Mashiach S, Dor J, Levron J, Farhi J. Zygote intrafallopian transfer may improve pregnancy rate in patients with repeated failure of implantation. *Fertil Steril* 1998; **69**:26–30.

40. Jansen RPS, Anderson JC, Sutherland PD. Non-operative embryo transfer to the fallopian tube. *N Engl J Med* 1988; **319**:288–291.

41. Fluer MR, Zouves CG, Bebbington MW. A prospective randomized comparison of zygote intrafallopian transfer and in vitro fertilization embryo transfer for non tubal factor infertility. *Fertil Steril* 1993; **60**:515–519.

42. Scholtes M, Roozenburg BJ, Verhoeff A, Zeihmuker GH. A randomized study of transcervical intrafallopian transfer of pronucleate embryos controlled by ultrasound versus intrauterine transfer of four to eight cell embryos. *Fertil Steril* 1994; **61**:102–104.

43. Asch RH, Balmaceda JP, Ellsworth LR, Wong PC. Preliminary experiences with gamete intrafallopian transfer (GIFT). *Fertil Steril* 1986; **45**:366–371

44. Ajossa S, Melis GB, Cianci A *et al.* An open multicenter study to compare the efficacy of intraperitoneal insemination and intrauterine insemination following multiple follicular development as treatment for unexplained infertility. *J Assist Reprod Genet* 1997; **14**:15–20.

15 Early pregnancy: normal and abnormal

Robert S Howe

Introduction

This chapter describes the ultrasound appearance of early human pregnancy and describes a method of evaluating the health of such pregnancies using the tools available to community physicians: a careful history, quantitative β-human chorionic gonadotropin (hCG) levels done on a 'stat' or daily basis, and transvaginal ultrasound (US) examinations performed on modern equipment capable of magnifying the image. This method is based upon 12 years' experience of evaluating hundreds of normal and abnormal pregnancies, most of which were of known gestational age.

Performing the early pregnancy scan

Transvaginal ultrasound is superior to transabdominal ultrasound in evaluating an early pregnancy, because the transducer is only 2–4 cm from the structures being imaged.[1] This allows the use of a higher frequency signal, with finer image resolution. Thus, intrauterine events can be noted earlier and with greater assurance on transvaginal studies.[2] The patient need not fill her bladder.

The ultrasound study is performed on a standard pelvic examination table. The patient is most comfortable with the head of the table raised so that she can see the monitor easily. This also maximizes the volume of pelvic fluid visible in the cul-de-sac, simplifying evaluation of the adnexa and of possible ectopic pregnancy. The patient is draped as for a pelvic examination. A chaperone is recommended for all physicians, to reassure the patient, help the examiner, and take notes as needed.

The US examination must not merely scan the uterus. Just as a radiologist studying chest films of a patient in heart failure may first look over the ribs for fractures, the clinician scanning an early pregnancy should proceed in a standard fashion, looking at the cervix, bladder, adnexa and cul-de-sac in addition to the uterus. The cervix is hidden during vaginal US scanning, as the transducer head usually moves past the external ostium into one of the vaginal fornices. Thus, the cervix is best seen as the transducer enters the mid-vagina. The rare cervical ectopic pregnancy will only be noted if it is sought; what the brain does not expect, the eye will not see.

The uterus is first briefly scanned and evaluated for fibroids, adenomyosis, endometrial development, and the presence or absence of a pregnancy. To minimize energy exposure to the embryo, use the lowest power output adequate to provide a satisfactory image and compensate as needed by increasing the gain. However, the clinician can be reassured that there are no known harmful effects on human pregnancy from ultrasound equipment in clinical use.[3,4]

Next, the adnexa are visualized and the corpus luteum measured. The tubes are invisible in a normal scan, but are sought by moving laterally from the uterine cornua towards the ovaries. An ectopic pregnancy must be carefully sought. As the cul-de-sac is scanned the character of any fluid is noted by boosting the power output to maximum; this will allow the sonographer to differentiate clear, physiologic peritoneal fluid from bloody fluid, which often has debris or layers of different density denoting settling out of the blood. If the volume of fluid seems excessive, three-dimensional measurement of this fluid pocket allows approximation of its volume by the formula:

$$\text{volume} = (\pi/6)\,(d1 \times d2 \times d3)$$

where d1, d2 and d3 are the diameters of the pocket measured in three mutually perpendicular axes.

All significant findings are examined under magnification, measured and recorded. An experienced sonographer may describe cervix, cul-de-sac, and the adnexa without the corpus luteum as 'normal' if no pathology is seen.

Ultrasonic and anatomic landmarks in early pregnancy

A succession of US findings correlate to normal embryologic development. Endometrial decidualization and edema correspond to the time of implantation. Appearance of the chorionic sac corresponds to omnidirectional growth of the trophoblast and expansion of the extra-embryonic coelom beyond 2 mm diameter. Appearance of the yolk sac correlates to growth of the trilaminar embryo. The appearance of the visible embryonic heart rate (EHR) occurs about 1 week after the beginning of cardiac activity. Appearance of the embryonic crown–rump length and visualization of the amnion surrounding the embryo correlate to further differentiation of the embryo.

A basic understanding of embryogenesis is essential to understand these images, although detailed descriptions are best left to standard textbooks. Gestational ages are described in this chapter using anatomists' nomenclature, as if measured from the day of fertilization. Obstetrical nomenclature, when used, assumes measurement from the first day of the last menstrual period (LMP) in an ideal menstrual cycle, with ovulation and fertilization on the 14th day.

Implantation

After fertilization occurs in the ampulla of the fallopian tube, the dividing conceptus is moved down the lumen of the tube into the endometrial cavity. In the uterus, the blastocyst lands on the decidualized endometrium about 1 week after fertilization (3 weeks LMP). Implantation most often is in the upper posterior fundus, placing the transvaginal scanner close to the implantation site.

Implantation is in process by day 8 from fertilization (22nd day LMP), with the blastocyst embedded in the endometrial stroma. The endometrium caps over the site of implantation, leaving the blastocyst in the superficial part of the endometrial stratum compactum, projecting marginally into the uterine cavity. The endometrium is now called 'decidua' and is divided into three distinct portions defined by their relationships to the implanted blastocyst: decidua capsularis, overlying the blastocyst; decidua basalis, underneath the blastocyst; and decidua parietalis, everywhere else in the uterine cavity.

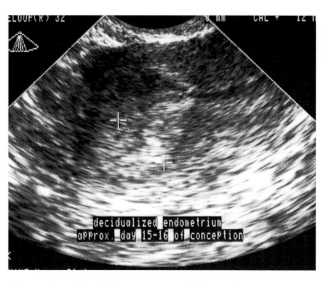

Figure 15.1 Typical appearance of the endometrium in a conception cycle, at the time of the missed menses. Urine hCG was positive.

This early stage of a pregnancy (days 8–14 from fertilization, days 22–28 LMP) has no definitive US signs, so a sensitive serum pregnancy test is a more reliable determinant of pregnancy than US at this point.[5,6] One paper has reported irregularity of the anterior endometrial–myometrial interface during the peri-implantational period,[7] but the validity and utility of this observation remain uncertain. Despite this, the early post-implantational endometrium has a characteristic appearance, with brighter, more echogenic tissue than is usually seen in the luteal phase (Fig. 15.1). There is a vague prominence to the arcuate vessels. With magnification of the image, blood flow in individual arcuate vessels can be noted before a chorionic sac is visualized. Although typical of a conception cycle, these findings are not diagnostic and may be seen in the secretory endometrium of a non-conceptional cycle. Visualization of a very decidualized, lush, edematous endometrium about the time of the expected menses suggests but does not diagnose pregnancy.

Chorionic sac

The chorionic sac is often called the gestational sac, which is not an anatomic term. Whatever nomenclature is used, the chorionic sac is the site of maternal–fetal nutrient exchange in the first trimester.[8] It can be seen as early as the 17th day of pregnancy,[9–11] is apparent to most observers a week after the missed period (day 21, or 5 weeks LMP),[12–14] and is the first sign of an intrauterine pregnancy. Sonographically, it appears as a bright, generally uniform echogenic ring—sometimes called the

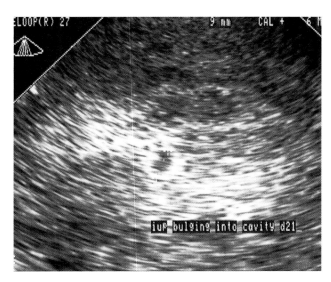

Figure 15.2 Chorionic sac as seen on the 21st day of pregnancy.

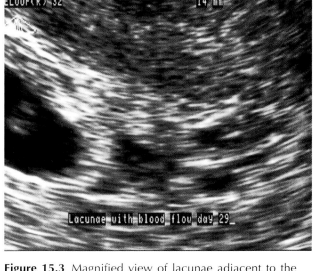

Figure 15.3 Magnified view of lacunae adjacent to the chorionic sac on day 29 of a healthy pregnancy. Blood flow is evident, even without Doppler imaging, as a shimmering in the fluid space.

'rind'—around a dark, round, sonolucent center. This latter is the fluid-filled chorionic cavity, containing the embryonic disc, amnion, secondary yolk sac, and extra-embryonic coelom. These structures are as yet too small to see on US even with maximal magnification, but the fluid of a normal sac surrounded by its characteristic echogenic rind allows for its ultrasonic recognition (*Fig. 15.2*).

The early chorionic sac may be inapparent. In a typical situation with implantation two-thirds of the way up the fundus, a 4 mm chorionic sac will subtend an arc of only 3–4° when imaged transvaginally. Care and persistence are needed to see such a structure, even when using magnification.

The appearance of the rind is the result of invasion of the primary villi into the maternal decidua. Some of these villi will grow and bud out, forming secondary villi, tertiary villi, chorion frondosum, and eventually the placenta. Others regress, resulting in creation of the chorion laeve. At this point, however, the villous projections are omnidirectional, creating a bright sonographic ring around the chorionic cavity. The trophoblast is thicker on the decidua basalis aspect of the implantation than on the decidua capsularis side, probably owing to decreased nutrition available on the capsularis side. This subtle finding is notable with magnification of the image, which will show that the rind is slightly eccentric to the bright line of the endometrial cavity, confirming the fact of implantation and capping off.

The chorionic sac can be reliably detected 20–22 days after ovulation (5 weeks LMP); hCG levels here may be as low as 1000 mIU/ml.[5,14] The early chorionic sac, visualized before the yolk sac becomes evident, will measure 3–5 mm (inner wall to inner wall) and will grow by 1–2 mm/day until the yolk sac, embryonic heart beat, and embryo become apparent.[15] Vascular lacunae are visible in a semicircular ring on the basalis side of the chorionic sac (*Fig. 15.3*). Flow is visible through these vessels, and is readily appreciated by patients in the scanning suite.

Cases of failed intrauterine or ectopic pregnancy may include the accumulation of clear, hydropic cysts in a decidualized endometrium. These must not be confused with a chorionic sac, from which they differ in appearance by lacking a well-defined rind. Fluid accumulations in the non-pregnant uterus can also be mistaken for a chorionic sac (*Fig. 15.4*).

Do not conform rigidly to published growth curves for the chorionic sac and for other early structures. The observer's visual acuity, the use of different equipment, the inability to scan in exactly the same plane twice, and normal biological variability make exact comparisons of measurements unreliable. A study of 107 healthy singleton pregnancies conceived after assisted reproductive treatments, in which the date of conception was precisely known, showed 7- to 10-fold variation of hCG values during days 13–16, and 2- to 3-fold variation in chorionic sac size during days 25–36.[16] Chorionic sac diameter and early crown–rump length correlated to newborn weight, suggesting the inherent biologic variability was being expressed as early as the first

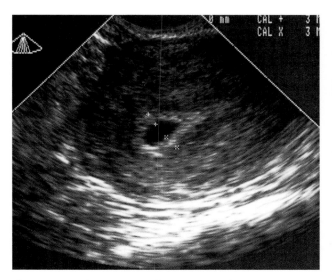

Figure 15.4 This is not a chorionic sac, but an accumulation of fluid in the endometrial cavity of a woman on menopausal estrogen therapy.

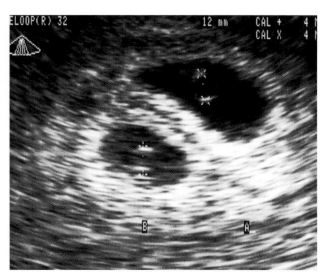

Figure 15.5 Yolk sacs on day 24 of a twin pregnancy. Note that the portions of the sacs parallel to the ultrasound beam are not visible.

weeks after conception. Thus, it is more reliable to scan a pregnancy twice, several days apart, and compare the results to look for appropriate growth, than to compare a single reading to a table derived from an author's experience in another city.

Visualization of the chorionic sac essentially rules out ectopic pregnancy, except in patients who conceive after ovulation induction or assisted reproductive techniques; the incidence of heterotopic pregnancy is greatly increased in such patients over the rate of 1:30 000 in naturally occurring pregnancies.[17–19] Visualization of a normal chorionic sac carries with it a miscarriage rate of 11–20%.[20]

Yolk sac

The next structure visible after the chorionic sac and the first reliable indication of a healthy pregnancy is the yolk sac.[21] This is generally imaged at days 22–24 (5.5 weeks LMP) with the appearance of a pair of parentheses located on the decidua basalis aspect of the chorionic sac, perpendicular to the US beam (*Fig. 15.5*). With growth of the yolk sac, its circular shape becomes apparent (*Fig. 15.6*).

The yolk sac is of embryonic origin and is extra-amniotic. The primary yolk sac was present at the blastocyst stage. The secondary yolk sac protrudes into the extra-embryonic coelom while the amnion develops around the embryo. Initially the yolk sac occupies much of the chorionic sac; typically, before the embryo itself or the embryonic heartbeat are visible the 2–3 mm yolk sac will fill about one-

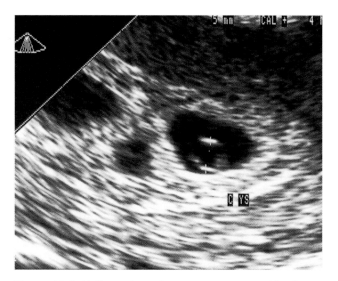

Figure 15.6 Yolk sac in a day 28 pregnancy, with almost the entire circumference of the sac visible.

third of the diameter of the chorionic sac. As the chorionic sac continues to grow and the amnion expands, a 'double bleb' may be noted around day 25 (5.5 weeks LMP), below the yolk sac, before the embryo is visible (*Fig. 15.7*). This finding disappears in only a day or two as the embryo becomes apparent.[22]

As the embryo grows and the yolk sac no longer occupies most of the chorionic sac, the amnion enlarges and envelops the embryo, pushing the yolk

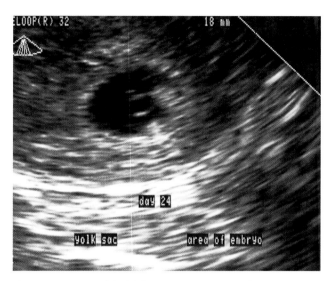

Figure 15.7 'Double bleb' sign as seen on day 24. The embryo, which is not discretely visible, is in the line between the upper bleb (the yolk sac) and the lower.

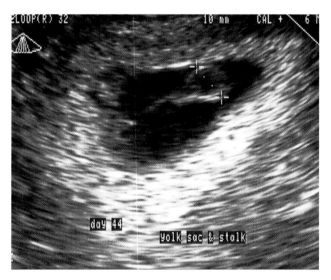

Figure 15.8 Yolk sac and stalk as seen on the 44th day of pregnancy.

sac to the side. The yolk sac grows to be a constant round structure of up to 6 mm in diameter, having a thin bright rim about a sonolucent center. It is connected to the base of the umbilical cord by the fine but unmistakable thread of the yolk stalk (*Fig. 15.8*). Through this stalk, germ cells and red cells migrate into the embryo. This author likes to point out to the parents that the germ cells that will ultimately become their grandchildren are present in the yolk sac. As the amnion grows and eventually fuses with the chorion, the yolk sac becomes

progressively lateral and obscure; by 9 weeks LMP it is actively degenerating in normal pregnancies.[23]

Visualization of the yolk sac precedes that of the embryo and its heartbeat by 3–7 days. The yolk sac allows more certain diagnosis of the chorionic sac by inexperienced sonographers and rules out a pseudosac, thus effectively ruling out ectopic pregnancy.[21] The presence of a normal yolk sac is associated with miscarriage in 8–15% of patients.[22]

Abnormal yolk sacs are uncommon. These can be large (> 6 mm diameter), irregular or infolded (reflecting collapse of the sac), free floating (implying death of the embryo and separation of the embryonic complex from the implantation site), or calcified sacs.[24] If the trophoblast is viable, these signs of embryonic demise will precede the fall in hCG levels. Although growth of the yolk sac is evident through the early first trimester, the size of the yolk sac is not indicative of outcome in cases of first trimester bleeding.[23]

Embryonic heartbeat

After the appearance of the yolk sac, the next sign seen by most observers is the pulsation of the embryonic heart (EHR). The embryo itself may be too small to be seen as a distinct structure until around day 28 (6 weeks LMP). The earliest pulsations of the EHR are visible to the careful observer, using magnification and perhaps M mode (*Figs 15.9* and *15.10*).

The EHR is initially imaged on real-time US as a shutter-like pulsation at the point where the yolk sac joins the wall of the chorionic sac. As the embryo becomes discretely visible after day 30, this enlarges into the pulsation of two parallel lines.[25]

The EHR is initially in the range 80–120 beats per minute (bpm) before day 28 (6 weeks LMP), probably representing impulse generation in the sinus venosus. EHR increases rapidly to 160– 190 bpm by day 47–50 (9 weeks LMP), reflecting the growing competency of the sinoatrial node, and continues in this range into the second trimester, slowing then to the 120–169 bpm range seen in the second and third trimesters.[25–27] This slowing is thought to represent early parasympathetic innervation of the SA node.

In normal pregnancies, EHR correlates with the crown–rump length (CRL) up to a CRL of 23 mm.[26] Until about day 50, serial scans should show a continued and definite increase in the rate of the EHR; a falling heart rate in the first trimester usually indicates a pregnancy destined to abort, both in

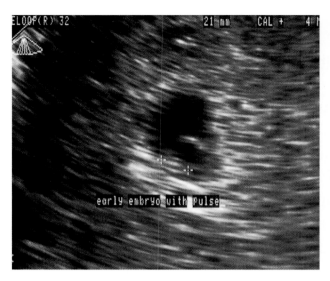

Figure 15.9 Day 27 pregnancy. The yolk sac is visible. The embryo, although inapparent against the wall of the chorionic sac, is made visible by the pulse, noted between the markers.

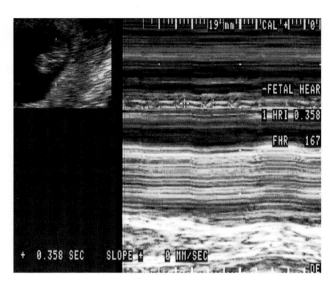

Figure 15.10 M-mode demonstration of the embryonic pulse.

human pregnancies and in animal models.[25,28–30] In the author's experience, this finding predates the fall in hCG values by 3–7 days. Falco et al analysed sonographic findings in cases of first trimester bleeding with a viable embryo, defined as the presence of an EHR.[31] They found that a heart rate < 1.2 SD below the mean of their data predicted abortion, as did discrepancies in the gestational sac size, and a CRL smaller than dates by > 1 week; the probability of death was 6% when none of these factors were present, and 84% when all were.

Multiple pregnancies with concordant increases in EHR between the embryos tend to be maintained as multiples, while those in which one or more embryos display falling heart rates will usually lose the 'bradycardic' embryos and reduce spontaneously to lower order gestations.[32]

The presence of an EHR by day 30 is associated with miscarriage in 10–16% of patients.[25,33] Several studies using abdominal ultrasound techniques showed that only 2–4% of pregnancies will miscarry if the EHR is noted at or after 8 weeks LMP.[34–36]

Crown–rump length

Also called the embryonic pole, fetal pole, early embryonic size, and (most correctly) the greatest embryonic length, the CRL is first noted as a small echogenic focus between the yolk sac and decidua basalis aspect of the chorionic sac, 3–7 days after the yolk sac is seen (*Fig. 15.11*). The EHR should be noted with earliest visualization of the CRL, which

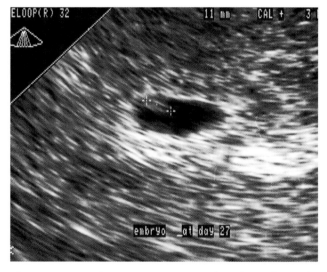

Figure 15.11 Embryonic crown–rump length on the 27th day of pregnancy; the yolk sac is not in the plane of the photograph.

can be distinguished reliably at a size of 2 or 3 mm. Several authors have shown that finding an embryo that is of a given CRL without the EHR being visible is diagnostic of embryonic death; these cut-off values for CRL are 3 and 4 mm, so it is reasonable to expect an EHR in all viable pregnancies of CRL ≥ 5 mm.[37,38] In other words, if an embryo is distinctly seen with CRL of ≥ 5 mm, the EHR should be seen, or the embryo is dead. In embryos of ≤ 4 mm CRL, the finding is non-diagnostic and should be reassessed in 3–7 days.

Early on, the CRL grows about 1 mm per day.[39] Sonographers can roughly date early pregnancies from the CRL using the formula: gestational age = CRL + 42, where gestational age is in days from LMP and CRL is in mm. Two standard deviations from the mean of these data comes to ± 3 days.[40,41] Studies of terminated pregnancies show that ultrasound measurements of CRL are imperfect,[42] and therefore any dates so derived must be viewed in the context of the clinical situation.

Goldstein's data show that the chance of miscarriage is 7.1% if the CRL is up to 5 mm; 3.3% if the CRL is 5–10 mm; and 0.5% if the embryo reaches 10 mm.[20] Thus, a live embryo of 10 mm CRL is extremely reassuring. Because these data may not apply to women with a history of recurrent miscarriage, the author scans such patients at 8–9 weeks LMP. By this time, the EHR should be above 160 bpm and the CRL > 10 mm. Patients who show such embryonic development miscarry < 5% of the time.

Amniotic sac

The amniotic sac develops around the embryo and grows outward in all directions. It displaces the yolk sac and eventually fuses with the chorionic sac. The extra-embryonic coelom is filled with a fluid, presumably derived from the chorionic villi which line it, whereas the amnionic fluid is essentially fetal urine. It is distinct by day 35 (7 weeks LMP (*Fig. 15.12*). Few detailed studies of the normal development of the amniotic sac are available;

however, failure of the sac to grow in all directions towards the chorion may be associated with embryonic bradycardia and death.[43] The presence of a well-defined amniotic sac without the embryo and EHR being visible is diagnostic of embryonic death.[44]

Twins and higher order multiple gestations

One benefit of early US evaluation of pregnancy is the ability to diagnose multiple gestation reliably before it becomes a hazard to the pregnancy and while it can be dealt with. Patients conceiving after ovulation induction or assisted reproductive techniques frequently conceive multiple gestations; one group noted 34 singletons, 11 twins, two triplets, one quadruplet and one quintuplet among 49 consecutive live IVF pregnancies.[45] Presumably, this led to a reconsideration of their transfer protocol! Because of this tendency for the ARTs to produce multiple gestations, most reproductive endocrinologists have had the experience of scanning an early pregnancy and finding three, four, or more sacs (*Fig. 15.13*).

When this occurs, scan the uterus from cornu to cornu, carefully counting sacs; then view from internal os to fundus, again counting sacs. The numbers should agree. A nomenclature should be devised and recorded, describing each sac as A, B, C, etc. according to its location in the uterus. Subsequent scans can be compared to determine which embryos

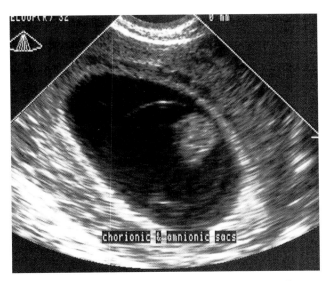

Figure 15.12 Chorionic sac, with amniotic sac inside and completely encircling the embryo. Only a portion of the embryo is visible in this view, taken on about day 44 of pregnancy.

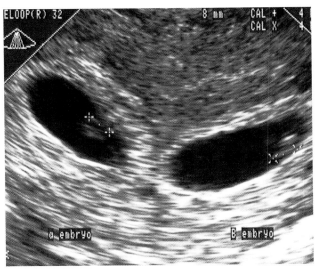

Figure 15.13 Dichorionic twins as seen at the first scan, day 27. Both chorionic sacs contain embryos with crown–rump lengths as marked. A healthy boy and girl were delivered at 37 weeks.

are growing normally and which may not be. These scans are extremely difficult to perform, as it is easy for the operator to lose their bearings and confuse sacs in a uterus littered with chorions. Do not forget to look for a heterotopic pregnancy in the cervix, tubes, and ovaries of these patients.

In some papers, discordant CRL or EHR between members of a multiple gestation predict the demise of the embryo which lags behind its siblings.[32,46,47] Other authors have reported considerable variability in the measurements of ultimately healthy twins and higher order multiples.[46,48] Similarly, the 'per embryo' incidence of embryonic demise has been reported as being higher in multiple pregnancies,[49] and as lower in multiple pregnancies;[47,50] the varying explanations for these observations tend to obscure the fact that with so few cases being reported per paper, random error is likely. Because of the lack of adequate data, it is not known whether the spontaneous loss rate per sac is truly increased or decreased in multiple gestation; however, rates of 5–20% have been reported, which are similar to the rate of loss of similarly aged singleton pregnancies.[32,47,49–51]

Whatever its incidence, the vanishing twin syndrome is real.[52] This is seen on US as one or more chorionic sacs growing normally with normal progression of the EHR and CRL. In another chorionic sac, the yolk sac may not appear, the EHR may not appear or may be slow or may fall off with time, and the CRL may not appear or will consistently lag. These latter chorionic sacs tend to stabilize at a diameter of 20–25 mm and regress in the second trimester (*Fig. 15.14*). This author always informs

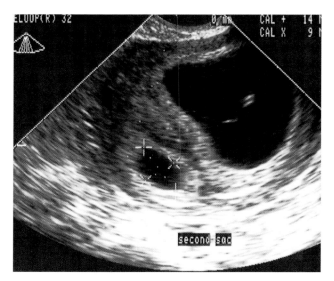

Figure 15.14 Empty chorionic sac in a woman with a vanishing twin.

women carrying triplets of the possibility of embryo reduction; however, since spontaneous embryonic loss is so common, detailed discussions of the ramifications of high order multiple pregnancies are delayed until further embryonic death is unlikely. Since 90% of vanishings occur by 7 weeks from LMP,[49] if an EHR is noted in three or more sacs at or after 7 weeks, the patient is offered counseling regarding embryo reduction.

Monoamniotic twins can be diagnosed after the amnions become evident around day 35 (7 weeks LMP); the normal expansion of the amnion is seen encompassing more than one CRL. This finding, which several authors claim is 100% accurate,[53,54] allows the diagnosis of monoamnionicity more than a month earlier than it can be made by transabdominal US.[55]

A clinical protocol

How can these observations be used to care for patients? This author divides patients into two groups: those in whom the gestational age is precisely known, and those in whom this is not the case.

Patients in whom the gestational age is precisely known include women conceiving on gonadotropins or clomiphene, after isolated acts of intercourse, after donor or intrauterine insemination, after IVF or similar techniques, and those who keep basal body temperature charts which record the dates of intercourse. In all these women, the date of ovulation, insemination, or fertilization is certain enough that the expected appearance of embryologic structures may be dated to within ±1–2 days. Most of these women have iatrogenically abnormal follicular phases, so the LMP should not be used to set the due date.

In patients of known gestational age, minimal effort will allow adequate evaluation of the health of the pregnancy. Knowing the gestational age allows the clinician to have a virtually exact expectation of what the pregnancy should look like on US on a given day. The women in this category usually have histories of infertility or recurrent miscarriage. Thus, the clinician must make every effort to avoid inducing anxiety.

In such patients, this author obtains a quantitative hCG level and serum progesterone with the initial pregnancy test, repeating the hCG 3 days later. If progesterone is normal and hCG has doubled in this time, an initial US is scheduled for day 24–27, by which time the yolk sac is easily visible, and the EHR is generally seen. A normal scan at this visit (i.e. a clear chorionic sac with a recognizable yolk sac) almost rules out ectopic pregnancy, although the rare possibility of heterotopic pregnancy must be considered. Early diagnosis of heterotopic pregnancy allows conservative treatment with preservation of the intrauterine embryos.[56]

If this scan is normal, it is repeated 2 weeks later. By this time the heart rate is easily imaged in the range 150–200 bpm, and embryonic anatomy has progressed to show the cranium and limb buds,[57] making a normal scan at this gestational age a treat for patients. The patient is then returned to the care of her obstetrician, after quoting her a 4% chance of a spontaneous miscarriage.[34–36] For patients with overwhelming anxiety or a history of a previous late first trimester loss, a final scan is obtained around day 50 (9 weeks LMP).

If any step in this evaluation is abnormal, it is repeated. Failure of the initial hCG increase to occur normally suggests an abnormal gestation, but does not define the location of that pregnancy. If further hCG levels fall or plateau, a failed intrauterine or extrauterine gestation is likely, and can usually be managed conservatively by following levels to zero. An US evaluation at day 21 helps to rule out ectopic pregnancy; if no intrauterine pregnancy is diagnosed, re-evaluation in 2–3 days is indicated, with dilation and curettage (D&C), laparoscopy or methotrexate as appropriate. Methotrexate can occasionally be used to treat the woman with an hCG plateau, in whom ectopic or intrauterine gestation is uncertain, thus avoiding D&C or laparoscopy.

If hCG levels have increased and the first scan at day 27 shows no obvious intrauterine pregnancy, an ectopic must be strongly suspected. If an ectopic is not visible in the adnexa, a repeat hCG is warranted to rule out the falling levels of a failed intrauterine pregnancy (IUP), and US 2–3 days later is indicated.

Certain signs are abnormal at any time in the first weeks.[58] These include a consistently falling EHR before around day 40; a chorionic sac > 12 mm mean diameter without a yolk sac; a yolk sac > 6 mm without an EHR or CRL; a CRL > 5 mm without an EHR; and a distinct amniotic sac without CRL. An abnormal scan on day 30 (having already established an IUP) can be defined by failure to note the heart rate, bradycardia (rates < 80 bpm),[25,28,29] or lack of an obvious embryo. Such patients are re-scanned 3–5 days later and action is taken if the pregnancy has not improved. Most early demises require no intervention, but a D&C may be offered in order to obtain chromosome studies and to end the period of waiting in anxious patients.

It is important, however, to keep a certain distance from the intrauterine events. Ultrasound scans carried out too frequently may provide information that is too detailed to interpret rationally. What is a normal US progression between day 28 and 29? Thus, re-evaluating asymptomatic patients of known gestational age, it is often best to let 5–7 days pass. Shorter intervals are appropriate if bleeding is noted and are mandatory if an ectopic is possible.

Patients without known dates of conception require a more elaborate evaluation, because the physician is less certain as to what should be seen at any given scan. What is normal at 25 days is quite abnormal at 35 days; thus, findings suggesting pregnancy failure can result in an erroneous diagnosis of non-viability when applied to an unselected patient population.[59,60] If there is any doubt about the health of an intrauterine pregnancy, give it a chance to prove itself by re-evaluating 3–7 days later. Do not offer termination of a wanted pregnancy based on a single ultrasound, unless it is very clearly non-viable.

To evaluate early pregnancies of uncertain gestational age, start by sitting down with a calendar and obtaining the patient's best estimate of the date of conception. Then, perform a scan and order a quantitative hCG. If these are consistent with the menstrual and sexual histories, assign a due date and introduce the patient into the paradigm for evaluating women of known conceptional age. If the menstrual and sexual histories are less certain, hCG is repeated in 3 days. If the hCG levels rise appropriately and the scan shows a definite intrauterine pregnancy, repeat the scan 7 days later and compare the two scans. Concordance between the scans makes it possible to assign the due date and settle into the paradigm described for women of known gestational age.

Patients in either group with significant bleeding are scanned immediately and have an hCG drawn. Bleeding is very common in early pregnancy, but carries a four-fold increase in the spontaneous abortion rate.[61] Subchorionic hemorrhage, a crescenteric sonolucent collection outside the chorionic sac, is seen in about 20% of live first trimester pregnancies presenting with bleeding[62] (*Figs 15.15* and *15.16*); 30–40% of such cases will miscarry.

If the scan is reassuring in a woman who is bleeding (i.e. normal CRL and EHR, no subchorionic hemorrhage noted), repeat it in 3–4 days if the bleeding continues or in a week if it does not. Patients who lose the presumptive symptoms of pregnancy (nausea, bloating, pelvic fullness) during the first trimester are, in this author's experience,

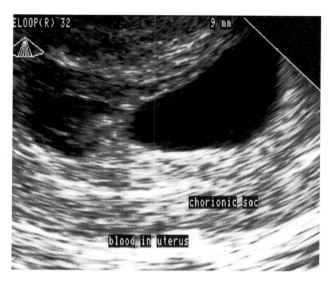

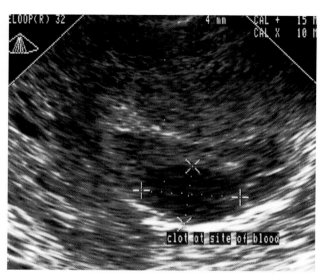

Figure 15.15 Subchorionic hemorrhage. The rind is seen to encompass a collection of clot and blood (left) and a normal-appearing extra-embryonic coelom (right). A healthy pregnancy ultimately delivered, but 5 weeks prematurely.

Figure 15.16 Another image of subchorionic hemorrhage. Fluid blood (outlined by cursors) with surrounding clot are contained within the rind. This view is from the same scan and is taken perpendicular to the view in Fig. 15.15.

virtually destined to miscarry; such a complaint is considered to be the equivalent of bleeding. However, because the transvaginal US examination may push the transducer firmly against the hyper-emic and potentially friable cervix, all pregnant patients are warned to expect slight red spotting on the day of the study and slight brown spotting for a day or two afterwards.

REFERENCES

1. Cullen MT, Green JJ, Reece EA, Hobbins JC. A comparison of transvaginal and abdominal ultrasound in visualizing the first trimester conceptus. *J Ultrasound Med* 1989; **8**:565–569.

2. Pennell RG, Needleman L, Pajak T *et al*. Prospective comparison of vaginal and abdominal sonography in normal early pregnancy. *J Ultrasound Med* 1991; **10**:63–67.

3. Brent RL, Jensh RP, Beckman DA. Medical sonography: reproductive effects and risks. *Teratology* 1991; **44**:123–146.

4. Yip YP, Capriotti C, Rosenthal MS, He BQ, Yip JW. Effect of ultrasound on axonal outgrowth in the sympathetic nervous system of the chick. *Ultrasound Med Biol* 1991; **17**:139–146.

5. Berneshek G, Rudelstorfer R, Csaicsich P. Vaginal sonography versus human chorionic gonadotropin in early detection of pregnancy. *Am J Obstet Gynecol* 1988; **158**:608–612.

6. Yeh HC, Goodman JD, Corr L *et al*. Intradecidual sign: an ultrasound criterion of early intrauterine pregnancy. *Radiology* 1986; **161**:463–467.

7. Dastidar SG, Dastidar KG. Earliest ultrasound finding of implantation? *J Assist Reprod Genet* 1997; **14**:148–151.

8. Campbell J, Wathen N, Perry G, Soneji S, Sourial N, Chard T. The coelomic cavity: an important site of materno-fetal nutrient exchange in the first trimester of pregnancy. *Br J Obstet Gynaecol* 1993; **100**:765–767.

9. Hay DL, de Crespigny LC, McKenna M. Monitoring early pregnancy with transvaginal ultrasound and choriogonadotrophin levels. *Aust NZ J Obstet Gynaecol* 1989; **29**:165–167.

10. Levi CS, Lyons EA, Lindsay DJ. Ultrasound in the first trimester of pregnancy. *Radiol Clin North Am* 1990; **28**:19–38.

11. Jurkovic D, Gruboeck K, Campbell S. Ultrasound features of normal early pregnancy development. *Curr Opin Obstet Gynecol* 1995; **7**:493–504.

12. Pellicer A, Calatayud C, Miró F *et al*. Comparison of implantation and early development of human embryos fertilized in vitro versus in vivo using transvaginal ultrasound. *J Ultrasound Med* 1991; **10**:31–35.

13. Goldstein SR, Snyder JR, Watson C, Danon M. Very early pregnancy detection with endovaginal ultrasound. *Obstet Gynecol* 1988; **72**:200–204.

14. Goldstein I, Zimmer EA, Tamir A, Peretz BA, Paldi E. Evaluation of normal gestational sac growth: appearance of embryonic heartbeat and embryo body movements using the transvaginal technique. *Obstet Gynecol* 1991; **77**:885–888.

15. Daya S, Woods S, Ward S, Lappalainen R, Caco C. Early pregnancy assessment with transvaginal ultrasound scanning. *Can Med Assoc J* 1991; **144**:441–446.

16. Dickey RP, Gasser RF. Ultrasound evidence for variability in the size and development of normal human embryos before the tenth post-insemination week after assisted reproductive technologies. *Human Reprod* 1993; **8**:331–337.

17. Rein MS, DiSalvo DN, Friedman AJ. Heterotopic pregnancy associated with in vitro fertilization and embryo transfer: a possible role for routine vaginal ultrasound. *Fertil Steril* 1989; **51**:1057–1058.

18. Dimitry ES, Subak-Sharpe R, Mills M, Margara R, Winston R. Nine cases of heterotopic pregnancy in 4 years of in vitro fertilization. *Fertil Steril* 1990; **53**:107–110.

19. Molloy D, Deambrosis W, Keeping D, Hynes J, Harrison K, Hennessey J. Multiple-site (heterotopic) pregnancy after in vitro fertilization and gamete intrafallopian transfer. *Fertil Steril* 1990; **53**:1068–1071.

20. Goldstein SR. Early detection of pathological pregnancy by transvaginal ultrasound. *J Clin Ultrasound* 1990; **18**:262–273.

21. Nyberg DA, Mack LA, Harvey D, Wang K. Value of the yolk sac in evaluating early pregnancies. *J Ultrasound Med* 1988; **7**:129–135.

22. Yeh HC, Rabinowitz JG. Amniotic sac development: ultrasound features of early pregnancy—the double bleb sign. *Radiology* 1988; **166**:97–103.

23. Jauniaux E, Jurkovic D, Henriet Y, Rodesch F, Hustin J. Development of the secondary human yolk sac: correlation of sonographic and anatomical features. *Human Reprod* 1991; **6**:1160–1166.

24. Harris RD, Vincent LM, Askin FB. Yolk sac calcification: a sonographic finding associated with intrauterine embryonic demise in the first trimester. *Radiology* 1988; **166**:109–110.

25. Howe RS, Isaacson KJ, Albert JL, Coutifaris CB. Embryonic heart rate in human pregnancy. *J Ultrasound Med* 1991; **10**:367–371.

26. Yapar EG, Ekici E, Gökmen O. First trimester fetal heart rate measurements by transvaginal ultrasound combined with pulsed Doppler: an evaluation of 1331 cases. *Eur J Obstet Gynecol Reprod Biol* 1995; **60**:133–137.

27. Rotsztejn D, Rana N, Dmowski WP. Correlation between fetal heart rate, crown–rump length, and beta-human chorionic gonadotropin levels during the first trimester of well-timed conceptions resulting from infertility treatment. *Fertil Steril* 1993; **59**:1169–1173.

28. Laboda LA, Estroff JA, Benacerraf BR. First trimester bradycardia, a sign of impending fetal loss. *J Ultrasound Med* 1989; **8**:561–563.

29. Achiron R, Tadmor O, Mashiach S. Heart rate as a predictor of first-trimester spontaneous abortion after ultrasound-proven viability. *Obstet Gynecol* 1991; **78**:330–334.

30. Howe RS, Burggren WW, Warburton SJ. Fixed patterns of bradycardia during late embryonic development in domestic fowl with C locus mutations. *Am J Physiol* 1995; **268**:H56–H60.

31. Falco P, Milano V, Pilu G et al. Sonography of pregnancies with first-trimester bleeding and a viable embryo: a study of prognostic indicators by logistic regresison analysis. *Ultrasound Obstet Gynecol* 1996; **7**:165–169.

32. Howe RS, Duncan DE, Hannigan SC, Wiczyk HW. Differences in heart rate as a predictor of early embryonic mortality in multiple pregnancies. *Fertil Steril* 1991; **56**:S133–S134.

33. Keenan JA, Rizvi S, Caudle MR. Fetal loss after early detection of heart motion in infertility patients. *J Reprod Med* 1998; **43**:199–202.

34. Simpson JL, Mills JL, Holmes LB et al. Low fetal loss after ultrasound-proved viability in early pregnancy. *JAMA* 1987; **258**:2555–2557.

35. Cashner KA, Christopher CR, Dysert GA. Spontaneous fetal loss after demonstration of a live fetus in the first trimester. *Obstet Gynecol* 1987; **70**:827–830.

36. MacKenzie WE, Holmes DS, Newton JR. Spontaneous abortion in ultrasonographically viable pregnancies. *Obstet Gynecol* 1987; **71**:81–84.

37. Goldstein SR. Significance of cardiac activity on endovaginal ultrasound in very early embryos. *Obstet Gynecol* 1992; **80**:670–672.

38. Brown DL, Emerson DS, Felker RE, Cartier MS, Smith WC. Diagnosis of early embryonic demise by endovaginal sonography. *J Ultrasound Med* 1990; **9**:631–636.

39. Evans J. Fetal crown–rump length values in the first trimester based upon ovulation timing using the luteinizing hormone surge. *Br J Obstet Gynaecol* 1991; **98**:48–51.

40. Goldstein SR. Embryonic ultrasonographic measurements: crown rump length revisited. *Am J Obstet Gynecol* 1991; **165**:497–501.

41. Silva PD, Mahairas G, Schaper AM, Schauberger CW. Early crown–rump length. A good predictor of gestational age. *J Reprod Med* 1990; **35**:641–644.

42. Harkness LM, Rodger M, Baird DT. Morphological and molecular characteristics of living human fetuses between Carnegie stages 7 and 23: ultrasound scanning and direct measurements. *Human Reprod Update* 1997; **3**:25–33.

43. Birnholz JC, Madares AE. Amniotic fluid accumulation in the first trimester. *J Ultrasound Med* 1995; **14**:597–602.

44. McKenna KM, Feldstein VA, Goldstein RB, Filly RA. The empty amnion: a sign of early pregnancy failure. *J Ultrasound Med* 1995; **14**:117–121.

45. Wax MR, Frates M, Benson CB, Yeh J, Doubilet PM. First trimester findings in pregnancies after in vitro fertilization. *J Ultrasound Med* 1992; **11**:321–325.

46. Dickey RP, Olar TT, Taylor SN et al. Incidence and significance of unequal gestational sac diameter or embryo crown–rump length in twin pregnancy. *Human Reprod* 1992; **7**:1170–1172.

47. Kol S, Levron J, Lewit N, Drugan A, Itskovitz-Eldor J. The natural history of multiple pregnancies after assisted reproduction: is spontaneous fetal demise a clinically significant phenomenon? *Fertil Steril* 1993; **60**:127–130.

48. Check JH, Chase JS, Nowroozi K, Goldsmith G, Dietterich C. Evidence that difference in size of fraternal twins may originate during early gestation: a case report. *Int J Fertil* 1992; **37**:165–166.

49. Manzur A, Goldsman MP, Stone SC, Frederick JL, Balmaceda JP, Asch RH. Outcome of triplet pregnancies after assisted reproductive techniques: how frequent are the vanishing embryos? *Fertil Steril* 1995; **63**:252–257.

50. Botchan A, Yaron Y, Lessing JB et al. When multiple gestational sacs are seen on ultrasound, 'take-home baby' rate improves with in-vitro fertilization. *Human Reprod* 1993; **8**:710–713.

51. Sampson A, de Crespigny LC. Vanishing twins: the frequency of spontaneous reduction of a twin pregnancy. *Ultrasound Obstet Gynecol* 1992; **2**:107–109.

52. Landy HG, Weiner S, Corson SL, Batzer FR, Bolognese RJ. The 'vanishing twin'. Ultrasonographic assessment of fetal disappearance in the first trimester. *Am J Obstet Gynecol* 1986; **155**:14–19.

53. Hill LM, Chenevey P, Hecker J, Martin JG. Sonographic determination of first trimester twin chorionicity and amnionicity. *J Clin Ultrasound* 1996; **24**:305–308.

54. Copperman AB, Kaltenbacher L, Walker B, Sandler B, Bustillo M, Grunfeld L. Early first-trimester ultrasound provides a window through which the chorionicity of twins can be diagnosed in an in vitro fertilization (IVF) population. *J Assist Reprod Genet* 1995; **12**:693–697.

55. Lee CY. Management of monoamniotic twins diagnosed antenatally by ultrasound. *Am J Gynecol Health* 1992; **2**:17–21.

56. Mantzavinos T, Kanakas N, Zourlas PA. Heterotopic pregnancies in an in-vitro fertilization program. *Clin Exp Obstet Gynecol* 1996; **23**:205–208.

57. Timor-Tritsch IE, Peisner DB, Raju S. Sonoembryology: an organ-oriented approach using a high-frequency vaginal probe. *J Clin Ultrasound* 1990; **18**:286–298.

58. Goldstein SR, Kerenyi T, Scher J, Papp C. Correlation between karyotype and ultrasound findings in patients with failed early pregnancy. *Ultrasound Obstet Gynecol* 1996; **8**:314–317.

59. Rowling SE, Coleman BG, Langer JE, Arger PH, Nisenbaum HL, Horii SC. First-trimester US parameters of failed pregnancy. *Radiology* 1997; **203**:211–217.

60. Tadmor OP, Achiron R, Rabinowiz R, Aboulafia Y, Mashiach S, Diamant YZ. Predicting first-trimester spontaneous abortion. Ratio of mean sac diameter to crown–rump length compared to embryonic heart rate. *J Reprod Med* 1994; **39**:459–462.

61. Dantas ZN, Singh AP, Karachalios P, Asch RH, Balmaceda JP, Stone SC. Vaginal bleeding and early pregnancy outcome in an infertile population. *J Assist Reprod Genet* 1996; **13**:212–215.

62. Goldstein SR. Subchorionic bleeding in threatened abortion. Sonographic findings and significance. *Am J Radiol* 1983; **141**:975–978.

16 Early pregnancy failure

Steven R Goldstein

Introduction

Imaging in the infertile couple is obviously an important component of proper diagnosis, therapy, and management in the ongoing quest for couples to achieve a successful pregnancy outcome. The chapter immediately preceding this one dealt with the role of sonography in the diagnosis of early pregnancy. This chapter deals with those less fortunate patients—those in whom conception takes place but the pregnancy is not ongoing and viable. For the purposes of this book this chapter will only deal with pregnancy failure through the embryonic period (70 days from the onset of the last menstrual period (LMP)). After that time, pregnancies would be expected to be turned back over to the obstetrical caregivers and pregnancy failure and imaging aspects of it are outside the scope of this book.

The natural history of early pregnancies, those that progress and those that fail, has long been of interest to obstetrician-gynecologists, and more specifically infertility specialists. In the early 1980s, the new-found ability to measure very low human chorionic gonadotrophin (hCG) levels resulted in numerous studies of the incidence of loss rates in clinically recognized pregnancies[1–3] as well as clinically unrecognized pregnancies that exhibited small and transitory increases in hCG.[4]

Reported pregnancy loss rates after a normal ultrasound study[5–7] using improved high-resolution abdominal ultrasound transducers have wide variations. The timing of scans in early pregnancy and indications for the ultrasound scans varied. In these early studies, findings were compared with menstrual dating rather than anatomic or embryonic structures. Transvaginal ultrasound probes allow assessment of anatomic and embryologic detail not previously appreciated.[8–10]

In a recent study,[11] 232 women with positive urinary pregnancy tests and no antecedent history of vaginal bleeding had endovaginal sonography performed at the initial visit and at subsequent visits as clinically indicated. Patients were followed until delivery, unless sonographic evidence of non-viability was seen, or spontaneous loss occurred.

Twenty-seven losses occurred during the embryonic period, four losses occurred in the fetal period, and there were 201 liveborns. If a gestational sac developed there was a subsequent loss of viability in the embryonic period of 11.5%; with yolk sac it was 8.5%, for an embryo up to 5 mm it was 7.2%, an embryo of 6–10 mm was 3.3%. The fetal loss rate after the embryonic period was 2.0%.

Thus, the rate of early pregnancy demise decreases successively with gestational age and most occur before the end of the embryonic period (70 days after onset of LMP). Subsequent pregnancy losses in the fetal period between 14 and 20 weeks are infrequent. This pattern of early pregnancy demise suggests there is a period of embryonic loss that is distinct from a period of fetal loss. The physiologic significance of the traditional boundary of the first trimester as an appropriate dividing timeline for early pregnancy may be questioned on the basis of these data.

The successful use of ultrasound requires an understanding of how to interpret the findings in early pregnancy failure. Threatened abortion is a clinical term. It is defined as a pregnancy of < 20 weeks with vaginal bleeding and a closed cervical os. In the past it has been the most common indication for a first trimester ultrasound request. It is important to realize, however, that all patients with positive pregnancy tests and vaginal bleeding are also 'r/o ectopic'.

Ultrasound findings in the majority of such patients will show a normal appearing intrauterine gestation (findings will depend on the age of the gestation) with no obvious reason for or source of the clinically apparent vaginal bleeding. If a definitive intrauterine gestation is identified based on the landmarks outlined earlier or the presence of embryonic cardiac activity, then sonography may not provide the clinician with the cause of the vaginal bleeding, but the normal findings should be reassuring to the anxious patient.

Occasionally on initial ultrasound examination the uterus shows no gestational sac and an obvious extrauterine pregnancy is diagnosed. This allows the clinician to proceed immediately to therapeutic intervention.

If initial ultrasound evaluation of the patient who is pregnant and bleeding fails to reveal a definitive intrauterine gestation, then the clinician must resort to following serial β-subunit determinations until they surpass a 'discriminatory zone' of hCG. It should be recognized that a subnormal rate of rise compared to the expected rate for hCG (66% every 48 hours) indicates either a failing intrauterine gestation or an ectopic gestation. At this point curettage and examination of tissue for the presence of villous material (fetal) versus 'decidua only' (maternal) is an important step in triage.

Once the diagnosis of an intrauterine gestation is firmly established by sonographic criteria, whether or not in combination with serial β-subunit determination, further questions may arise regarding the normalcy of that particular gestation.

Intrauterine pregnancy failure

Previously a blighted ovum was thought of as an anembryonic pregnancy. Sonographically this was represented by a gestational sac with a mean sac diameter > 25 mm without embryo (measured by transabdominal techniques). This comes from the classic work by Nyberg et al[12] on the major and minor criteria of abnormal gestational sacs. The vaginal probe has further refined these definitions. In particular, once the sac gets above a mean diameter of 8–10 mm (measurement including only the sonolucent portion of the chorionic cavity) a yolk sac should be visualizable (*Fig. 16.1*). However, the important question is not how early a yolk sac can be seen (threshold level), but rather at what point is the lack of such a structure *absolutely* pathognomonic of non-viable pregnancy, especially allowing for variability in equipment, biology, and measuring error.

Similarly a 'missed abortion' was previously defined as an embryo of some agreed-upon crown–rump length (usually 15 mm) without cardiac activity but not yet spontaneously passed. Cardiac activity

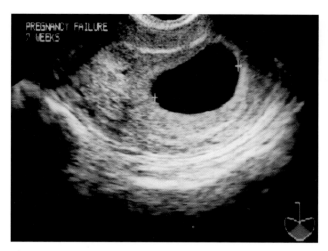

Figure 16.1 Transvaginal sonogram in the long axis reveals a gestational sac of 28 mm (calipers). Patient is 7 weeks from last menstrual period. Failure to develop yolk sac or embryonic structures in a sac of such size is pathognomonic of intrauterine pregnancy failure.

begins 21 days after conception and is actually present before the embryonic structure is large enough to be imaged. This is why M-mode can often detect a cardiac signal from the lateral edge of the visualized yolk sac. Once again the question is not how early can cardiac activity be detected, but at what point is its absence *absolutely* indicative of failed pregnancy. An embryo measuring 5 mm or more with no cardiac activity indicates a failed pregnancy.

Embryonic resorption

The vaginal probe allows the realization that many so-called 'blighted ova' that previously gave the appearance of an empty sac in the days of transabdominal ultrasound are really cases of intrauterine pregnancy failure with subsequent 'embryonic resorption' (*Fig. 16.2*). What is seen sonographically will depend on: (1) at what point in development viability is lost and the resorption process begins, and (2) at what point in that resorption process the patient is studied. Certainly this explains the process by which the multiple pregnancy is spontaneously reduced to a singleton (previously called the vanishing twin). This is also the process by which many singletons become 'blighted ova'. The vaginal probe has often shown a small embryonic structure at 2, 3 or 4 mm demonstrating cardiac activity only to have the patient return 2 weeks later and then demonstrate what appears to be a large empty sac, with or without the ability to see the dead embryo.

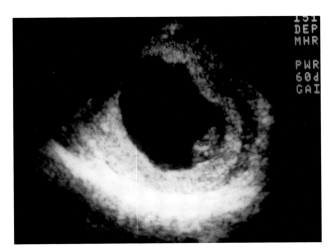

Figure 16.2 Transvaginal sonogram reveals embryonic structure somewhat amorphous in appearance measuring 11 mm. No cardiac activity is discernible. Patient presented with vaginal bleeding in a closed cervical os; 9 days prior, transvaginal sonogram had revealed a 13 mm embryo and cardiac activity present. This is an example of embryonic demise with resorption. In the past such cases viewed transabdominally often appeared to show an 'empty sac'. However, this is not an anembryonic pregnancy and the term blighted ovum should be eliminated.

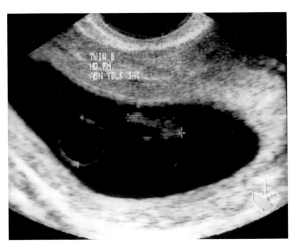

Figure 16.3 Transvaginal sonogram showing an example of hydropic yolk sac measuring 8.8 mm (solid calipers). This was associated with a twin pregnancy in which embryonic demise had occurred. The embryo shown here measuring 11 mm (open calipers) had no cardiac activity.

The incidence of chromosomal abnormalities is generally reported to be increased in cases of early pregnancy failure. Sonographic abnormalities may be seen in cases prior to embryonic visualization, but after the yolk sac has become apparent. Often the yolk sac may be enlarged (*Fig. 16.3*), 'floating', or poorly formed. Remember that the yolk sac, embryonic disc, and amnion are present in the earliest gestational sac, but they are too small to be imaged even by vaginal probe techniques. The yolk sac portion of this complex is imaged first as the complex enlarges, partially because its sonolucent center and echogenic rim make it appear very bright and distinct, as opposed to the early ambiguous echogenic thickening of the embryo which is best recognized by its cardiac pulsations. The endothelial heart tube has folded on itself by 21 days postconception and the cardiovascular system is the first organ system formed in the developing embryo. It too is there and beating, before it can be imaged by current techniques.

hCG levels in pathologic pregnancies—whether they are rising or falling and at what rate—will be a function of the condition of trophoblastic tissue, not the embryonic structures. Sonographically this is depicted by the echogenic rind (trophoblastic decidual reaction). Many cases of intrauterine pregnancy

failure will have high levels of hCG and seemingly normal appearing villi at the time of curettage. Others will have much lower hCG levels associated with very poor trophoblastic decidual reaction. This may represent separate etiologies with mechanisms such as poor implantation, inadequate blood supply, or poor flow versus a 'fetal factor' such as abnormal chromosomal number or poor embryonic cleavage. However, such cases may also represent the same process merely observed at different points along a naturally occurring 'timeline'.

Ectopic pregnancy

Ectopic pregnancy is a complex subject. From a sonographic perspective the presence of a definitive intrauterine pregnancy virtually excludes ectopic pregnancy. Heterotopic pregnancy (a simultaneous intra- and extra-uterine pregnancy) is said to occur in 1:30 000 spontaneous pregnancies.[13] However, in women undergoing reproductive assistance this will increase to about 1:6000.[14,15] The ability to definitely diagnose an intrauterine pregnancy will rely on the milestones outlined above. When no intrauterine gestation is seen on ultrasound the quantitative hCG level must be determined and the concept of a discriminatory level (already described above both for transvaginal and transabdominal ultrasound) employed. If the hCG level is less than the discriminatory level then the concept popularly known as serial β-subunit determination must be employed. hCG will rise by 66% every 48 hours or effectively double every 3 days in a normal pregnancy. Once the hCG level surpasses a discriminatory level an intrauterine gestation should be imaged. The absence of an intrauterine gestation suggests that the pregnancy is not capable of continuing, i.e. it represents either a failing intrauterine gestation or an extrauterine pregnancy. Similarly a subnormal rate of rise of hCG also indicates a failing intrauterine gestation or extrauterine pregnancy. In such cases, since ongoing normal pregnancy has been excluded, curettage and examination of tissue for the presence or absence of chorionic villi may be useful as a next step in triage. The presence of chorionic villi proves an intrauterine gestation. The presence of decidual tissue only raises the index of suspicion for ectopic, although, especially with previous bleeding, complete abortion (possibly tubal as well) can account for such findings. Follow-up quantitative hCG level, whether rising or plateauing or falling, may help to distinguish ectopic from completed abortion. Some intrauterine fluid collections may look like gestational sacs. The presence of the yolk sac precludes a diagnosis of such pseudosacs. If any doubt exists about the legitimacy or normalcy of a gestational sac prior to yolk sac or embryo being present, a follow-up ultrasound scan is warranted.

Extrauterine findings on ultrasound will reflect in vivo findings. In all, 15–28% of ectopics will develop to the point of yolk sac and/or cardiac activity[16–18] (*Fig. 16.4*). Obviously such pregnancies will often follow the normal doubling times of hCG. Furthermore, the familiar gestational sac appearance with its sonolucent center will be seen more easily on ultrasound. This will be especially true if cardiac activity is present. Likewise, not all sonolucent or complex adnexal structures will be extrauterine gestations. The ovaries should be identified on the side in question to avoid calling a corpus luteum or corpus luteum cyst an extrauterine gestation. Finally free fluid in the cul-de-sac may be helpful but is not pathognomonic—it is present in 41–83% of extrauterine pregnancies.[17,18]

New considerations for pregnancy failure

Increasingly pregnancies are being and will be diagnosed as having failed prior to spontaneous passage. There may indeed be a role for cytogenetic analysis as a first step in triage to determine if any further workup is indicated.

Chromosomal pregnancy failure

Various studies show that up to 70% of spontaneous abortions will exhibit abnormal chromosomes.[19] Byrne et al[20] attempted to correlate gross morphology of abortus material with its karyotype and found that various developmental levels could be associated with the various chromosomal anomalies. Thus trisomies 13, 18, and 21, unlike other trisomies, were more often associated with fetuses and less often with tissue fragments. Focal malformations were multiple and severe in abortuses with triploidy, trisomies 13 and 18, and monosomy X, but tended to be and were mild in trisomy 21.

A more recent study[21] utilized endovaginal ultrasound transducers of 5–7.5 MHz. This was the first study to utilize more current concepts of ultrasound landmarks of normal pregnancy and ultrasound indications of definitive pregnancy failure.[21]

The ultrasound appearance of early pregnancy failure in terms of furthest anatomic landmark reached appears not to be significantly different in cases of normal or abnormal karyotypes. However, it does appear that an abnormal and/or enlarged yolk sac is a non-specific finding of failed pregnancy and does not seem to correlate with karyotypic status. Presumably such an anatomic appearance of the yolk sac is secondary to hydropic change.

It also appears that some karyotypic abnormalities (trisomy 22, mosaics, monosomy X) seem to develop further prior to embryonic demise than do others (trisomy 16, multiple trisomies, and other unusual variants). Perhaps in the future such information may help to show which chromosomes are involved

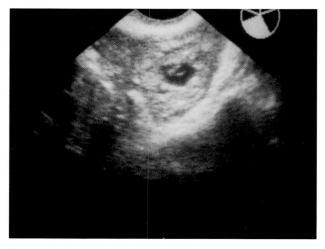

Figure 16.4 Transvaginal pelvic scan of a patient with a right ectopic pregnancy at 45 days from the last menstrual period. Such ectopics that ultimately form a gestational sac with yolk sac and embryo will be the ones that also display normal doubling times of hCG.

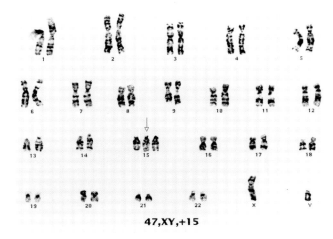

47,XY,+15

Figure 16.5 Karyotype of a patient with intrauterine pregnancy failure. Curettage and examination of the tissue for karyotypic analysis revealed trisomy 15.

in the clinical expression of different developmental defects.

The majority of these chromosomal abnormalities are numerical owing to errors occurring during gonadogenesis (chromosomal non-dysjunction during meiosis) (*Fig. 16.5*), fertilization (triploidy from dispermy), or the first division of the fertilized ovum (tetraploidy or mosaicism). Of the overall abnormalities two-thirds will be autosomal trisomies, followed by monosomy X and structural rearrangements. Thus, except for a very small percentage of parental balanced translocations or inversions, the overwhelming majority of these women whose failed pregnancies have abnormal karyotypes would not be expected to show repetitive pregnancy failure.

Non-chromosomal failure

The reasons for non-chromosomal pregnancy failure include uterine abnormalities, luteal phase defects, immunologic factors, infectious agents, alcohol, and smoking, as well as occasional molecular genetic abnormalities lethal to the embryo.

New approach

With the first failed pregnancy cytogenetic analysis of the conceptus will be helpful in subsequent management. If the chromosomes of the conceptus are normal the couple can undergo evaluation of the various other causes discussed above. However, if the chromosomes of the conceptus are abnormal, then no further workup or evaluation should be necessary at that time and the likelihood of recurrent loss is very small (unless multiple factors are at play).

Increasingly failed pregnancies can and should be offered chromosomal analysis. There are two advances that make such an approach possible. First, high resolution endovaginal ultrasound transducers have enhanced the understanding of early pregnancy and its normal milestones. This yields an ability to consistently diagnose pregnancy failure prior to spontaneous passage. Ultrasound is employed at the first examination after the missed menses, usually with a positive home monoclonal antibody pregnancy test. The patient is then reassessed every 2 weeks until the embryo is > 10 mm with cardiac activity. The embryonic loss rate at that point is < 1%. If intrauterine pregnancy failure is diagnosed sonographically, then elective dilatation and curettage are carried out the following day prior to the patient's cramping, bleeding, and spontaneous passage.

The second advance is the routine examination of tissue from curettage for the presence or absence of chorionic villi versus maternal decidua. While initially done to diagnose unsuspected ectopic pregnancy at the time of elective termination, such examination of tissue in cases of failed intrauterine pregnancy allows a portion of chorion and attached villi to be separated from maternal decidua and submitted for chromosomal study. This avoids the maternal contamination (46XX) that precludes merely submitting 'products of conception' for such chromosomal studies. Also, since normal cells will grow better in tissue culture, it seems plausible that some of the spontaneous abortion material karyotyped in old studies may well have represented false negative cases with contamination of maternal decidua.

Increasingly, pregnancy failure is and will be diagnosed prior to spontaneous passage. Increasingly, clinicians who have spent 4 months in gynecologic pathology as residents will be able to distinguish chorion and attached villi from maternal decidua. Such embryonic tissue can easily be used for cytogenetic evaluation. The cases with abnormal karyotypes require no further evaluation and should conceive again as soon as possible. The failed pregnancies with normal karyotypes need not await subsequent loss, but can immediately be evaluated as for lupus anticoagulant and anticardiolipin antibodies, luteal phase deficiencies, endometrial (and possible cervical) *Ureasplasma urealyticum* infection, congenital Müllerian abnormalities, and submucous myomas.

Summary

Early pregnancy can be best divided into embryonic and fetal periods (dividing line 70 days LMP) which more naturally reflect developmental changes, morphologic appearance, loss rates, and concerns about teratogens. Newer endovaginal probes and a better understanding of anatomic landmarks and expected growth rates can improve clinical management and patient counseling. Karyotyping of failed pregnancy can often give families a definite diagnosis and identify couples at risk for recurrence.

REFERENCES

1. Miller JF, Williamson E, Glue J et al. Fetal loss after implantation: a prospective study. *Lancet* 1980; **ii**:554–556.

2. Edmonds DK, Lindsay KS, Miller JF et al. Early embryonic mortality in women. *Fertil Steril* 1982; **38**:447–453.

3. Whittaker PG, Taylor A, Lind T. Unsuspected pregnancy loss in healthy women. *Lancet* 1983; **i**:1126–1127.

4. Wilcox AJ, Weinberg CR, O'Connor JF et al. Incidence of early pregnancy loss. *N Engl J Med* 1988; **319**:189–194.

5. Gilmore DH, McNay MB. Spontaneous fetal loss rate in early pregnancy. *Lancet* 1985; **i**:107–109.

6. Wilson RD, Kendrick V, Wittmann BK et al. Spontaneous abortion and pregnancy outcome after normal first trimester ultrasound examination. *Obstet Gynecol* 1986; **67**:352–355.

7. Simpson JL, Mills JL, Holmes LB et al. Low fetal loss rates after ultrasound-proved viability in early pregnancy. *JAMA* 1987; **258**:2555–2557.

8. Goldstein SR, Snyder JR, Watson C, Danon M. Very early pregnancy detection with endovaginal ultrasound. *Obstet Gynecol* 1988; **72**:200–204.

9. Fine C, Cartier M, Doubilet P. Fetal heart rates: values throughout gestation. *J Ultrasound Med* 1988; **7**:S105–S106.

10. Timor-Tritsch I, Peisner D, Raju S. Sonoembryology: an organ oriented approach using a high frequency vaginal probe. *J Clin Ultrasound* 1990; **18**:286–298.

11. Goldstein SR. Embryonic demise in early pregnancy: a new look at the first trimester. *Obstet Gynecol* 1994; **84**:294–298.

12. Nyberg DA, Filly RA, Filho DL, Laing FC, Mahony BS. Abnormal pregnancy: early diagnosis by ultrasound and serum chorionic gonadotropin levels. *Radiology* 1986; **158**:393–396.

13. DeVoe RW, Pratt JH. Simultaneous intrauterine and extrauterine pregnancy. *Am J Obstet Gynecol* 1948; **56**:1119–1126.

14. Gamberdella FR, Marrs RP. Heterotopic pregnancy associated with assisted reproductive technology. *Am J Obstet Gynecol* 1989; **160**:1520–1524.

15. Dimitry ES, Subak-Sharpe R, Mills M, Margara R, Winston R. Nine cases of heterotopic pregnancies in 4 years of in vitro fertilization. *Fertil Steril* 1990; **53**:107–110.

16. Stiller RJ, de Regt RH, Blair E. Transvaginal ultrasonography in patients at risk for ectopic pregnancy. *Am J Obstet Gynecol* 1989; **161**:930–933.

17. Fleischer AC, Pennell RG, McKee MS et al. Ectopic pregnancy: features at transvaginal sonography. *Radiology* 1990; **174**:375–378.

18. de Crespigny LC. Demonstration of ectopic pregnancy by transvaginal ultrasound. *Br J Obstet Gynaecol* 1988; **95**:1253–1256.

19. Ohno M, Maeda T, Matsunobo A. A cytogenetic study of spontaneous abortions with direct analysis of chorionic villi. *Obstet Gynecol* 1991; **77**:394–398.

20. Byrne J, Warburton D, Kline J et al. Morphology of early fetal deaths and their chromosomal characteristics. *Teratology* 1985; **32**:297–315.

21. Goldstein SR, Kerenyi T, Scher J, Papp C. Correlation between karyotype and ultrasound findings in patients with failed early pregnancy. *Ultrasound Obstet Gynecol* 1996; **8**:314–317.

17 Ectopic pregnancy

Mary C Frates

Ectopic pregnancy (EP) is defined as the implantation and growth of products of conception outside the uterus. It occurs in 1–2% of all pregnancies in the general population,[1] and more frequently in patients undergoing treatment for infertility. EP results in significant morbidity for women of childbearing age. In the USA, complications from EP are the leading cause of pregnancy-related death during the first trimester. Despite a 22-year increase in the rate of EP,[1] the morbidity and mortality associated with these pregnancies has decreased over the same time period. Much of this decrease is related to early, prompt diagnosis. Ultrasonography is at the forefront of evaluating patients for ectopic pregnancy, with transvaginal imaging of particular importance. This chapter will review the use of ultrasound in the diagnosis of EP, present ways to optimize imaging technique, review several of the more unusual forms of ectopic pregnancy, and, finally, consider the role of ultrasound in treatment.

with a transabdominal approach through a physiologically distended bladder. However, transabdominal scanning is often inconclusive, except when a live intrauterine embryo is seen. Transvaginal sonography is more likely to diagnose an early intrauterine or ectopic pregnancy.[4,5] A normal intrauterine gestational sac can be identified as early as 5 weeks menstrual age with transvaginal sonography (*Fig. 17.1*). The examination is rapid and well tolerated by patients. Transvaginal sonography may provide added benefit in symptomatic patients who prove to have intrauterine gestations, by localizing the source of pain.

Once a normal or abnormal intrauterine pregnancy has been identified at transvaginal sonography, the diagnosis of EP is virtually excluded in the general population, owing to the extremely low frequency of heterotopic pregnancy (1:7000).[6] However, the rate of occurrence of heterotopic pregnancy is signifi-

Sonographic evaluation

The classical presentation of patients with EP is the triad of pain, vaginal bleeding, and an adnexal mass. However, these components are all non-specific and most patients with this presentation are not pregnant.[2] Because of this, a pregnancy test should be part of the initial workup of any woman of childbearing age with pelvic symptoms. If the pregnancy test is positive, symptomatic patients should proceed to ultrasound for further evaluation. Pregnant patients with known risk factors for EP, such as assisted fertilization, pre-existing tubal disease, prior tubal surgery, DES exposure, or previous EP, should also undergo early first trimester sonography to establish the intrauterine location of the gestational sac, even if they are asymptomatic.[3]

The sonographic examination is typically performed transvaginally. Prior to the development of transvaginal probes, pelvic sonography was performed

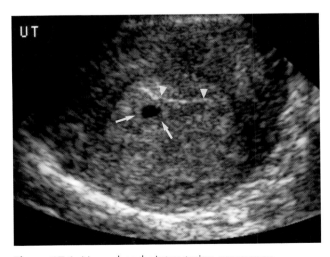

Figure 17.1 Normal early intrauterine pregnancy. Longitudinal transvaginal sonogram of the uterus shows the intradecidual location of a normal 5-week intrauterine pregnancy (arrows), just posterior to the thin echogenic endometrial stripe (arrowheads).

cantly higher following assisted reproduction.[7] Therefore, even when an intrauterine gestation has been identified, careful evaluation of the adnexa is required, particularly in patients complaining of pain or following fertility treatment.

If no identifiable intrauterine gestational sac is found in a patient with a positive pregnancy test, there are three diagnostic alternatives: a recent spontaneous abortion, an early intrauterine pregnancy too small for sonographic identification, or an EP. In this situation, quantitative analysis of the serum β-human chorionic gonadotropin (β-hCG) may be useful. β-hCG is produced by trophoblastic tissue beginning 8 days after conception,[8] and in a normal gestation it doubles approximately every 48 hours. A normal intrauterine gestational sac can usually be seen by transvaginal sonography with a β-hCG value of ≥ 1000 mIU/ml (International Reference Preparation (IRP)).[9] If the β-hCG is < 1000 mIU/ml (IRP), an early normal intrauterine pregnancy may not be visible sonographically. In this instance, serial quantitative β-hCG levels along with serial transvaginal sonography should be performed until the pregnancy is identified. When no intrauterine sac is found with a β-hCG level above 1000 mIU/ml and there is no history of products of conception being passed, the possibility of an ectopic pregnancy is high. However, in some of these cases, a normal intrauterine gestation is found at later transvaginal sonography.[10] Therefore, before treating a patient with a desired but as yet unidentified pregnancy with an intervention that could jeopardize an intrauterine gestation, additional close follow-up is warranted.

The most common sonographic finding in a patient at risk for EP is an intrauterine pregnancy. In a normal pregnancy, a yolk sac can be identified during transvaginal sonography when the mean gestational sac diameter (MSD) is 8 mm, or at approximately 5.5 weeks gestational age. By 6.0 weeks, cardiac activity is usually seen. Likewise, cardiac activity is usually visible if the MSD is ≥ 16 mm (6.5 weeks gestational age), and absence of a heart beat at this sac size has been considered by many sonologists as synonymous with pregnancy failure.[11] The diagnosis of pregnancy failure should be made carefully. Some patients with MSDs of ≥ 16 mm and absent cardiac activity can subsequently develop an embryo with a heartbeat and have normal outcomes.[12] This important fact indicates that follow-up examinations are warranted in many such cases before diagnosing pregnancy failure in an individual patient.

If an intrauterine fluid collection is identified which is not a normal gestational sac, the finding may represent an abnormal intrauterine pregnancy or a

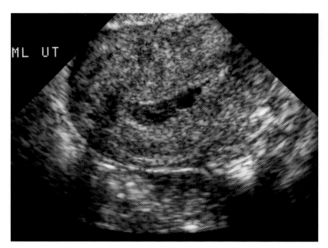

Figure 17.2 Pseudogestational sac. An intrauterine pseudogestational sac may be found in association with an ectopic pregnancy. In this patient, the sonogram shows a complex intrauterine fluid collection with internal debris, located within the endometrial cavity. The sonographic appearance of a pseudogestational sac is extremely variable.

pseudosac related to an ectopic pregnancy. While at times it can be difficult to differentiate a pseudosac from an early gestational sac, particularly an abnormal one, several criteria can be useful. A normal early gestational sac is round, has a thick, smooth echogenic margin, and is intradecidual in location. It often contains a yolk sac (see *Fig. 17.1*). A pseudosac is typically elongated, somewhat irregular in shape, and located within the endometrial cavity (*Fig. 17.2*).[13] It rarely has the thick, smooth, echogenic margin seen with a normal intrauterine sac. Pseudosacs result from prominent decidual reaction surrounding centrally located endometrial fluid. They may be found in 5–10% of patients with EP.[4,14] A pseudosac may contain internal debris that mimics embryonic tissue. If a pseudosac cannot be differentiated from an abnormal intrauterine gestation, it may be necessary to perform uterine dilatation and curettage once there is no possibility of a normal gestation. This procedure can confirm the intrauterine location of the pregnancy with retrieval of chorionic villi. Absence of villi suggests a persistent EP. While examining the uterus of a pregnant patient in the absence of a gestational sac or pseudosac, evaluation of the endometrial stripe may be of help. Both a multilayered appearance of the endometrium and a thin (< 8 mm) endometrial stripe have been reported as suggestive for ectopic pregnancy in small series.[15,16]

As the sonographic search for an ectopic pregnancy moves to the adnexa, the ovary can be used as a starting point. The ovary can most often be found just medial to the iliac vessels. Once the ovary has been localized and evaluated, the surrounding tissues should be carefully scanned for the presence of a mass or ring-like structure created by an EP within the fallopian tube. The ampullary portion of the tube is the most frequent site of ectopic implantation,[17] and it is located immediately adjacent to the ovary in most patients. Lack of peristalsis should help differentiate a mass from a loop of bowel. Overlying bowel gas that could obscure a mass can be displaced if either the examiner or the patient applies firm steady pressure over the patient's right or left lower quadrant. Any area that is particularly sensitive or painful for the patient during the examination should be considered suspicious and examined carefully, as the tenderness may correspond to the location of the EP. Most EPs are found between the ovary and uterus; however, because they can be located anywhere in the pelvis, the examination should always include the cul-de-sac as well as the superior and lateral margins of the pelvis. A brief transabdominal examination should be added if the EP cannot be identified with transvaginal sonography.[18]

The appearance of an adnexal ectopic pregnancy varies widely at transvaginal sonography. In up to 71% of patients, an echogenic ring surrounding an anechoic center can be identified, the so-called adnexal or tubal ring (*Fig. 17.3*).[19] With close observation, the ring can be seen to contain a fetal pole or yolk sac in a number of patients. In 8–15% of patients with a tubal ring, cardiac activity is found (*Fig. 17.4*).[19–22] A hematosalpinx may be seen in

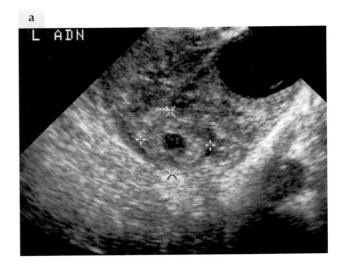

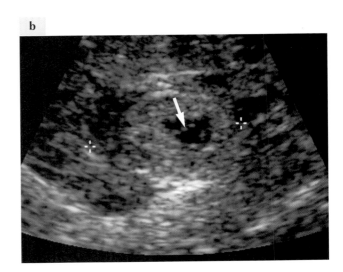

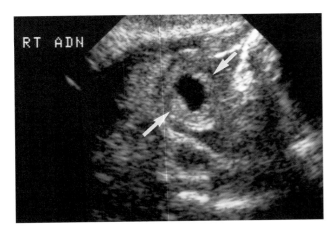

Figure 17.3 Adnexal ring of an ectopic pregnancy. Transvaginal sonogram in a patient with right-sided pelvic pain, a positive pregnancy test and no intrauterine pregnancy. Coronal image of the right adnexa shows an adnexal ring with an anechoic center and a bright echogenic periphery (arrows). This mass was clearly separate from the right ovary (not shown).

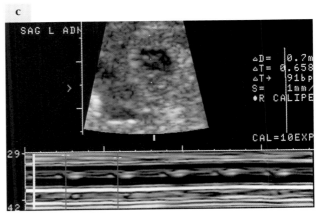

Figure 17.4 Adnexal ring with yolk sac and cardiac activity. While the adnexal ring of an ectopic pregnancy is often empty, close observation may reveal a yolk sac, embryo, or cardiac activity. (a) A well-defined echogenic tubal ring is outlined by calipers in the left adnexa. (b) Further imaging in the same patient revealed a yolk sac (arrow) within the ring. (c) Cardiac activity at 91 beats per minute (bpm) could also be appreciated.

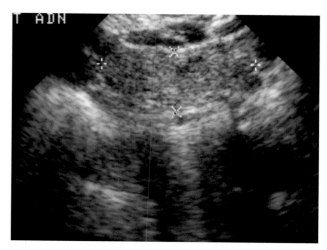

Figure 17.5 Hematosalpinx. In this transvaginal examination of a patient with no intrauterine gestation, a solid, tubular echogenic mass (calipers) representing a blood-filled fallopian tube was found in the right adnexa. Any non-cystic, non-ovarian mass should be considered as highly suspicious for ectopic pregnancy in the appropriate clinical situation.

some patients, filled with echogenic debris from blood or products of conception (*Fig. 17.5*). Rarely, ectopic trophoblastic tissue is identified within the enlarged tube (*Fig. 17.6*). In other patients, the finding is simply a complex adnexal mass of mixed echogenicity with poorly defined borders. This appearance is likely to represent a hematoma that

may or may not contain the ectopic trophoblastic tissue. In these cases, meticulous scanning can sometimes reveal the bright, echogenic ring of trophoblastic tissue buried deep in the mass, confirming the diagnosis of EP (*Fig. 17.7*).

If the adnexal mass of an ectopic pregnancy is small in size, it may be quite subtle as well as non-tender. This limits the ability of transvaginal sonography to diagnose ectopic pregnancy, particularly in patients undergoing treatment for infertility, because this group is typically studied at 5–6 gestational weeks. While early scanning may allow detection of an asymptomatic EP, optimal scanning technique as well as a high level of suspicion are required to demonstrate a subtle finding such as a tiny tubal ring. Follow-up examinations and serial β-hCG levels are frequently useful in this patient population.

The identification of a complex intraovarian lesion should not be considered suspicious for an EP. Simple ovarian cysts are typically unruptured follicular cysts, and complex intraovarian lesions usually represent the corpus luteum. True ovarian pregnancies constitute < 1% of all EPs,[23] and may not be diagnosable at sonography without central identifying characteristics such as a yolk sac, embryonic pole, or cardiac activity. The laterality of the corpus luteum (right versus left) does not provide useful information for the site of an EP, since up to one-third of ectopic pregnancies implant on the opposite site from the corpus luteum.[24]

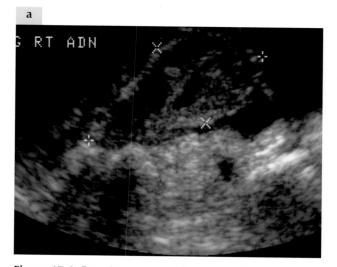

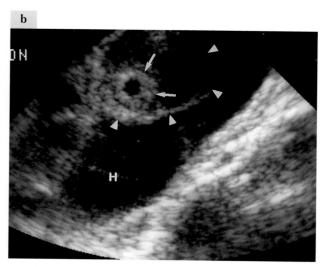

Figure 17.6 Ectopic pregnancy localized within the fallopian tube. The examiner may rarely appreciate an extrauterine gestational sac implanted within the wall of a dilated fallopian tube. (a) In this sagittal transvaginal sonogram of the right adnexa, a dilated fallopian tube with internal debris is outlined by calipers. (b) Coronal imaging of the tube demonstrates the echogenic trophoblast implanted on the internal wall of the tube (arrows). The lumen of the tube is filled with echoes, consistent with blood. The outer margins of the tube (arrowheads) are clearly defined by the surrounding hemoperitoneum (H).

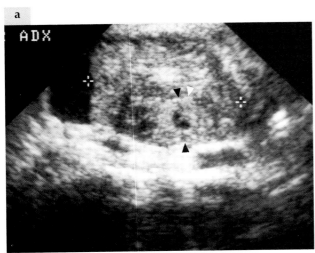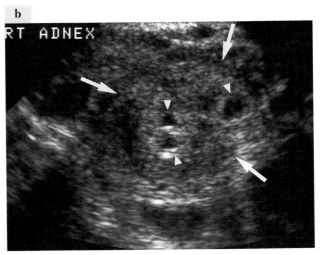

Figure 17.7 Large mass with central tubal ring. The adnexal mass of an ectopic pregnancy often appears complex. With careful scanning, additional characterization of the mass is sometimes possible. (a) Coronal sonogram of the right adnexa shows a 3.6 cm heterogeneous mass (outlined by calipers). Within the mass, a tubal ring (arrowheads) containing a yolk sac can be seen. (b) Sagittal image of the right adnexa in a different patient. There is a large, poorly defined, heterogeneous mass (arrows). Meticulous scanning of the mass reveals three small adnexal rings (arrowheads) that each contain a central yolk sac. This patient had recently undergone embryo transfer. Three of the embryos implanted into the fallopian tube at a single site.

Because of the wide range of transvaginal sonographic criteria used to diagnose ectopic pregnancy,[9,19–20,22,25] the reported accuracy of this examination varies considerably. The specificity ranges from 100% for an extrauterine gestational sac with a yolk sac or embryo (sensitivity of 15–20%) to 93–99.5% for a complex adnexal mass (sensitivity of anywhere from 21–84%) to a low of 69% for free intraperitoneal fluid.[22,25] In an attempt to determine the performance characteristics for these diagnostic criteria, the results of 10 previously reported studies were recently combined and analysed.[22] The results of this meta-analysis suggest that in patients clinically suspected to have an EP, the best diagnostic criterion was the identification of any non-cystic, extraovarian adnexal mass. This criterion included living ectopic pregnancies, tubal rings, and complex cystic or solid masses, and had both a high specificity (98.9%) and high positive predictive value (96.3%). The sensitivity of 84.4% and negative predictive value of 94.8% were also acceptable. In summary, in a pregnant patient without an intrauterine gestation, EP should be diagnosed when any non-simple non-ovarian adnexal lesion is identified at transvaginal sonography.

In up to one-third of women with EP, an adnexal mass cannot be found despite optimal sonographic technique.[14,21,25] In these patients, free intraperitoneal fluid may be helpful for suggesting the diagnosis. Any amount of cul-de-sac fluid more than a trace should be considered abnormal. It is important to examine the upper abdomen in these instances, to evaluate for large quantities of free fluid. While the least specific criterion for diagnosing EP is free intraperitoneal fluid in the absence of an adnexal mass, isolated free fluid is found in approximately 15% of patients with proven EP.[25] The free fluid associated with ectopic pregnancy is most often blood, the sources of which include tubal rupture, tubal abortion (spontaneous extrusion of the products of conception from the free end of the tube) and active bleeding from the fimbriated end of the fallopian tube.[21,25] Rarely, the fluid originates from a leaking or ruptured corpus luteum.

While any free fluid increases the likelihood of EP, fluid with internal echoes is of particular concern, because it suggests hemoperitoneum (*Fig. 17.8*). Echogenic free fluid is reported in 28–56% of patients with EP.[21,25] The echoes can be subtle, and optimal gain settings are required. If the gain control is adjusted to a level that is just beneath introducing artifactual echoes into urine within the bladder, echoes or even a fluid/debris level may be appreciated within the intraperitoneal fluid. Clotted blood can appear as a poorly defined echogenic mass or masses, separate from the mass of the EP. These clots frequently settle into the cul-de-sac. Alternatively, hemoperitoneum may appear completely anechoic.[25]

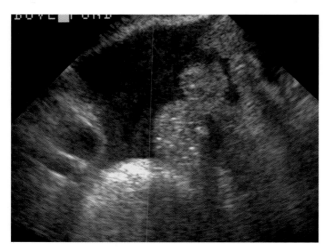

Figure 17.8 Echogenic free fluid. Free fluid containing internal echoes is of particular concern, as it most often represents hemoperitoneum. It is reported in more than half of patients with ectopic pregnancy. Transvaginal sonogram of the region just superior to the uterine fundus shows echogenic free fluid indicative of intraperitoneal blood in this patient with a live adnexal ectopic (not shown).

Infrequently, despite careful transvaginal and transabdominal imaging, there are no positive findings and the examination results are entirely normal. The negative predictive value of transvaginal sonography is approximately 95%.[22] However, in patients at risk for EP, this statistic should not be considered reassuring. A recent series reported four patients with entirely normal sonograms who had surgically proved EP and fallopian tube rupture within 24 hours of the ultrasound.[21] In a high risk population, continued clinical and sonographic monitoring is necessary until the pregnancy location is established. In patients with large uterine fibroids, pre-existing adnexal disease, or morbid obesity, the diagnostic accuracy of sonography for ectopic pregnancy can be quite limited, and caution should be used in interpreting negative sonographic results.[24]

With the addition of color and pulsed Doppler imaging capabilities to the vaginal probe, several different applications for Doppler sonography have been proposed, with the hope of increasing diagnostic accuracy for ectopic pregnancy. The reader is referred to Chapter 19 for a complete discussion on this topic.

Following the diagnosis of ectopic pregnancy, further characterization of the adnexal mass has been attempted, in an effort to determine whether the involved fallopian tube is intact or ruptured.

This information would be useful in situations in which medical management of the EP is being considered, because non-surgical management of a tubal gestation requires an intact tube prior to and during treatment.[26–29]

Several authors consider the finding of a tubal ring, with or without a yolk sac, embryo, or cardiac activity, indicative of an intact fallopian tube.[20,30] Others disagree, reporting that rupture may coexist with a tubal ring.[31] In one recent retrospective study of 132 patients with surgically proved EP, fallopian tube rupture was found in 38% of patients with tubal rings. Additionally, in 21% of patients lacking an adnexal mass, tubal rupture was evident at surgery.[21]

Negative findings at sonography, such as the absence of a large amount of intraperitoneal fluid, have also been used to infer an intact tube.[26,28,29,32] While this is often true, the lack of free fluid cannot be considered equivalent to the absence of tubal rupture, as rupture was found at surgery in 21% of the patients with no fluid or a trace of fluid in one series. While the frequency of tubal rupture rises with increasingly larger volumes of free fluid, over one-third of patients with a large hemoperitoneum have an intact tube.[21]

These results suggest that preoperative determination of fallopian tube status with transvaginal sonography is not reliable. Neither sonographic appearance of an adnexal mass nor the presence or volume of free fluid can be used to determine fallopian tube status with an EP.

Unusual forms of ectopic pregnancy

Interstitial pregnancies result when the gestational sac implants within the interstitial or intramural portion of the fallopian tube.[23,33] While these unusual EPs make up only 2–4% of all ectopics, the incidence is even higher in patients undergoing assisted reproduction following bilateral salpingectomy. As many as one-quarter of ectopic pregnancies in this high risk population are interstitial.[34] Interstitial pregnancies are associated with significantly higher morbidity and mortality than those in the isthmic or ampullary portions of the fallopian tube. With an interstitial pregnancy, a portion of the expanding gestational sac is surrounded by myometrium. This allows the sac to enlarge painlessly for a longer period of time as compared with a more distal tubal EP. Symptoms develop acutely in most patients with interstitial EPs when uterine rupture results in massive hemorrhage

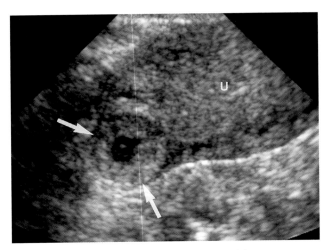

Figure 17.9 Interstitial pregnancy. Interstitial pregnancy can be diagnosed when there is an incomplete mantle of myometrium seen around a gestational sac situated at the edge of the uterus. In this patient with an interstitial pregnancy, a coronal sonogram of the uterus (U) shows the eccentrically located gestational sac that lacks myometrium around its lateral margins (arrows).

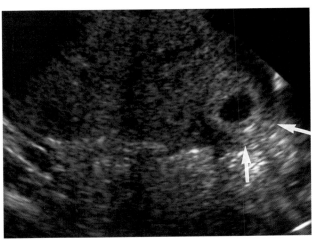

Figure 17.10 Eccentrically located gestational sac. A coronal transvaginal sonogram of a patient with a septate uterus demonstrates a gestational sac located at the far left edge of the uterus. In this instance, a rim of myometrium can be identified around the sac (arrows). This patient was able to carry this intrauterine pregnancy to term. Close sonographic follow-up of eccentric gestational sacs is often useful to differentiate an interstitial ectopic from an eccentric intrauterine sac.

during the late first or early second trimester. The frequently employed term cornual pregnancy, often used synonymously with interstitial pregnancy, should be reserved for pregnancies located within a rudimentary uterine horn.[23]

The diagnosis of interstitial pregnancy can be difficult. At transvaginal sonography, an interstitial EP should be suspected when the gestational sac is eccentrically located and there is thinning or absence of a portion of the myometrium surrounding the sac (*Fig. 17.9*). At times, it may not be possible to diagnose an early interstitial EP, because myometrium may be visible surrounding the tiny gestational sac. The interstitial line sign has been proposed as a useful diagnostic sign in this latter group of patients.[33] If a thin echogenic line can be found extending from the edge of the endometrial canal to the periphery of the interstitial gestational sac, it suggests that the sac is implanted in the interstitial portion of the fallopian tube, an interstitial pregnancy.[33] In combination with an incomplete myometrial mantle and eccentric placement of the sac, the interstitial line sign may aid in the early diagnosis of interstitial pregnancy.

One reason why interstitial EPs are so difficult to diagnose sonographically is the overlap that occurs with normal pregnancies that are either laterally situated in the normal uterus or located on one side of a septate uterus (*Fig. 17.10*). If the possibility of

an interstitial pregnancy is raised during the first trimester in a clinically stable patient, sonographic monitoring of the location of the sac as the pregnancy progresses is often useful.

Cervical pregnancy is an unusual form of ectopic pregnancy. Cervical pregnancies represent approximately 0.15% of EPs,[35] and are potentially life-threatening owing to the uncontrollable hemorrhage that occurs when the sac detaches from the cervix. Predisposing risk factors for cervical pregnancy include in vitro fertilization,[36] fibroids, an indwelling IUD, previous uterine curettage, and previously treated Asherman syndrome.[23] These factors have in common some disruption or scarring of the endometrial canal. The diagnosis of a cervical ectopic should be made at sonography when a well-formed gestational sac that contains a yolk sac, embryo, or cardiac activity is found within the cervix (*Fig. 17.11*). The echogenic trophoblastic ring of the ectopic is typically slightly asymmetrically located within the cervix, adjacent to but not within the cervical canal. These features help differentiate a cervical pregnancy from a spontaneous abortion in progress, in which the sac is irregular in shape, never contains cardiac activity, and is located directly within the canal. An abortion in progress can often be seen to change in shape during the examination, and serial sonograms will demonstrate altered appearance and position within the canal. While the location of a cervical pregnancy is identical to that of a mucous-filled

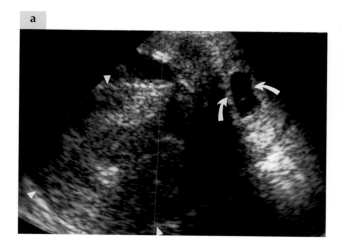

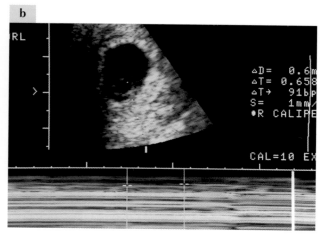

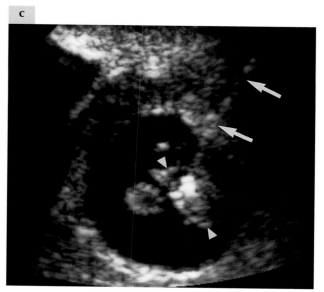

Figure 17.11 Cervical EP. When cervical pregnancy is diagnosed at an early gestational age, early intervention guided by transvaginal sonography may prevent life-threatening hemorrhage. (a) In this patient with vaginal bleeding, a sagittal transvaginal sonogram shows an empty uterus (arrowheads) and a gestational sac (curved arrows) with a yolk sac within the cervix. (b) Cardiac activity could be seen within the cervical sac. (c) Magnified image of a cervical gestational sac in a different patient. Under transvaginal sonographic guidance a needle (arrows) was inserted into the embryo (arrowheads) and KCl was injected. Cardiac activity ceased immediately. The patient subsequently passed a small amount of products of conception without significant hemorrhage.

nabothian cyst, the cyst lacks an echogenic rim, yolk sac, and embryo. Color Doppler interrogation of a questionable sac may provide useful information, as a cervical pregnancy has trophoblastic blood flow around the margins of the sac.

The uncontrollable hemorrhage associated with cervical EP invariably required hysterectomy in the past, as most patients presented during the late first or early second trimester already bleeding. With transvaginal sonography, cervical pregnancies can now be diagnosed at < 7 menstrual weeks, and treated promptly. Several alternative treatments have been proposed, all of which have been successful in controlling hemorrhage and preserving the uterus, thus maintaining the patient's fertility. These options include potassium chloride (KCl) injection directly into the pregnancy,[37] systemic methotrexate,[38] or preoperative uterine artery embolization prior to dilatation and evacuation.[39]

Sonographically guided termination of cervical pregnancy with KCl is the treatment of choice. This is performed in the ultrasound suite as an outpatient procedure, with mild intravenous sedation for discomfort as needed. Using the needle guide on the vaginal probe, a needle is placed into the cervical sac and KCl is injected into the embryo (if cardiac activity is present) or sac (in early cases with small sac size). This technique is a successful one which preserves the uterus, allowing patients to subsequently conceive.[37] The proven effectiveness and low complication rate of conservative treatment makes this the optimal means of therapy for cervical ectopic pregnancy.

Even more uncommon than cervical and interstitial ectopics are intra-abdominal pregnancies. These entities need to be carefully considered in patients undergoing infertility treatment, who may be at an increased risk for the more unusual forms of EP. In one case report, a microscopic fistulous tract in the uterus was postulated to be the source of an intra-abdominal pregnancy following IVF in a patient with bilateral salpingectomies.[40] In another patient, an ectopic pregnancy developed within a cesarean section scar, also via a presumed microscopic tract of scar dehiscence.[41] Continued search for the location of a pregnancy in an infertility patient with a positive β-hCG is necessary until the gestational sac is unequivocally identified, and even longer if symptoms suggesting heterotopic pregnancy persist.

The role of sonography in treatment

EP can now be diagnosed earlier and with more confidence, using high resolution vaginal sonography in combination with sensitive serological tests for early pregnancy. Early diagnosis allows prompt intervention, even before some patients become symptomatic. While most patients are treated surgically with salpingostomy or salpingectomy, alternative medical therapeutic options are increasing in frequency. Medical regimens often use the chemotherapeutic agent methotrexate, which may be administered intramuscularly or injected directly into the ectopic sac with sonographic or laparoscopic guidance. Transvaginal sonography provides useful information for patients undergoing non-operative treatment by monitoring the adnexal mass for change in size. Sonography is also invaluable in the evaluation of potential complications such as hemorrhage both during and after therapy.

Following methotrexate injection either into the ectopic or systemically, an adnexal mass may persist at transvaginal sonography for > 3 months, even if the β-hCG declines to zero. Increased Doppler flow or even transient enlargement of the mass are not uncommon findings immediately following medical therapy.[27,32] Reported complications of methotrexate injection into an EP include acute hemoperitoneum and pain requiring rehospitalization.[42] The β-hCG levels continue to rise in up to one-third of patients, and additional systemic injections of methotrexate may be required.[42]

Expectant management of EP is one of the most controversial areas of conservative treatment. In two small series of patients with declining or stable β-hCG levels, small adnexal masses, and no symptoms, who were followed without intervention, a successful outcome resulted in 69% and 100% of cases.[28,29] A similar spontaneous resolution rate of 69% was found in another series of larger EP masses (up to 5 cm) in patients with decreasing β-hCG and minimal symptoms.[43] In all of these series, the patients were carefully selected, and followed with repeated transvaginal sonography, β-hCG levels, and close clinical monitoring. Not surprisingly, the safety and efficacy of this management option has been questioned.[44] The potential role of color and pulsed Doppler in helping to identify EPs with low vascularity and absent trophoblastic activity that may respond successfully to expectant management remains to be determined.

In a population of patients suffering from infertility, other factors may contribute to the choice of treatment. Several reports have found surgical therapy to be more successful than local methotrexate injection, with failure defined as requiring a return to surgery, repeat injection of drug, or increased rate of hemoperitoneum.[45,46] Regardless of the type of treatment chosen, all patients with ectopic pregnancy have a subsequent reduced fertility rate.[47] Of particular concern in any patient is a delay in the diagnosis of EP. When ectopic pregnancies are 'missed' at first evaluation, salpingectomy is required more often than when the diagnosis is made early in the gestation.[48] This may in turn reduce the likelihood of future pregnancy even further. The ability to make an early and accurate diagnosis of ectopic pregnancy with transvaginal sonography therefore remains critical when caring for patients struggling with infertility.

REFERENCES

1. Centers for Disease Control. Ectopic pregnancy – United States, 1990–1992. *MMWR* 1995; **44**:46–48.

2. Schwartz RO, Di Pietro DL. β-hCG as a diagnostic aid for suspected ectopic pregnancy. *Obstet Gynecol* 1980; **56**:197–203.

3. Ankum WM, Mol BWJ, Van der Veen F, Bossuyt PMM. Risk factors for ectopic pregnancy, a meta-analysis. *Fertil Steril* 1996; **65**:1093–1099.

4. Thorsen MK, Lawson TL, Aimain EJ *et al.* Diagnosis of EP: endovaginal vs. transabdominal sonography. *Am J Roentgenol* 1990; **155**:307–310.

5. Cacciatore B, Stenman UH, Ylostalo P. Comparison of abdominal and vaginal sonography in suspected ectopic pregnancy. *Obstet Gynecol* 1989; **73**:770–774.

6. Hann LE, Bachman DM, Mcardle CR. Coexistent intrauterine and ectopic pregnancy: a reevaluation. *Radiology* 1984; **152**:151–154.

7. Goldman GA, Fisch B, Ovadia J, Tadir Y. Heterotopic pregnancy after assisted reproductive technologies. *Obstet Gynecol Survey* 1992; **47**:217–221.

8. Derman R. Early diagnosis of pregnancy: a symposium. *J Reprod Med* 1981; **26**:149.

9. Cacciatore B, Stenman UH, Ylostalo P. Diagnosis of ectopic pregnancy by vaginal ultrasonography in combination with a discriminatory serum hCG level of 1000 IU/L [IRP]. *Br J Obstet Gynaecol* 1990; **97**:904–908.

10. Mehta TS, Levine D, Beckwith B. Treatment of ectopic pregnancy: is a human chorionic gonadotropin level of 2000 mIU/ml a reasonable threshold? *Radiology* 1997; **205**:569–573.

11. Levi CS, Lyons EA, Lindsay DJ. Early diagnosis of nonviable pregnancy with endovaginal US. *Radiology* 1988; **167**:383–385.

12. Rowling SE, Coleman BG, Langer JE, Arger PH, Nisenbaum HL, Horii SC. First-trimester US parameters of failed pregnancy. *Radiology* 1997; **203**:211–217.

13. Yeh HC, Goodman JD, Carr L, Rabinowitz JG. Intradecidual sign: a US criterion of early intrauterine pregnancy. *Radiology* 1986; **161**:463–467.

14. Russel SA, Filly RA, Damato N. Sonographic diagnosis of ectopic pregnancy with endovaginal probes: what really has changed? *J Ultrasound Med* 1993; **3**:145–151.

15. Lavie O, Boldes R, Neuman M, Rabinowitz R, Algur N, Beller U. Ultrasonographic 'endometrial three-layer' pattern: a unique finding in ectopic pregnancy. *J Clin Ultrasound* 1996; **24**:179–183.

16. Spandorfer SD, Barnhart KT. Endometrial stripe thickness as a predictor of ectopic pregnancy. *Fertil Steril* 1996; **66**:474–477.

17. Droegemueller W. Ectopic pregnancy. In: Danforth DN, ed. *Obstetrics and Gynecology* 4th edn. Philadelphia, PA: Harper & Row, 1982:407–409.

18. Zinn HL, Cohen HL, Zinn DL. Ultrasonographic diagnosis of ectopic pregnancy: importance of transabdominal imaging. *J Ultrasound Med* 1997; **16**:603–607.

19. Rempen A. Vaginal sonography in ectopic pregnancy. *J Ultrasound Med* 1988; **7**:381–387.

20. Fleischer AC, Pennel RG, McKee MS *et al.* Ectopic pregnancy: features at transvaginal sonography. *Radiology* 1990; **174**:375–378.

21. Frates MC, Brown DL, Doubilet PM, Hornstein MD. Tubal rupture in patients with ectopic pregnancy: diagnosis with transvaginal US. *Radiology* 1994; **191**:769–772.

22. Brown DL, Doubilet PM. Transvaginal sonography for diagnosing ectopic pregnancy: positivity criteria and performance characteristics. *J Ultrasound Med* 1994; **13**:259–266.

23. Fredericks CM, Hotz G. Nontubal ectopic pregnancy. In: Fredericks CM, Paulson JD, Holtz G, eds. *Ectopic Pregnancy*. New York, NY: Hemisphere Publishing, 1989:193–206.

24. Berry SM, Coulam CB, Hill LM, Breckle R. Evidence of contralateral ovulation in ectopic pregnancy. *J Ultrasound Med* 1985; **4**:293–295.

25. Nyberg DA, Hughes MP, Mack LA, Wang KY. Extrauterine findings of ectopic pregnancy at transvaginal US: importance of echogenic fluid. *Radiology* 1991; **178**:823–826.

26. Stovall TG, Ling FW, Gray LA, Carson SA, Buster JE. Methotrexate treatment of unruptured ectopic pregnancy: a report of 100 cases. *Obstet Gynecol* 1991; **77**:749–753.

27. Brown DL, Felker RE, Stovall TG, Emerson DS, Ling FW. Serial endovaginal sonography of ectopic pregnancies treated with methotrexate. *Obstet Gynecol* 1991; **77**:406–409.

28. Ylostgalo P, Cacciatore B, Sjoberg J, Kaariainen M, Tenhunen A, Stenman UH. Expectant management of ectopic pregnancy. *Obstet Gynecol* 1992; **80**:345–348.

29. Atri M, Bret PM, Tulandi T. Spontaneous resolution of ectopic pregnancy: initial appearance and evolution at transvaginal US. *Radiology* 1993; **186**:83–86.

30. Cacciatore B. Can the status of tubal pregnancy be predicted with transvaginal sonography? A prospective comparison of sonographic, surgical and serum hCG findings. *Radiology* 1990; **177**:481–484.

31. Atri M, deStempel J, Bret PM. Accuracy of transvaginal ultrasonography for detection of hematosalpinx in ectopic pregnancy. *J Clin Ultrasound* 1992; **20**:255–261.

32. Atri M, Bret BM, Tulandi T, Senterman MK. Ectopic pregnancy: evolution after treatment with transvaginal methotrexate. *Radiology* 1992; **185**:749–753.

33. Ackerman TE, Levi CS, Dashefsky SM, Holt SC, Lindsay SJ. Interstitial line: sonographic finding in interstitial [cornual] ectopic pregnancy. *Radiology* 1993; **189**:83–87.

34. Agarwal SK, Wisot AL, Garzo G, Meldrum DR. Cornual pregnancies in patients with prior salpingectomy undergoing in vitro fertilization and embryo transfer. *Fertil Steril* 1996; **65**:659–660.

35. Jones HW, Cobton AC, Brunett LS. *Novak's Textbook of Gynecology* 11th edn. Baltimore, MD: Williams & Wilkins, 1988:499.

36. Ginsburg ES, Frates MC, Rein MS, Fox J, Hornstein M, Friedman AJ. Early diagnosis and treatment of cervical pregnancy in an in vitro fertilization program. *Fertil Steril* 1994; **61**:966–969.

37. Frates MC, Benson CB, Doubilet PM *et al.* Cervical ectopic pregnancy: results of conservative treatment. *Radiology* 1994; **191**:773–775.

38. Stovall TG, Ling FW, Smith WC *et al.* Successful nonsurgical treatment of cervical pregnancy with methotrexate. *Fertil Steril* 1988; **50**:672–674.

39. Meyerovitz MF, Lobel SM, Harrington DP, Bengston JM. Preoperative uterine artery embolization in cervical pregnancy. *J Vasc Interv Radiol* 1991; **2**:95–97.

40. Fisch B, Peled Y, Kaplan B, Zehavi S, Neri A. Abdominal pregnancy following in vitro fertilization in a patient with previous bilateral salpingectomy. *Obstet Gynecol* 1996; **88**:642–643.

41. Godin P-A, Bassil S, Donnez J. An ectopic pregnancy developing in a previous caesarian section scar. *Fertil Steril* 1997; **67**:398–400.

42. Fernandez H, Benifla JL, Lelaidier C, Baton C, Frydman R. Methotrexate treatment of ectopic

pregnancy: 100 cases treated by primary transvaginal injection under sonographic control. *Fertil Steril* 1993; **59**:773–777.

43. Cacciatore B, Korhonen J, Stenman U-H, Ylostalo P. Transvaginal sonography and serum hCG in monitoring of presumed ectopic pregnancies selected for expectant management. *Ultrasound Obstet Gynecol* 1995; **5**:297–300.

44. Zacur HA. Expectant management of ectopic pregnancy. *Radiology* 1993; **186**:11–12.

45. Yao M, Tulandi T, Falcone T. Treatment of ectopic pregnancy by systemic methotrexate, transvaginal methotrexate, and operative laparoscopy. *Intl J Fertil* 1996; **41**:470–475.

46. Shalev E, Peleg D, Bustan M, Romano S, Tsabari A. Limited role for intratubal methotrexate treatment of ectopic pregnancy. *Fertil Steril* 1995; **63**:20–24.

47. Korell M, Albrich W, Hepp H. Fertility after organ-preserving surgery of ectopic pregnancy: results of a multicenter study. *Fertil Steril* 1997; **68**:220–223.

48. Robson SJ, O'Shea RT. Undiagnosed ectopic pregnancy: a retrospective analysis of 31 'missed' ectopic pregnancies at a teaching hospital. *Aust NZ J Obstet Gynaecol* 1996; **36**:182–185.

18 Multifetal pregnancy reduction procedures

Jodi P Lerner and Ilan E Timor-Tritsch

Recent advances in the assisted reproductive technologies have done much to improve the plight of many couples affected with long-standing infertility problems. Use of these techniques has been associated with increased rates of multiple gestations as a result of multiple ovulation, from overstimulation with FSH and LH, or, in the case of in vitro fertilization, from the transfer of large numbers of embryos. Unfortunately, these multiple gestations are not limited to twins, but often include higher order multiples, including a substantial number of triplets and quadruplets, and, less commonly, multifetal pregnancies of even higher order. As the number of fetuses in a pregnancy increases, there is a proportional increase in the chance of premature contractions and delivery. The sad irony is that many of these women with long-standing infertility now have too many fetuses to carry safely to viability. In the past, these unfortunate women with multifetal pregnancies of high order had one of two options: either carry the grand order multiple gestation with its high likelihood of miscarriage or serious neonatal morbidity and mortality, or terminate the entire pregnancy and start anew, in the hope that fewer fetuses will implant during the next cycle.

In the mid-1980s, several groups began performing first trimester transcervical suction aspiration of a fetus or fetuses in a grand order multiple pregnancy in an attempt to decrease the number of fetuses to a more acceptable number, thereby optimizing the chance for that pregnancy to remain intact to a later gestational age.[1-6] Since that time, the technique known as multifetal pregnancy reduction (MFPR) has been modified and improved. It is performed by many groups around the world during the latter first trimester using either transabdominal or transvaginal approaches.

In contrast to first trimester MFPR as described above, the procedure of second trimester multifetal pregnancy reduction, sometimes referred to as selective reduction, is usually performed for the selective termination of an abnormal fetus in a multiple gestation, to improve outcome for the remaining fetus or fetuses. This is usually performed in the mid-second trimester, after a major structural abnormality is detected sonographically, or after an abnormal genetic karyotype is found. In both first trimester multifetal pregnancy reduction and second trimester selective reduction, patient counseling is an important component of the treatment algorithms.

This chapter summarizes procedures of MFPR as they have evolved over the last decade. Little by little, knowledge and experience accumulated by individual centers and by the combined registry tracking the results of MFPR have made it possible to draw clinically meaningful conclusions for the benefit of these patients.

First trimester multifetal pregnancy reduction

The first published technique for multifetal pregnancy reduction was transcervical suction aspiration.[7] However, this procedure was quickly abandoned because if was associated with a high miscarriage rate. Since that time, the majority of the centers which perform MFPR have used ultrasound-guided transabdominal or transvaginal injection of potassium chloride solution into the area of the fetal heart until cardiac asystole occurs. Although the specific technique varies from institution to institution, several controversial issues have arisen over the last 10 years which deserve more detailed discussion.

(1) MFPR, can it be done?
(2) Which is the better approach for MFPR, the transabdominal route or the transvaginal route?

(3) Is MFPR an option for triplet gestations?

(4) Are monochorionic gestations candidates for multifetal pregnancy reduction?

(5) What are the ethical and psychological considerations?

(6) When should chorionic villus sampling or amniocentesis be performed with respect to the MFPR?

(7) What is the place of maternal serum α-feto-protein screening?

(8) What is the role of the automated puncture device in MFPR?

Multifetal pregnancy reduction: can it be done?

There are many reports in the literature describing the technique of first and second trimester multifetal pregnancy reduction and outcome for individual institutional series.[1-6,8-24] Comparisons among studies are difficult, because different techniques are used and different outcome measures are reported. In 1993, Evans et al[25] published the initial collaborative data, in an attempt to establish the relative safety of the multifetal pregnancy reduction procedure, especially when compared to the high morbidity and mortality associated with multifetal pregnancies. This initial report covered the years 1988 to early 1991, and included all cases performed transabdominally, with insertion of a needle and potassium chloride injection into the fetal thorax. The data showed an overall 16.4% pregnancy loss rate through 24 completed weeks' gestation.[25]

The second collaborative report focused on cases between mid-1991 and 1993,[26] and demonstrated a significant drop in the overall pregnancy loss rate. This was the first report that compared transabdominal versus transcervical or transvaginal multifetal pregnancy reduction. The data included over 1000 completed pregnancies. In general, the transabdominal procedures were performed at a slightly later gestational age than the transvaginal ones. Both methods were found to be relatively safe and efficient for improving outcome in multifetal pregnancies: of the cases performed transabdominally, the loss rate was 8% in this series, and the transvaginal/transcervical cases had a loss rate of approximately 13%. The percentage of patients having very early premature deliveries, in the range 25–28 weeks gestation, was 5.5% for both approaches. Approximately 10% of the patients delivered at 29–32 weeks, and nearly 50% of patients reached 37 weeks gestation or beyond. They found that the greater the starting number of fetuses, the higher the pregnancy loss rate and the earlier the gestational age at delivery. There is a cost to iatrogenic multifetal pregnancies, even if multifetal pregnancy reduction can be performed successfully.

The latest collaborative data, published in 1996,[27] confirm the results of the first two collaborative studies. Data were obtained from nine centers in five countries and included 1789 completed cases: this nearly doubled the number of cases and two new centers were added to the consortium. The authors' hope was, that with the additional data, enough cases in each category would be available to develop relatively reliable risk estimates for most clinical situations. The overall pregnancy loss rate in this last series was 11.7%, but ranged from a low of 7.6% for reduction of triplets to twins to a high of 22.9% for sextuplets or higher.

Transabdominal versus transvaginal approach

Most centers have a preferred technique for multifetal pregnancy reduction. Although reductions performed by the transvaginal route are usually performed slightly earlier in gestation, usually at 10–11 weeks, there does not appear to be a distinct advantage to either approach. Appropriate patient selection and an experienced operator are the most important variables. The obese patient with a multifetal pregnancy of grand order presents a great challenge for the transabdominal approach, and these particular patients are often referred to centers that specialize in the transvaginal approach.

Whether the transabdominal or the transvaginal route is employed, basic information is given to the patient regarding the technique and the risks and benefits, and information is obtained from the patient, including concurrent medical problems and blood type. When the transvaginal route is employed, as for most of the procedures performed at this institution, patients are asked to have group B streptococcal and chlamydial cultures of the cervix prior to the procedure. If any of the vaginal or cervical cultures is positive, the patient is treated and a repeat culture is obtained prior to the procedure. Patients undergoing the transabdominal approach do not require these tests. Patients with Rhesus negative blood type are given a Rhogam injection intramuscularly, by the same protocol as after an amniocentesis is performed.

Most patients present to the institution on the day of the procedure for both their counseling session and procedure, but some patients ask for a separate counseling session with prereduction scan well before the procedure itself. Whether the mapping scan is done on a date prior to the procedure, and/or immediately before the procedure, a detailed ultrasound evaluation of the pregnancy is a very important aspect of the multifetal pregnancy reduction algorithm (*Figs 18.1* and *18.2*). This scan is performed in order to obtain important information,

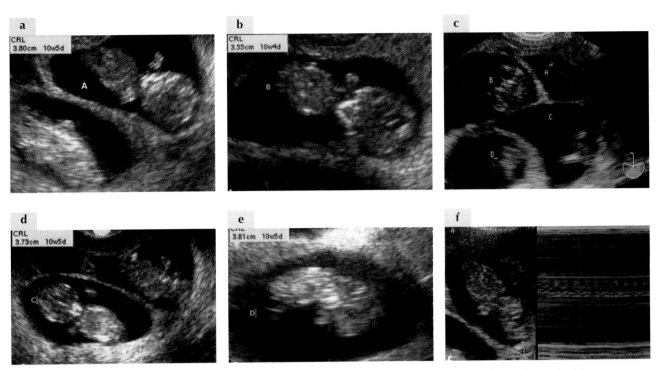

Figure 18.1 Pre-reduction scan. A transvaginal scan of a quadruplet pregnancy at 10 weeks is pictured with concordant crown–rump lengths (a, b, d, e). (c) A scan of the quadruplet pregnancy as an overview. (f) The positive fetal heart rate by M-mode of one of the quadruplets as an example.

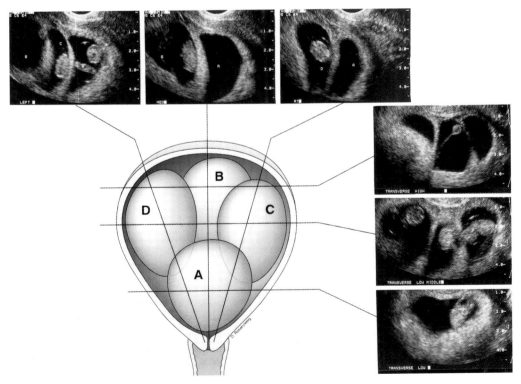

Figure 18.2 Schematic of mapping scan. The central drawing represents a quadruplet pregnancy. The scans across the top represent the sonographic views seen in the longitudinal plane when the transducer is pointed towards the right, median, and left aspects of the uterus, respectively. The scans along the right side of the figure represent the sonographic views seen in the transverse plane when the transducer is placed across the upper, middle, and lower aspects of the uterus, respectively.

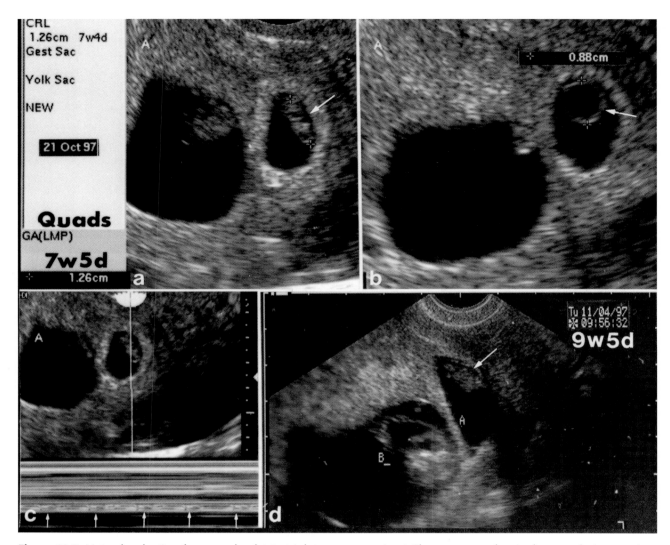

Figure 18.3 Natural reduction from quadruplet to triplet pregnancy. (a–c) The presence of a singleton early intrauterine demise within a quadruplet pregnancy at 7 weeks 5 days (arrow), with a hydropic yolk sac (b), and lack of cardiac activity as seen on M-mode (c). When the patient returned for her MFPR appointment at 9 weeks 5 days, the demised fetus A (d, arrow) was noted and a three to two reduction was performed on fetus B only.

including the actual number of live embryos/fetuses, their chorionicity and amnionicity, their position in the uterus and location with respect to the internal os and lateral uterine blood vessels, and the location of the placentas. Each fetus is measured, and the presence of a fetal heartbeat is confirmed. Occasionally, a smaller number of viable fetuses is encountered at the time of the mapping scan than was anticipated by either history or previous ultrasound findings (*Fig. 18.3*). This is sometimes termed a 'natural reduction'. The counseling and plan must be altered to reflect the newest findings. Fetuses scanned at this institution are labeled alphabetically as they appear starting at the level of the internal os and continuing towards the fundus (*Fig. 18.4*). As long as consistency is maintained throughout the scan and procedure, any identification system may

be employed. However, it is important to document the location of the sacs and their interrelationships by several well annotated images or by a drawing.

In addition to number of fetuses and presence of fetal heartbeats, the detailed mapping scan performed prior to the reduction procedure also provides information regarding a preliminary structural evaluation of each fetus. Certainly, only gross structural abnormalities may be sonographically visualized at 9–11 weeks gestation, and the patients and their referring physicians should understand that only an extremely small number of significantly gross anomalies may be seen at this gestational age. This evaluation is usually limited to a view of the posterior contour to detect an abnormally large nuchal translucency, the anterior contour to detect

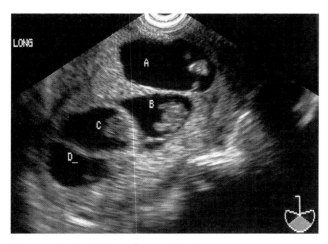

Figure 18.4 Labeling of a quadruplet pregnancy as seen on transvaginal scan from cervix to fundus.

a liver containing omphalocele or other large abdominal fusion defect or a major structural anomaly such as a body stalk anomaly, and the cranium to detect a large defect of the skull such as acrania or exencephaly (*Fig. 18.5*).

Reduction of triplet gestations: do the benefits outweigh the risks?

Although there is little controversy regarding the risks versus benefits of the multifetal pregnancy reduction of a grand order pregnancy such as quintuplets or septuplets, when a triplet pregnancy is encountered the best course of action is much less clear cut. The current preference appears to be to keep triplet pregnancies intact, because neonatal care in the late 1990s has improved so much that a preterm delivery of triplets secures a better outcome than the risk of miscarriage from a triplet gestation reduced to twins.[28-35] These data have been derived mainly from anecdotal reports of triplets which

claim that the mean gestational age at delivery of triplets is approximately 33 weeks.[30-37] In several of the studies, however, exclusion of pregnancies delivered at < 24 weeks gestation or fetuses weighing < 500 g may in fact bias the conclusions inappropriately. Recently, several articles have appeared in the literature that compare the outcomes of unreduced triplets, triplets reduced from three to two, and unreduced twins. Macones et al[38] published the results of their group in 1993: they compared the perinatal outcomes of each of the three groups described above. They found that for all the following variables, mean gestational age at delivery (weeks), mean birthweight, per cent of neonates requiring intensive care nursery admission, per cent of neonates requiring ventilatory support, stillbirth rate, and perinatal mortality rate, non-reduced triplets did worse than three to two reductions. The three to two reductions, when compared to non-reduced twins, did not fare significantly worse in any of the variables; the mean birthweight for the reduced triplets was actually higher than for the non-reduced twins, albeit not significantly. *Table 18.1* shows these results. Sassoon et al[30] also investigated the comparison of non-reduced to reduced triplets for several similar variables and also found improved outcomes in the reduced group including a perinatal mortality rate seven-fold less in the reduced group compared with non-reduced triplets. Lipitz et al[39] found that, in general, the outcome of triplet pregnancies reduced to twins did not differ significantly from those of the naturally occurring twin pregnancies. Haning et al[40] investigated the outcomes of in vitro fertilization pregnancies, and concluded that multifetal pregnancy reduction in pregnancies with three or more fetuses was beneficial and increased the duration of the gestation. This group found that each viable fetus found at the eighth week ultrasound scan could be expected to reduce the length of the gestation by 3.6 weeks, and each fetus reduced could be expected to prolong the gestation by approximately 3 weeks as well. Although all these studies confirm that

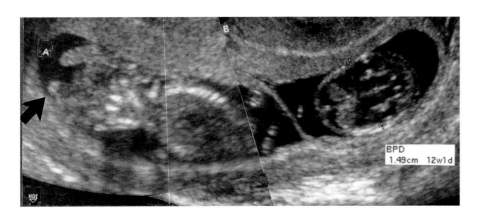

Figure 18.5 Dichorionic diamniotic twins at 11 weeks with a major anomaly (acrania) of fetus A (arrow). Fetus A was selectively reduced.

Table 18.1 **Neonatal outcome.**

Parameter	Non-reduced triplets	Reduction three to two	Non-reduced twins
Mean gestational age at delivery (weeks)	31.2 ± 4.9	35.6 ± 2.8	34.8 ± 4.5
Mean birthweight (g)	1593	2279	2293
Intensive care nursery admission (%)	85	36	30
Ventilatory support (%)	51	14	23
Stillbirth rate (per 1000)	47	10	8
Perinatal mortality rate (per 1000)	210	30	40

This table illustrates the differences between non-reduced triplets, reduced triplets to twins, and non-reduced twins for several important obstetrical parameters. The results for reduced triplets approach those for non-reduced twins in all variables. Modified from Macones et al.[38]

reduction of triplet gestations to twins is a viable option, patient counseling and selection remain critical determinants in making this difficult decision. Some authors challenge the medical validity of reduction of triplets based on their results.[41]

Monochorionic pregnancies and multifetal reduction

If two or more fetuses are identified within one chorionic sac during the scanning procedure of a multifetal gestation (*Fig. 18.6*), these fetuses will need special consideration with respect to reduction. Because of the strong possibility of vascular connections between the two (or occasionally three or four) monochorionic fetuses, the decision on selection to reduce specific fetuses may be limited and must be considered for the group as a whole. The decision must be to reduce all the fetuses within the chorionic sac or leave alone all the fetuses within the sac. It may be surmised by understanding of the vascular connections as well as by direct clinical experience that in monochorionic

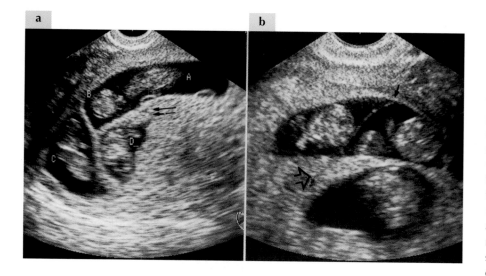

Figure 18.6 Monochorionic twin set within a trichorionic-quadramniotic quadruplet pregnancy. (a) The overview of the pregnancy with the 'twin peaks' or 'lambda' sign (arrows) separating the monochorionic set from the other two quadruplets. (b) A close-up of the differentiation between the thin membranes separating the monochorionic set (closed arrow) and the thicker membranes plus chorion separating one of the other quads (open arrow).

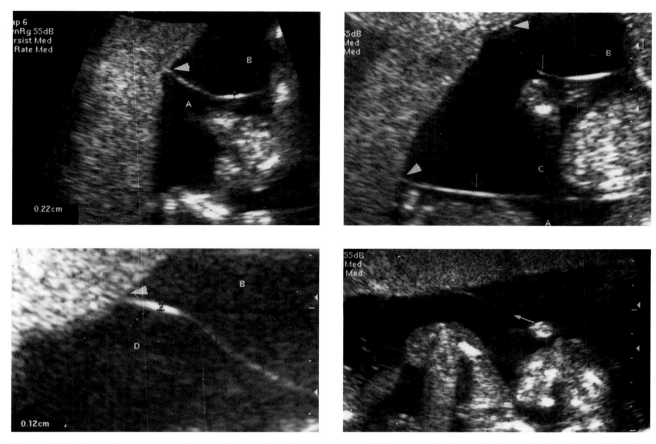

Figure 18.7 Monochorionic quadramniotic quadruplet pregnancy. All four panels show the interrelationships of the four amniotic sacs and their insertions into the chorion or each other as depicted by the short and long arrows.

twins where one is reduced and one left alone, the demise of the non-reduced twin will inevitably occur.

At times, owing to the presence of certain chorionicity and amnionicity, the procedure itself has to be canceled, as in the example of a monochorionic/quadramniotic pregnancy that presented to the author's group for proposed reduction (*Fig. 18.7*). In this situation, the reduction was deferred as there was strong suspicion that vascular anastomoses were present between at least two of the four fetuses.[42]

In addition to limiting the accessibility and/or desired final number of fetuses after a multifetal pregnancy reduction, monochorionic fetuses may be considered targets for reduction owing to the fact that monochorionic pregnancies have higher complication rates throughout gestation, with possible abnormal vascular connections leading to twin–twin transfusion syndrome or other adverse sequelae.

There are few data available regarding the comparable outcomes for the reduction of multifetal pregnancies which contain a monochorionic set versus those that do not contain any monochorionic fetuses, although these authors found anecdotally, that in a set of 495 multifetal pregnancy reductions, the 26 monochorionic twin-containing pregnancies had a higher loss rate than the remaining pregnancies that did not contain any monochorionic sets. This conclusion is preliminary and needs to be investigated with larger monchorionic patient numbers as well as matched case-controls.

Ethical considerations and psychological aspects

Certainly, any discussion regarding the controversial topic of multifetal pregnancy reduction must consider ethical aspects and inclusion of patients' desires regarding the decisions to be made. First and foremost, the name given for the procedure has finally become universally termed 'multifetal pregnancy reduction'.[43] The term 'selective' reduction is reserved for the situation where there is an abnormality or anomaly of a specific fetus that is targeted for reduction. These procedures are usually performed in the second trimester.

One article that specifically addressed the ethical issues of multifetal pregnancy reduction reflected on Jewish law and ethics,[44] which regard the procedure as a morally acceptable procedure, although care should be taken to reduce the minimum number of fetuses that will reasonably assure that the remaining fetuses will be born healthy and alive.

The American College of Obstetricians and Gynecologists addressed the ethical and psychological aspects of multifetal pregnancy reduction in a committee opinion published in 1991.[45] The committee did not make any statements regarding censure of those assisted reproductive technologies responsible for creating these multiple pregnancies of grand order, but suggested that the infertility centers must exercise a high degree of diligence to minimize the problem. The committee opinion continues that the ethical issues should be discussed with the patient before initiation of any infertility treatment. The committee opinion correctly emphasizes that even for some patients, who do not believe that abortion is acceptable, multifetal pregnancy reduction could be justified ethically, if the risks of carrying the pregnancy are considerably higher than that for a reduced number of fetuses.

Several articles in the literature have evaluated the short- and long-term psychological effects for patients undergoing multifetal pregnancy reduction.[46–48] The general conclusions from all of them could have been expected: while the reduction decision and procedure were experienced as stressful and distressing, when the pregnancy outcome was successful, the medical intervention did not appear to put patients at significant risk for long-term affective disorders or worsened psychiatric symptoms. Shreiner-Engle et al described the acute and persistent psychological reactions of the first 100 women who underwent first trimester multifetal pregnancy reduction at Mount Sinai Hospital in New York.[48] The outcome measures described included reproductive loss, catastrophic fears, and lingering depressive feelings. More than 65% of the sample recalled acute feelings of emotional pain, stress, and fear, and mourning for the lost fetuses was reported by 70% of the patients. Over 90% of the patients said that they would come to the same decision again. The patients at risk for being most affected were the younger and more religious patients, and those who had seen the multifetal pregnancy on ultrasound more often.

Chorionic villus sampling before and genetic amniocentesis after MFPR

Frequently the multifetal pregnancy occurs in a woman who will be 35 years or older at the time of delivery, making her a candidate for prenatal diagnosis by either prereduction chorionic villus sampling (CVS) or post-reduction second trimester genetic amniocentesis. Although the ideal setting would be for CVS to be performed in the first trimester followed by selective multifetal pregnancy reduction if an abnormality is encountered, this option is limited because CVS is not readily available in many places. Second trimester amniocentesis has the advantage of being technically easier and available at most facilities.

Prereduction first trimester CVS avoids the potential for a later selective reduction. In a series of 745 multifetal pregnancy reductions performed by Wapner and Weinblatt at Thomas Jefferson Medical College in Philadelphia, 254 had a pre-procedure CVS.[49] Abnormal chromosome results were encountered in approximately 2–3% of pregnancies and the abnormal fetus was terminated as part of the reduction procedure. The pregnancy loss rate to 24 weeks gestation of those having a pre-procedure CVS was 5.5% compared to 5.6% loss rate in those having the reduction alone.

Brambati et al[50] published their group's experience of 100 CVS procedures performed before MFPR of two or three fetuses. The total loss before 24 weeks was 7% and no significant relationship was found with the final number of fetuses and CVS. Diagnostic error due to incorrect sampling was reported in 1.5% of cases. Their data indicate that fetal reduction can be preceded by CVS without a significant increase in the loss of pregnancy.

At present the trend in several centers in the USA is to offer CVS before MFPR. This may delay the timing of the reduction by several days to one week. However, the presently available laboratory tests such as the FISH (fluorescence in situ hybridization) enable a fast and acceptably reliable return of the results to permit a minimal delay in performing the reduction.

Even though Coffler et al[51] advocate an early (7–8 weeks) MFPR by an aspiration technique with a low (2.6%) pregnancy loss rate if the starting number is 4 or more, this technique becomes less attractive if a prereduction CVS cannot be offered for patients in need of karyotyping.

In another article, DeCatte et al[52] report no fetal losses in 32 cases of MFPR in which CVS was performed. Although this series is small, the result seems to reinforce the safety of CVS before MFPR.

Although multifetal pregnancy reduction followed by second trimester amniocentesis[55] is the more readily available option, it would necessitate a second reduction procedure if an abnormality were detected. These cases should be infrequent, since even at 40 years of age there is only a 2% risk that one of the remaining fetuses will be aneuploid. Tabsh and Theroux report on their experience in 53 women who elected to reduce their higher order multifetal pregnancies to twins and subsequently underwent genetic amniocentesis.[53] Five of these patients lost their entire pregnancy following the procedure: all pregnancies were lost within 2–14 days following the amniocentesis; however, some patients began experiencing adverse symptoms, including rupture of membranes, sooner than this. In this reported series, the pregnancy loss rate for genetic amniocentesis following multifetal pregnancy reduction was 9.4%. Although there appears to be no obvious etiology for the increased loss rate following genetic amniocentesis in these patients, the authors hypothesize that the multifetal reduction procedure causes some alteration in the intrauterine environments that then predisposes the patient to a higher risk of spontaneous rupture of the membranes and/or infection following genetic amniocentesis.

Three recent studies have evaluated the added risk of amniocentesis on top of the risk of MFPR. Selam et al[54] evaluated 127 patients who underwent genetic amniocentesis after MFPR. These were compared to a group of 167 patients who did not have genetic amniocentesis after MFPR. The pregnancy losses were 3.1% and 7.2%, respectively ($p > 0.05$). The data suggest that genetic amniocentesis after MFPR does not increase the risk of pregnancy loss over that observed in association with the reduction itself. This reinforces the earlier observation by McLean et al[55] based on data from three centers performing amniocentesis after MFPR in 79 patients. The loss rate was 5.1% in this group. In the control group from the collaborative study the loss rate after only MFPR was 11.4%. These loss rates were not statistically different.

In the authors' series of MFPR, patients had post-reduction amniocenteses.[56] The loss rate was not significantly different from the general loss rate of the entire reduction group. The authors speculate, and with good reason, that it is safe to perform CVS before and genetic amniocentesis after MFPR when clinically indicated.

Recently, Monni et al[57] have stressed the importance of nuchal translucency thickness measurements before MFPR.

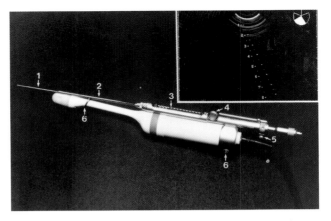

Figure 18.8 The main components of the automated puncture device attached to the transvaginal probe: (1) needle, (2) needle guide shaft, (3) centimeter depth scale, (4) trigger release, (5) safety knob, (6) for attachment (screw for attachment to probe). The inset shows the centimeter depth scale which is seen on the ultrasound monitor screen.

Role of α-fetoprotein testing after multifetal pregnancy reduction

Maternal serum α-fetoprotein (MSAFP) testing has become a staple within the antepartum screening armamentarium, usually drawn in the 15–20 weeks gestation range. Although aneuploidy rates do not appear to be higher for twins than for singletons,[58] there are several studies in the literature which describe an elevated rate of anencephaly and encephalocele in twin gestations,[59,60] which would then make multifetal pregnancies excellent candidates for MSAFP testing. However, it has been described first by Grau et al in 1990,[61] then confirmed by Lynch and Berkowitz,[62] that MSAFP values are consistently elevated in patients after multifetal pregnancy reduction and therefore this is not an informative test in these patients. Grau et al found that this elevation may last as long as 7 weeks after the reduction procedure, although no plausible explanation for this has yet been elaborated based on the understanding of the pharmacokinetics of α-fetoprotein itself.

Lynch and Berkowitz[62] found elevated MSAFP levels in their first several patients undergoing multifetal pregnancy reduction, which then prompted follow-up amniocentesis to be performed; in all cases, the amniotic fluid α-fetoprotein levels were normal. In a later study, they were able to correlate the elevated α-fetoprotein values and the number of dead fetuses, and a negative correlation was not found with the time elapsed since the performance of the reduction.

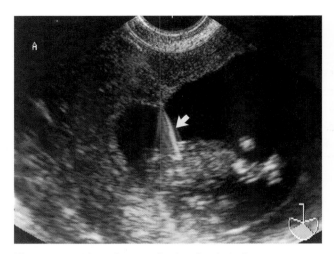

Figure 18.9 First trimester fetal reduction. A cross-sectional view of a reduction performed at 10 weeks with the needle (arrow) within the fetal chest.

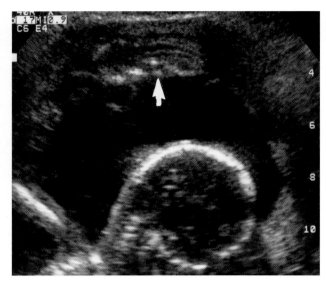

Figure 18.11 Visualization of fetal remnant after first trimester MFPR. The reduced fetus can still be seen (arrow) on this 19 week transabdominal scan, 8 weeks after the MFPR was performed.

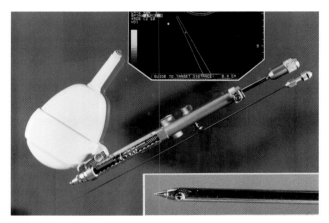

Figure 18.10 Automated puncture device (APD) adapted for transabdominal use. This photograph shows the APD mated to the transabdominal probe. The lower inset shows a close-up of the needle; the upper inset shows the needle guide as seen on the ultrasound monitor.

Use of the automated puncture device

Before describing the use of the automated puncture device, the general differences between the transabdominal and transvaginal approaches should be briefly described. The transabdominal approach is performed freehand, much as a second trimester amniocentesis is performed, usually with a 22 gauge or similar needle, relying on the operator's eye and hand coordination to keep the entire length of the needle within the scanning plane. Using the transabdominal approach, a quick readjustment corrects any inability to image the full length of the needle or needle tip. By the transvaginal approach, the limited mobility of the probe and the needle makes such adjustment impossible. Therefore, a needle-guide attached to the vaginal probe shaft should always be used; this keeps the entire length of the needle within the scanning plane at all times and allows control over the needle tip.

During the past 8–9 years, the authors have employed the use of an automated puncture device (APD), which is a spring-loaded instrument mated to the shaft of the vaginal probe.[19] The main components of the APD (Labotext, Gottingen, Germany) used are depicted in *Fig. 18.8*. Software-generated double dotted lines seen on the ultrasound monitor show the needle path direction and measure the depth needed for accurate needle penetration; then the depth setting on the APD is adjusted appropriately. After releasing the safety and trigger, the needle is propelled by a powerful spring into the desired structure, both accurately and painlessly (*Fig. 18.9*). After injection of the potassium chloride solution and observation for 2–5 minutes, the needle is removed, and then the procedure is repeated using new, sterile needles, for as many fetuses as will be reduced.

In order to duplicate the technique used transvaginally of employing the APD, the authors have developed a modified version of the APD mated to the abdominal ultrasound probe (*Fig. 18.10*). This puncture device is attached to the transabdominal transducer by a plastic bracket. A new needle was constructed by Labotect with one basic modification

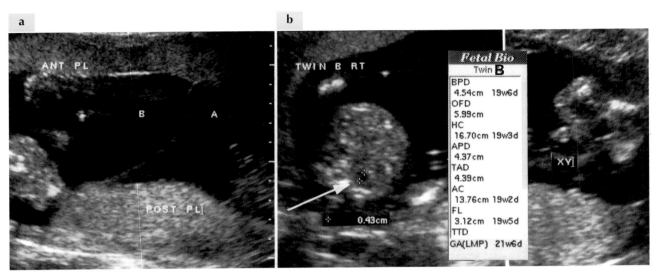

Figure 18.12 Selective second trimester MFPR in a dichorionic twin pregnancy with Down's syndrome. (a) A transabdominal scan labeling the fetuses. (b) The abnormal fetus was confirmed to be the fetus for intended selective reduction by sex typing (XY), a sonographically evident anomaly (pyelectasis, see arrow), and short biometry measurements.

from those used via the transvaginal route: the sharp penetrating tip of these new needles is now located on a stylet. With the needle in place, the stylet is removed, leaving behind a blunt tip which avoids harm to even the most delicate organs. A side hole assures free flow of fluid should the tip get obstructed by any structure draped across it.

The APD has been used successfully to perform several MFPRs via the transabdominal route in the first trimester, second trimester selective reductions, and punctures of obstructed and dilated fetal bladders and kidneys in utero with excellent results. The value of this new use of the 'old' device is that it is extremely accurate, virtually painless, and enables easy teaching and mastery of the technique.

Whether using the transabdominal or transvaginal approach, sonographic visualization of the reduced fetuses may be seen for many weeks after the MFPR procedure (*Fig. 18.11*).

Selective termination of a multifetal pregnancy

In contrast to the previously discussed situation of multifetal pregnancy reduction, where the inherent problem is purely of fetal number, the term selective reduction or selective termination of an abnormal twin or triplet fetus is a unique problem with its own issues and controversies. As early as 1978, Aberg et al[63] reported on a case of cardiac puncture of a twin fetus with Hurler syndrome. In 1981, Kerenyi and Chitkara[64] reported on a selective reduction of one twin with Down's syndrome when the mother threat-

ened to abort both the normal and abnormal twins. Despite the emotionally charged cases and the ethical issues these situations raise, several authors have reported on selective second trimester termination to prevent the birth of an abnormal child and permit the birth of a normal one.[63–67]

The differences between multifetal pregnancy reduction and what is termed 'selective termination' are several: in most situations one abnormal twin is encountered in a naturally occurring twin pregnancy and not in a couple after infertility treatment, and in most cases these abnormalities are discovered in the second trimester, not the first. The technique of selective termination is similar to that of first trimester multifetal pregnancy reduction, but the KCl injection must be performed directly into the fetal heart in order to achieve asystole. The dose of KCl required increases with gestational age,[58] but rarely exceeds 3 ml.

The selective termination of a fetus with a congenital abnormality is a specific problem with additional issues: namely correct identification of the affected fetus is required, sometimes weeks after the initial diagnostic procedure. Identification of the abnormal fetus may be obtained using either: (1) drawings from the time of the prenatal diagnostic procedure, (2) the presence of a detectable structural malformation, or (3) fetal sex if discordant and sonographically discernible (*Fig. 18.12*). If identification is at all uncertain, further diagnostic testing by either cordocentesis, placental biopsy, or amniocentesis should be performed prior to the reduction procedure.[8] Weinblatt et al reported on their experience with second trimester selective reduction.[8] In cases where the selective reduction was performed for a cytogenetic or biochemical abnormality, a sample of fetal blood and/or amniotic fluid was obtained from the injected fetus and analysed for confirmation. Eight pregnancies had selective termination between 13 and 20 weeks of gestation for a fetal abnormality. Four procedures in twins were performed for abnormal CVS results, two sets of twins for abnormal amniocentesis results, and one twin for hydrocephalus and neural tube defect. One triplet set was reduced to twins for a fetus with thanatophoric dysplasia. One twin to singleton reduction had a 14 week pregnancy loss 2 days after the procedure, the remaining pregnancies continued and delivered between 32 and 33 weeks gestation in two pregnancies and > 37 weeks gestation in five pregnancies.

Berkowitz et al[9] recently reported their findings regarding the first 100 patients who underwent second trimester selective reduction at their institution during the years 1986–1996. The technique was successful in all cases and the group encountered a 4% overall loss rate. Three of the four losses occurred within 3–4 weeks of the procedure, the patients presenting with either spontaneous rupture of membranes or labor. Of the 96 completed pregnancies, 95 delivered after 28 weeks gestation. Overall, 85% of their cases delivered after 32 weeks gestation and 14% between 28 and 32 weeks gestation. There were many indications for the selective reductions, including 40 fetuses with Down's syndrome.

Selective termination of a fetus with a lethal malformation is only indicated if the continued presence of such a defect presents greater hazards to the co-existing pregnancy than does the risk of termination. Selective termination in these situations would potentially improve the outcome by eliminating the probability of significant polyhydramnios and premature delivery.[68]

The short-term complications following second trimester multifetal pregnancy reduction are rare, and seem to be limited to the consistent finding of an elevated maternal serum α-fetoprotein, as has been described after first trimester procedures.[61,62] There appears to be a low probability of maternal coagulopathy secondary to retained fetal products. Despite the observed low risk, coagulation screening following second trimester procedures is felt to be justified by some authors until more data are collected.[69,70]

Second trimester selective reduction is a viable alternative in a multiple pregnancy where there is an abnormal fetus, usually carrying a non-lethal anomaly. As in the situation of first trimester reduction, patient selection and appropriate informed consent are key. In the unique situation of selective reduction for a fetus with an abnormality, correct identification of the affected fetus must be assured before the procedure is performed. Once these criteria are met, the chance for successful outcome is optimized.

Summary and conclusions

The use of multifetal pregnancy reduction to improve perinatal outcome has become an accepted component of reproductive medicine. The experience gained in performing the technique over the last 10 years has allowed reasonably objective conclusions to be made, although several issues remain controversial. The multifetal pregnancy reduction procedure itself has been modified and improved and, whether performed via the transabdominal or the transvaginal route, shows very little maternal risk and stabilized loss rates. Loss rates appear to be best with a lower starting fetal number and proportionately increase with increasing starting number. Reducing a pregnancy to a final number of two appears to be the ideal final number in most settings, but final numbers of three or one may be decided upon by the individual patient. The decision to reduce triplets remains controversial, although there are now several well performed studies in the literature that confirm that the decision to reduce triplets is a reasonable option and may improve perinatal outcome. Monochorionic multifetal pregnancies necessitate a unique approach, both in the decisions as to which fetuses to target, and the future complications that may occur if a monochorionic set remains intact, such as twin–twin transfusion syndrome. It has been well established that maternal serum α-fetoprotein testing is not of any value in reduced pregnancies, and the role for CVS and/or genetic amniocentesis is becoming better understood. It seems from the recent literature that CVS before and amniocentesis after MFPR are safe and do not increase the loss rate over that observed in association with the reduction itself. The automated puncture device mated to the vaginal probe has become an indispensable tool in the performance of multifetal pregnancy reduction in the authors' laboratory.

Second trimester selective reductions are performed for an entirely different set of criteria and, although the technique is similar to that of the transabdominal first trimester MFPR, its selective nature keeps it unique. Finally, any counseling session must include detailed discussion regarding ethical and psychological issues and inclusion of patients' beliefs. Both first and second trimester multifetal pregnancy reduction procedures provide an important alternative for patients with complicated multifetal pregnancies. Appropriate patient selection assures maximization of a successful outcome.

REFERENCES

1. Brandes JM, Itskovits J, Timor-Tritsch IE, Drugan A, Frydman R. Reduction of the number of embryos in multiple pregnancies in the first trimester. *N Engl J Med* 1988; **318**:1042–1047.

2. Berkowitz RL, Lynch L, Chitkara U, Wilkins IA, Mehalek KE, Alvarez E. Selective reduction of multifetal pregnancies in the first trimester. *N Engl J Med* 1988; **71**:289–296.

3. Evans MI, Fletcher JH, Zador IE et al. Selective first-trimester termination in octuplet and quadruplet pregnancies: clinical and ethical issues. *Obstet Gynecol* 1988; **71**:289–296.

4. Itskovitz J, Boldes R, Thaler I, Bronstein M, Erlik Y, Brandes JM. Transvaginal ultrasonography-guided aspiration of gestational sacs for selective abortion in multiple pregnancy. *Am J Obstet Gynecol* 1989; **160**:215–217.

5. Itskovitz J, Boldes R, Thaler I, Levron Y, Rottem S, Brandes JM. First trimester selective reduction in multiple pregnancy guided by transvaginal sonography. *J Clin Ultrasound* 1990; **18**:323–327.

6. Shalev E, Frenkel Y, Goldenberg M, Shalev J. Selective reduction in multiple gestations: pregnancy outcome after transvaginal and transabdominal needle-guided procedures. *Fertil Steril* 1989; **52**:416–420.

7. Martene-Duplan J, Aknin AJ, Alamowitch R. Aspiration embryonnaire partielle au cours de grossesses multiples. *Contracept Fertil Sexual* 1983; **11**:745–748.

8. Weinblatt V, Wapner R, Davis G et al. Fetal reduction and selective termination in multifetal pregnancy: outcomes, ethical and counseling issues. *Birth Defects* 1990; **26**:81–94.

9. Berkowitz RL, Stone JL, Eddleman KA. One hundred consecutive cases of selective termination of an abnormal fetus in a multifetal gestation. *Obstet Gynecol* 1997; **90**:606–610.

10. Dumez Y, Oury JF. Method for first trimester selective abortion in multiple pregnancy. *Contrib Gynecol Obstet* 1986; **15**:50.

11. Salat-Baroux J, Aiknin J, Antoine JM, Alamowitch R. The management of multiple pregnancies after induction for superovulation. *Human Reprod* 1988; **3**:399–401.

12. Dommergues M, Nisand I, Mandelbrot L, Isfer E, Radunovic N, Dumez Y. Embryo reduction in multifetal pregnancies following infertility therapy: obstetrical risks and perinatal benefits are related to operative strategy. *Feril Steril* 1991; **55**:805–811.

13. Tabsh KA. A report of 131 cases of multifetal pregnancy reduction. *Obstet Gynecol* 1993; **81**:57–60.

14. Berkowitz RL, Lynch L, Lapinski R, Bergh P. First trimester transabdominal multifetal pregnancy reduction: a report of two hundred completed cases. *Am J Obstet Gynecol* 1993; **169**:17–21.

15. Lipitz S, Yaron Y, Shalev J, Achiron R, Zolti M, Mashiach S. Improved results in multifetal pregnancy reduction: a report of 72 cases. *Fertil Steril* 1994; **61**:59–61.

16. Donner C, McGinnis, Simpon P, Rodesch F. Multifetal pregnancy reduction: a Belgian experience. *Eur J Obstet Gynecol Reprod Biol* 1990; **38**:183–187.

17. Wapner RJ, Davis GH, Johnson A et al. Selective reduction of multifetal pregnancies. *Lancet* 1990; **335**:90–93.

18. Boulot P, Hedon B, Pelliccia G et al. Multifetal pregnancy reduction: a consecutive series of 61 cases. *Br J Obstet Gynecol* 1993; **100**:63–68.

19. Timor-Tritsch IE, Peisner DB, Monteagudo A, Lerner JP, Sharma S. Multifetal pregnancy reduction by transvaginal puncture: evaluation of the technique used in 134 cases. *Am J Obstet Gynecol* 1993; **168**:799–804.

20. Donner C, McGinnis, Simon P, Rodesch F. Multifetal pregnancy reduction: a Belgian experience. *Eur J Obstet Gynecol Reprod Biol* 1990; **38**:183–187.

21. Poreco RP, Burke MS, Hendrix ML. Multifetal reduction of triplets to pregnancy outcome. *Obstet Gynecol* 1991; **78**:335–339.

22. Radestad A, Bui TH, Nygren KG. Multifetal pregnancy reduction in Sweden. *Acta Obstet Gynecol Scand* 1994; **73**:403–406.

23. Tanniradorn Y, Pharosaviasdi S. Transabdominal fetal reduction in quadruplet pregnancy during first trimester: a case report. *J Med Assoc Thailand* 1994; **77**:52–56.

24. Bollen N, Camus M, Tournaye H, Wisanto A, Van Steinteghem AC, Devroey P. Embryo reduction in triplet pregnancies after assisted procreation: a comparative study. *Fertil Steril* 1993; **60**:504–509.

25. Evans MI, Dommergues M, Wapner RJ et al. Efficacy of transabdominal multifetal pregnancy reduction: collaborative experience among the world's largest centers. *Obstet Gynecol* 1993; **82**:61–66.

26. Evans MI, Dommergues M, Timor-Tritsch I et al. Transabdominal versus transcervical and transvaginal multifetal pregnancy reduction: international collaborative experience of more than one thousand cases. *Am J Obstet Gynecol* 1994; **170**:902–909.

27. Evans MI, Dommergues M, Wapner RJ et al. International, collaborative experience of 1789 patients having multifetal pregnancy reduction: a plateauing of risks and outcomes. *J Soc Gynecol Invest* 1996; **3**:23–26.

28. Melgar CA, Rosenfield DL, Rawlinson K, Greenberg M. Perinatal outcome after multifetal reduction to twins compared with nonreduced multiple gestations. *Obstet Gynecol* 1991; **78**:763–767.

29. Atlas R, Bolognese RJ. Perinatal outcome of triplets: is there a place for selective reduction? In: *Proceedings of the American College of Obstetricians and Gynecologists Junior Fellows District 3 Meeting*. Atlantic City, NJ: ACOG, 1992: 16–32.

30. Sassoon DA, Castro LC, Davis JL, Hobel CJ. Perinatal outcome in triplet versus twin gestations. *Obstet Gynecol* 1990; **75**:817–820.

31. Lipitz S, Reichman B, Paret G. The improving outcome of triplet pregnancies. *Am J Obstet Gynecol* 1989; **161**:1279–1284.

32. Gonen R, Heyman E, Asztalos EV et al. The outcome of triplet, quadruplet, and quintuplet pregnancies managed in a perinatal unit: obstetric, neonatal, and follow up data. Am J Obstet Gynecol 1989; **162**:454–459.

33. Ron-el R, Caspi E, Schreyer P et al. Triplet and quadruplet pregnancies and management. Obstet Gynecol 1981; **57**:458–463.

34. Manzur A, Goldsman MP, Stone SC, Frederick JL, Balmadceda JP, Asch RH. Outcome of triplet pregnancies after assisted reproductive techniques: how frequent are vanishing embryos. Fertil Steril 1995; **63**:252–257.

35. Collins JW Jr, Merrick D, David RJ, Ameli S, Ogata ES. The Northwestern University triplet study III: neonatal outcome. Acta Genet Med Gemellol 1988; **37**:77–80.

36. Caspi E, Ronen J, Schreyer P, Goldberg MD. The outcome of pregnancy after gonadotropin therapy. Br J Obstet Gynaecol 1976; **83**:967.

37. Botting BJ, Davies IM, MacFarlane AJ. Recent trends in the incidence of multiple births and associated mortality. Arch Dis Child 1987; **62**:941–950.

38. Macones GA, Schemmer G, Pritts E, Weinblatt V, Wapner RJ. Multifetal reduction of triplets to twins improves perinatal outcome. Am J Obstet Gynecol 1993; **169**:982–986.

39. Lipitz S, Uval J, Achiron R, Schiff E, Lusky A, Reichman B. Outcome of twin pregnancies reduced from triplets compared with nonreduced twin gestations. Obstet Gynecol 1996; **87**:511–514.

40. Haning RV Jr, Seifer DB, Wheeler CA, Frishman GN, Silver H, Pierce DJ. Effects of fetal number and multifetal reduction on length of in vitro fertilization pregnancies. Obstet Gynecol 1996; **87**:964–968.

41. Kadhel P, Olivennes F, Fernandez H, Vial M, Frydman R. Are there still obstetric benefits for selective embryo reduction of triplet pregnancies? Human Reprod 1998; **13**:3555–3559.

42. Timor-Tritsch IE, Fleischer A, Monteagudo A, Valderrama E. Monochorionic quadramniotic quadruplets: sonographic workup. Fetal Diagn Ther 1997; **12**:363–367.

43. Berkowitz RL, Lynch L. Selective reduction: an unfortunate misnomer. Obstet Gynecol 1990; **75**: 273–274.

44. Grazi RV, Wolowelsky JB. Multifetal pregnancy reduction and disposal of in transplanted embryos in contemporary Jewish Law and ethics. Am J Obstet Gynecol 1991; **165**:1268–1271.

45. Multifetal pregnancy reduction and selective fetal termination. ACOG committee opinion. Committee on Ethics #94, April 1991. Int J Gynecol Obstet 1992; **38**:140–142.

46. Kanhai HHH, de Haan M, van Zanten LA, Geerinck-Vercammen C, van der Ploeg HM, Gravenhorst JB. Follow up of pregnancies, infants, and families after multifetal pregnancy reduction. Fertil Steril 1994; **621**:955–959.

47. McKinney M, Downey J, Timor-Tritsch IE. The psychological effects of multifetal pregnancy reduction. Fertil Steril 1995; **64**:51–61.

48. Schreiner-Angle P, Walther VN, Mindes J, Lynch L, Berkowitz RL. First trimester multifetal pregnancy reduction: acute to persistent psychologic reactions. Am J Obstet Gynecol 1990; **172**:541–547.

49. Weinblatt V, Wapner RJ. Chorionic villus sampling and amniocentesis in multifetal pregnancy. In: Monteagudo A, Timor-Tritsch IE, eds. Ultrasound and Multifetal Pregnancy. New York: Parthenon, 1998: 209.

50. Brambati B, Tului L, Baldi M, Guercilena S. Genetic analysis prior to selective fetal reduction in multiple pregnancy: technical aspects and clinical outcome. Human Reprod 1995; **10**:818–825.

51. Coffler MS, Kol S, Drugan A, Itskovitz-Eldor J. Early transvaginal embryo aspiration: a safer method for selectvie reduction in high order multiple gestations. Human Reprod 1999; **14**:1875–1878.

52. DeCatte L, Camus M, Bondvelle M, Liebaers I, Foulon W. Prenatal diagnosis by chorionic villus sampling in multiple pregnancies prior to fetal reduction. Am J Perinatal 1998; **15**:339–343.

53. Tabsh KMA, Theroux NL. Genetic amniocentesis following multifetal pregnancy reduction to twins: assessing the risk. Prenat Diagn 1995; **15**:221–223.

54. Selam B, Török O, Lembert A, Stone J, Lapinski R, Berkowitz RL. Genetic amniocentesis after multifetal pregnancy reduction. Am J Obstet Gynecol 1999; **180**:226–230.

55. McLean LK, Evans MI, Carpenter RJ Jr, Johnson MP, Goldberg JD. Genetic amniocentesis following multifetal pregnancy reduction does not increase the risk of pregnancy loss. Prenat Diagn 1998; **18**:186–188.

56. Stephen J, Timor-Tritsch I, Lerner J, Monteagudo A, Alonso CM. Amniocentesis following multifetal pregnancy reduction: is it safe? Am J Obstet Gynecol 2000; **182**:962–965.

57. Monni G, Zoppi MA, Cau G, Loni R, Baldi M. Importance of nuchal translucency measurement in multifetal pregnancy reduction. Ultrasound Obstet Gynecol 1999; **13**:377–378.

58. MacGilvray I. Malformations and other abnormalities in twins. In: MacGilvray I, Nylander PPS, Corney G, eds. Human Multiple Reproduction. London: WB Saunders, 1975:165–175.

59. Windham GC, Sever LE. Neural tube defects among twin births. Am J Human Genet 1982; **34**:988–998.

60. Windham GC, Bjerkedal T, Sever LE. The association of twinning and neural tube defects: studies in Los Angeles, California, and Norway. Acta Genet Med Gemellol 1982; **31**:165–172.

61. Grau P, Robinson L, Tabsh K, Crandall BF. Elevated maternal serum alpha-fetoprotein and amniotic fluid alpha-fetoprotein after multifetal pregnancy reduction. Obstet Gynecol 1990; **76**:1042–1045.

62. Lynch L. Berkowitz RL. Maternal serum alpha-fetoprotein and coagulation profiles after multifetal pregnancy reduction. Am J Obstet Gynecol 1993; **169**:987–990.

63. Aberg A, Miterian F, Cantz M et al. Cardiac puncture of fetus with Hurler's disease avoiding abortion of unaffected co-twin. Lancet 1978; **ii**:990–991.

64. Kerenyi T, Chitkara U. Selective birth in twin pregnancy

with discordancy for Down's syndrome. *N Engl J Med* 1981; **304**:1525–1527.

65. Rodeck CH, Mibashan RS, Abramowicz J, Campbell S. Selective feticide of the affected twin by fetoscopic air embolism. *Prenat Diagn* 1982; **2**:189–194.

66. Evans MI, Littmann L, King M, Fletcher JC. Multiple gestation: the role of multifetal pregnancy reduction and selective termination. *Clin Perinatol* 1992; **19**:345–356.

67. Chitkara U, Berkowitz RL, Wilkins IA, Lynch L, Mihalek KE, Alvarez M. Selective second trimester termination of the anomalous fetus in twin pregnancies. *Obstet Gynecol* 1989; **73**:690–694.

68. Romero R, Duffy DP, Berkowitz RL, Chang E, Hobbins JC. Prolongation of a preterm pregnancy complicated by death of a single twin in utero and disseminated intravascular coagulation. *N Engl J Med* 1984; **310**:772–774.

69. Jackson L, Wapner R, Barr M. Evaluating the safety and cytogenetic diagnostic rate of chorionic villus sampling. *Am J Human Genet* 1987; 826 (abstract).

70. Skelly H, Marivate M, Norman R. Consumptive coagulopathy following fetal death in a triplet pregnancy. *Am J Obstet Gynecol* 1982; **142**:595–596.

19 Color and pulsed Doppler in early pregnancy

Mary C Frates

The addition of color and pulsed Doppler capabilities to the vaginal probe has prompted extensive investigation into the role of Doppler imaging in the assessment of early pregnancy. Studies have examined blood flow in vessels that supply structures including the uterus and ovary, as well as the developing gestation. This research has led to greater understanding of the physiology of normal and abnormal early pregnancies, which, in turn, may help investigators to find ways of using Doppler imaging to improve diagnostic accuracy in the first trimester.

Any discussion of the use of color and pulsed Doppler sonography during early pregnancy must begin by considering the risks and benefits of Doppler interrogation for the early developing embryo. While gray scale sonography is considered safe for use in pregnancy at all gestational ages, the addition of Doppler changes the parameters of the examination sufficiently to merit further consideration prior to its indiscriminate use. The energy used for combined Doppler and sonographic interrogation routinely exceeds that used for gray scale sonography alone. The major concern, therefore, is that the increased energy will cause the temperature to rise in the tissues exposed, thereby causing developmental abnormalities in the fetus. The Federal Drug Administration (FDA) has set standards for equipment that is used for ultrasound and Doppler imaging of pregnancies. Examiners who use Doppler sonography to study the embryo and fetus are obligated to confirm that their equipment is maintained at power levels approved by the FDA (< 720 mW/cm^2, spatial peak temporal average intensity) to prevent excessive temperature increases.[1,2] Information about the energy intensity levels generated by each probe is supplied by the manufacturer.

In order to minimize exposure of the embryo or fetus, Doppler should only be used when clinically indicated to answer a question that could not be resolved with gray scale ultrasound alone. Color Doppler should be used first to localize the vessel of interest, and then pulsed Doppler focally applied for waveform analysis. Those patients in whom the use of Doppler sonography is for research purposes only must provide informed consent before the examination. In all instances, the amount of time Doppler is in use should be kept to a minimum, particularly when the embryo or fetus is within the field of view.

In this chapter, after an introduction to the physiology of uteroplacental circulation, the proposed uses of color and pulsed Doppler in first trimester patients will be discussed. This will include Doppler evaluation of the early gravid uterus, including intrauterine fluid collections and how to categorize them. It will be followed by a discussion of the use of color and pulsed Doppler in predicting pregnancy outcome, in the evaluation of gestational trophoblastic diseases, and in the evaluation and treatment of ectopic pregnancy. The potential role of Doppler in clinical practice will be considered in each of these areas.

The uterus in normal early pregnancy

Knowledge of the anatomy and physiology of uterine blood flow is critical to defining the role of Doppler in evaluating early pregnancy. During the course of pregnancy there is a progressive fall in uterine vascular resistance and an increase in blood flow to the uterus, with a concurrent increase in maternal blood volume and cardiac output. A constant forward flow of maternal blood through the uterus is required to support the developing fetus. This blood flow originates from the paired uterine arteries, which arise from the anterior division of the

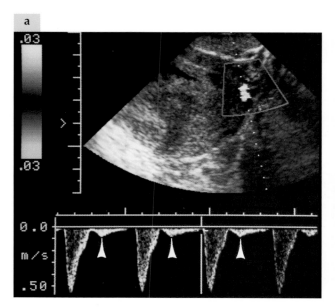

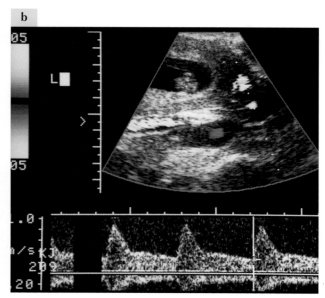

Figure 19.1 First trimester uterine artery waveforms. (a) Transvaginal sonography and Doppler image of the left uterine artery at 7.0 weeks gestational age (GA) demonstrates the typical high resistance waveform with a well-defined diastolic notch (arrowhead) of a uterine artery. (b) Transabdominal sonogram of the left uterine artery in a different patient at 10.3 weeks GA shows absence of the diastolic notch, a normal variant.

internal iliac artery. Each uterine artery arrives at the uterus at the level of the uterocervical junction, ascends along the lateral wall giving off multiple penetrating branches, then finally anastamoses with branches of the ovarian artery at the level of the fallopian tube. Pulsed Doppler of the uterine arteries in early pregnancy typically demonstrates high resistance flow with a prominent diastolic notch. Occasionally, the notch will be absent in a normal patient (*Fig. 19.1*). The diastolic notch usually disappears during the second trimester,[3] sometimes as early as 13 weeks gestation.[4]

Inside the uterus, the subchorionic vessels, or spiral arteries, are located at the junction of the echogenic trophoblast and the myometrium. Flow in these vessels is typically pulsatile and low resistance (*Fig. 19.2*). Flow in the intervillous space, at the site of eventual placental development, is non-pulsatile, with a more venous-like waveform (*Fig. 19.3*). In very early pregnancy (< 10 weeks gestation), true intervillous flow can only be identified with Doppler from the chorion frondosum, which arises from the decidua basalis and subsequently forms the placenta.[5] This site may be very difficult or impossible to localize. Furthermore, even later in the first trimester, when the placenta has formed, intervillous flow may be difficult to identify because of its extremely low velocities.

The creation of side-by-side maternal and fetal circulations to nurture the developing fetus begins

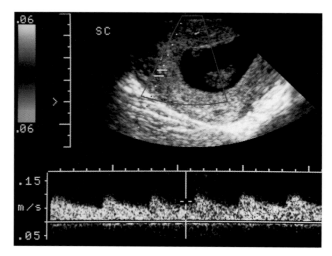

Figure 19.2 In this patient at 8.8 weeks gestational age, transvaginal scanning demonstrates the typical low resistance, pulsatile flow found in the subchorionic vessels. These vessels are located at the junction of the echogenic trophoblastic tissue and the more hypoechoic myometrium (Doppler gate).

at the time of implantation in the uterus, when trophoblastic cells attach to and invade the decidualized endometrium. These cells create the chorionic villi, which produce a framework that will surround the developing embryo. The trophoblastic cells extend into the decidualized endometrium and

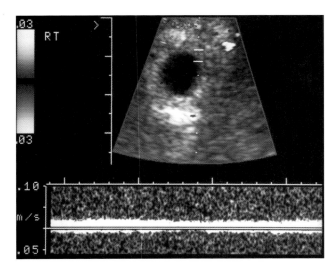

Figure 19.3 In some patients, careful scanning may reveal intervillous flow. This extremely low velocity, venous-type waveform is optimally obtained from the echogenic chorion frondosum, the site of eventual placental development. In this patient, intervillous flow was identified at transvaginal sonography at 6.0 weeks gestational age. The pregnancy outcome was normal.

form plugs within the maternal spiral arteries, which have simultaneously invaded the intervillous space. Exactly how early in the first trimester the intervillous space becomes perfused by the spiral arteries is not known; however, by the second trimester, this process is complete, and the intervillous space is fully perfused by maternal blood.

Partly as a result of studies on first trimester gravid hysterectomy specimens that demonstrated no communication between the maternal and fetal circulations,[6] it has been hypothesized that the intervillous spaces in early pregnancy are filled with clear fluid, possibly representing filtered maternal plasma. These fluid-filled intervillous spaces provide a hypoxic environment that protects the developing embryo by preventing superoxide dismutase and other potentially harmful substances from reaching it.[7] By the end of the first trimester, the trophoblastic plugs within the spiral arteries have dissolved or dislodged, and maternal blood then fills the intervillous spaces. Once this happens, there is a marked increase in uterine blood flow, which is evident as increased systolic velocities and decreased resistance in the uterine vessels. This hypothesis maintains that intervillous flow is therefore absent until the end of the first trimester.[4,5,8–12]

An alternative hypothesis proposes that the transformation of the intervillous space from fluid to blood-filled is gradual, occurring over the entire first trimester. Consequently, slow venous flow should

be identifiable with sensitive Doppler techniques within the intervillous space during the first trimester. Indeed, slow intervillous flow has been reported as early as 5.5 gestational weeks at transvaginal Doppler interrogation (*Fig. 19.3*).[13–16] This latter hypothesis is supported by studies that have shown a gradual decrease in uterine artery resistance during the first trimester,[3,4,17] as well as by sonographic contrast studies performed in animals.[18] Further investigation of early uteroplacental circulation is necessary to improve understanding of this process.

The assessment of early pregnancy with Doppler imaging

Doppler imaging may prove useful for evaluating first trimester gestations in those patients in whom the serum human chorionic gonadotropin (β-hCG) is positive, yet no definitive gestational sac can be identified by transvaginal sonography. These patients could have nothing in the uterus or they could have a non-specific intrauterine fluid collection.

In patients with empty uteri, Doppler can be used to interrogate the myometrium just beneath the endometrium, in the region of the spiral arteries. The demonstration of sparse amounts of flow by color Doppler, combined with extremely low peak systolic velocities of < 8 cm/s and low to absent end-diastolic flow, suggests that the pregnancy is not in the uterus and should raise concern regarding an ectopic pregnancy (*Fig. 19.4*).[19] In contrast, a gravid

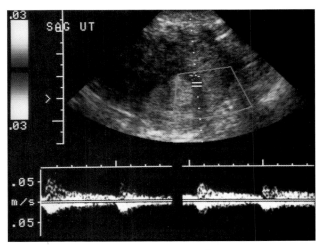

Figure 19.4 In a pregnant patient with an empty uterus, sparse flashes of low velocity flow (< 8 cm/s) suggest that the pregnancy is extrauterine in location. This appearance has been termed a 'cold' uterus.

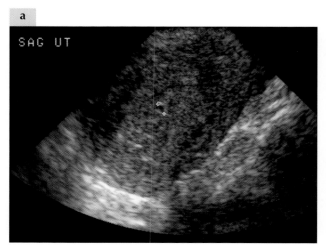
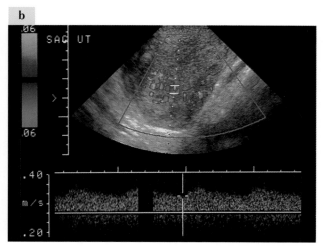

Figure 19.5 Pregnant patient with an indeterminate intrauterine fluid collection. (a) At transvaginal sonography of the uterus, a 3 mm fluid collection (calipers) is seen within the decidualized endometrium. (b) Following the addition of Doppler, multiple flashes of color are visible throughout the uterus. Pulsed Doppler tracing shows typical low resistance pulsatile waveform of subchorionic vessels, helping to confirm the fluid collection as an IUP.

uterus is usually 'warm' on color Doppler, with multiple flashes of myometrial color. This appearance suggests a very early intrauterine gestation (< 5.0 weeks) or a recent spontaneous miscarriage. Pulsed Doppler interrogation of the color flashes in a gravid uterus typically shows 'peritrophoblastic' arterial flow in the spiral arteries. This flow is characterized by peak systolic velocities of > 8 cm/s, with a high diastolic component (*Fig. 19.5*). More stringent criteria are often used with greater certainty, such as a peak systolic velocity of > 15 cm/s together with a resistive index (RI) of < 0.55 in the spiral arteries to diagnose an intrauterine pregnancy (IUP).[20]

When the uterus contains a non-specific fluid collection, it should be possible to differentiate a pseudosac associated with an ectopic pregnancy from a normal or abnormal intrauterine gestational sac. A pseudosac should have absent or only minimal low velocity flow around it (< 8 cm/s peak systolic velocity) (*Fig. 19.6*),[21] while flow around an intrauterine gestational sac should show relatively high velocity and low resistance. The blood flow around an abnormal IUP is not significantly different from that around a normal early gestational sac.[22–24] Unfortunately, very little information is available about the use of Doppler for the evaluation of pseudosacs. Therefore, in patients with an intrauterine fluid collection without an adnexal mass or definite IUP at first sonogram, sonographic and clinical follow-up is recommended rather than interrogation with Doppler. Within 1–2 weeks, normal IUPs will develop a chorionic rim, yolk sac,

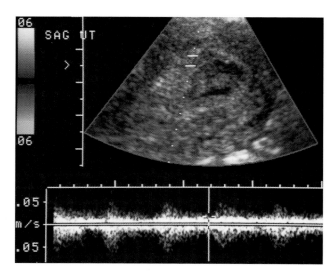

Figure 19.6 In this patient with proven ectopic pregnancy and an intrauterine pseudosac, interrogation of the complex intrauterine fluid collection shows sparse, low velocity tracings. (Note similarity in tracing to Fig. 19.4)

and cardiac activity. Failed IUPs will become more apparent by failing to progress normally both clinically and sonographically. Follow-up studies should also lead to the correct diagnosis in the presence of an ectopic pregnancy. Because Doppler has not been shown to improve diagnosis in this clinical setting, its use should be avoided, to prevent unnecessary and potentially harmful exposure of an early embryo.

Predicting pregnancy outcome

The loss rate for first trimester pregnancies ranges from 5% to 20%, depending on a multitude of factors, including presence and rate of embryonic cardiac activity, maternal age, and the gestational age at the time of the sonographic examination.[25,26] With the ultimate goal of improving prediction of pregnancy outcome, researchers are now examining the relationship between early pregnancy blood flow and pregnancy outcome.

Studies of uterine artery blood flow in early pregnancies have found no correlation between the uterine artery waveform or its progressive changes during the first trimester and pregnancy outcome.[17,27] Therefore, uterine artery tracings cannot be used to predict first trimester pregnancy outcome.

Some studies of subchorionic vessels and pregnancy outcome have suggested that normal pregnancy outcome is associated with an RI of $\leqslant 0.55$.[10,28] Others, however, have found no significant difference in pregnancy loss rates with subchorionic RIs above as compared to those below 0.55.[17,27]

Vascular spaces around the periphery of the gestational sac are occasionally seen as prominent hypoechoic areas with visible venous flow (*Fig. 19.7*). These are sometimes called venous lakes, and should not be confused with intervillous flow during early pregnancy. Slow flow within the vascular spaces around a sac is often visible with gray scale sonography when high gain settings are

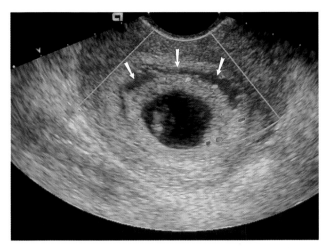

Figure 19.7 Small venous lake. Coronal transvaginal color Doppler image of a live 7.4 week embryo and sac, showing a hypoechoic, crescentic collection (arrows) surrounding the anterior portion of the gestational sac. Although no flow is demonstrated within the collection at color Doppler, it was easily appreciated with gray scale sonography at high gain settings.

used, but this flow can be difficult to document with color or pulsed Doppler owing to its low velocity. Because the flow can be subtle, the vascular spaces may be misinterpreted as subchorionic hematomas. Some reports suggest that the appearance of these vascular spaces is an ominous sign in early pregnancy;[24,28] however, others disagree (*Fig. 19.8*). Because of the uncertainty about the clinical

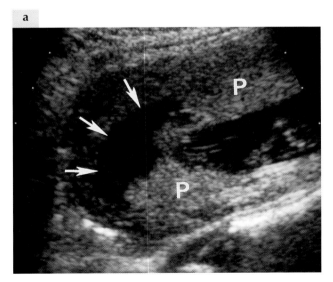

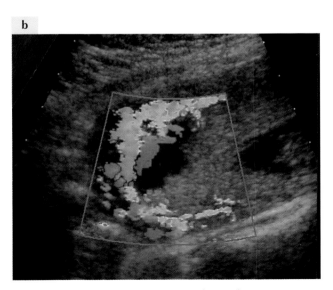

Figure 19.8 Large venous lake. (a) Sagittal sonogram of the uterine fundus at 11 weeks gestational age shows an anechoic collection (arrows) between the sac and the myometrium, that appears to lift the placenta (P). This was incorrectly diagnosed as a subchorionic hematoma. (b) With the addition of color Doppler, prominent flow can be seen within the collection, indicating its vascular nature. The outcome of this pregnancy was normal.

significance of this finding, close sonographic follow-up is probably warranted.

The corpus luteum and pregnancy outcome

The corpus luteum is an intraovarian structure found during the first trimester. It is responsible for the production of progesterone, required to support the developing gestation until the placenta is formed.[29] It has been hypothesized that a non-functioning or 'suboptimal' corpus luteum may result in pregnancy loss. Exactly what constitutes a 'suboptimal' corpus luteum, however, has not been defined.

The sonographic appearance of the corpus luteum is quite variable. The most common sonographic appearance is a thick-walled cyst, which may or may not contain internal echoes (*Fig. 19.9*). Another common appearance is a hypoechoic or isoechoic lesion which may be difficult to localize without color Doppler to delineate the margins (*Fig. 19.10*). Infrequently, the corpus luteum may appear as a simple cyst. Despite the wide range of sonographic appearances, no relationship between corpus luteum appearance and pregnancy outcome has been found.[30,31]

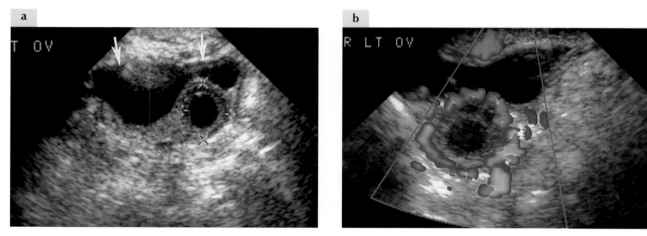

Figure 19.9 Corpus luteum. (a) A thick-walled cystic corpus luteum within the left ovary is outlined by calipers. A simple follicular cyst is seen anteriorly (arrows). (b) With the addition of color Doppler, a well defined ring of color is seen around the margins of the corpus luteum.

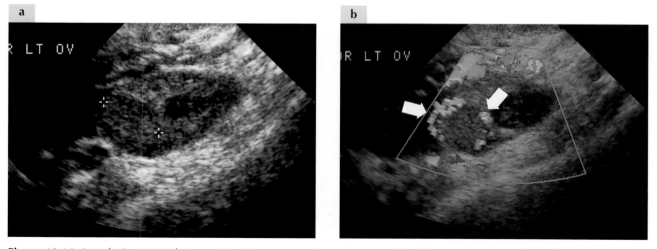

Figure 19.10 Isoechoic corpus luteum. (a) At transvaginal sonography of the left ovary, a nearly isoechoic corpus luteum is marked with calipers. (b) Color Doppler produces a distinct ring of vascularity (arrows), making the corpus luteum easier to appreciate.

Corpora lutea typically have a prominent ring of flow that is almost universal at color Doppler interrogation, and it has been postulated that inadequate vascularization of the corpus luteum may cause suboptimal progesterone synthesis. This, in turn, may result in pregnancy loss. Preliminary investigations have shown no correlation between pregnancy outcome and the RI of corpus luteal vessels.[31] Once the pregnancy has failed, however, the RI may be elevated.[32,33]

Rarely, the corpus luteum cannot be identified with gray scale or color Doppler sonography. The absence of the corpus luteum is associated with an increased pregnancy loss rate.[30,31] It is possible that patients with normal early pregnancies and no visible corpus luteum might benefit from supplemental progesterone therapy.

At this time, there are no definitive Doppler criteria that can be used to predict pregnancy outcome. While certain Doppler patterns may suggest a somewhat better or somewhat worse prognosis for an individual pregnancy, no pattern can supersede the value of visualizing embryonic cardiac activity and appropriate fetal growth. The use of Doppler in early pregnancy is an area of ongoing research, and, as such, should not be considered part of the standard first trimester ultrasound examination.

Molar pregnancy

Gestational trophoblastic diseases are a spectrum of chorionic tumors that arise from the placental tissues. They range from benign hydatidiform mole to choriocarcinoma. Most complete moles have a 46XX karyotype, with both sets of chromosomes of paternal origin. In contrast, most partial moles have a triploid karyotype (69 chromosomes) with one maternal and two paternal haploid sets. Hydatidiform moles are found in 0.1–0.2% of pregnancies.[34] Persistent or invasive trophoblastic disease occurs in approximately 20–30% of patients with complete moles, and can be diagnosed by persistently elevated β-hCG levels following treatment of the molar pregnancy. Choriocarcinoma, occurring in approximately 4% of molar pregnancies,[35] leads to invasive growth of the trophoblast with absence of villi. Metastases are common.[36]

The diagnosis of a molar pregnancy can be suggested by gray scale sonography. At transvaginal sonography, the uterine cavity is distended and filled with an echogenic mass containing multiple cystic spaces. No fetus is identified. The cystic structures range in size from 1 to 30 mm, and represent clear vesicles and vascular spaces within the chorionic villi.[36] These structures become more prominent as the gestational age increases, and correlate with increasing levels of β-hCG. Flow within molar tissue is typically low resistance.

Because trophoblastic tumors are extremely vascular, high velocity, low resistance flow can easily be found with color and pulsed Doppler within the complex endometrial material (*Fig. 19.11*). The overall blood supply to the uterus is dramatically increased in the presence of gestational trophoblastic disease, with elevations in both systolic and diastolic velocities in the uterine arteries.[37] The RI

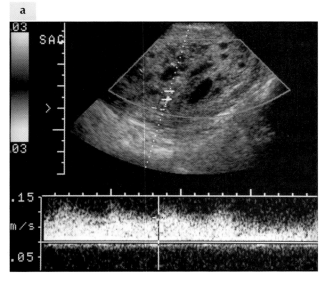
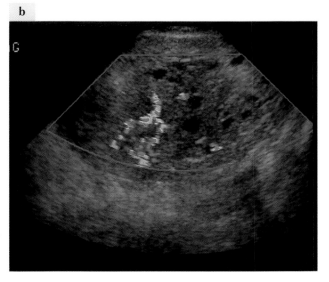

Figure 19.11 Benign hydatidiform mole. (a) A complex intrauterine collection composed of multiple small fluid-filled spaces is seen. Doppler interrogation reveals typical pulsatile, low resistance flow pattern. (b) Prominent vessels within the mole are identified with color Doppler.

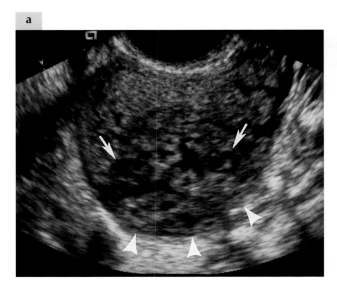
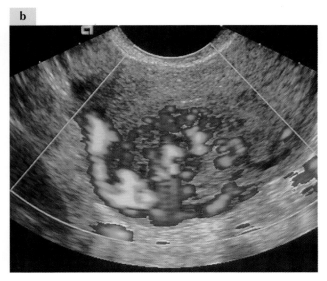

Figure 19.12 Invasive mole. (a) Sagittal gray scale sonogram of the uterus shows a heterogeneous mass with central cystic components (arrows) extending to the edge of the myometrium (arrowheads). (b) Addition of power Doppler shows marked vascularity extending to the surface of the myometrium, an appearance highly suspicious for invasion.

in all branches of the uterine artery is significantly lower than in normal pregnancy.[22,38] Focal areas of prominent color flow within the myometrium, with concurrent high velocity, low resistance Doppler tracings, are highly suggestive of myometrial invasion, and may indicate the need for additional therapy beyond curettage (*Fig. 19.12*). Color Doppler can be helpful in identifying residual or recurrent tissue in patients with persistently elevated β-hCG levels following treatment of molar pregnancy. The presence of focal myometrial flow suggests local intramural recurrence.

Role of Doppler with ectopic pregnancy

Several different applications for Doppler sonography in the evaluation of ectopic pregnancy have been proposed, with the hope of increasing diagnostic accuracy for ectopic pregnancy. With pulsed Doppler interrogation, the RI of an adnexal lesion can be obtained. With color Doppler, overall vascularity of the ectopic pregnancy can be assessed. However, the usefulness of color Doppler sonography for diagnosing ectopic pregnancy remains unproven. Transvaginal studies that compare gray scale and color Doppler imaging are limited in number[19,39] and the results are disparate as a result of variation in the study designs. Studies that employ very strict gray scale diagnostic criteria and

loose criteria for color Doppler cannot be compared to studies that employ less stringent but proven gray scale criteria. Sensitivities for diagnosing ectopic pregnancy with gray scale sonography are well established and high at 87–94%.[40–43] One hope was that color Doppler sonography would improve the sensitivity for early ectopic pregnancies, by identifying an extraovarian region of increased vascularity where no mass could be found with gray scale imaging. However, improvement beyond the well-documented high sensitivity of gray scale sonography alone has not been found.

A wide range of RIs are found in ectopic pregnancies, and considerable overlap exists between the RIs of an ectopic pregnancy and a corpus luteum (*Fig. 19.13*). The intraovarian location of the corpus luteum should be used to differentiate it from an ectopic pregnancy.[39] Other adnexal lesions such as pelvic inflammation or pedunculated fibroids may display similar Doppler findings to an ectopic pregnancy, thus increasing the chance of false positive results if Doppler is relied upon to diagnose an ectopic.

One potential use for color and pulsed Doppler could be in those patients with a known ectopic pregnancy in whom an adnexal mass is visible. In this group, Doppler may provide a means of monitoring trophoblastic activity within the mass, potentially helping to determine appropriate therapy. Absent trophoblastic flow around an adnexal mass on color Doppler interrogation may

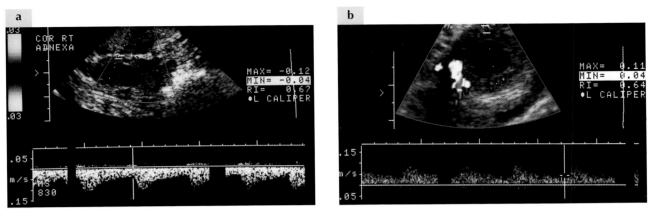

Figure 19.13 Considerable overlap exists between the RI of an ectopic pregnancy and that of a corpus luteum. (a) Coronal sonogram of a right adnexal ectopic pregnancy. Pulsed Doppler tracing shows an RI of 0.67. (b) Pulsed Doppler interrogation of the corpus luteum in a different patient shows a similar waveform, with an RI of 0.64.

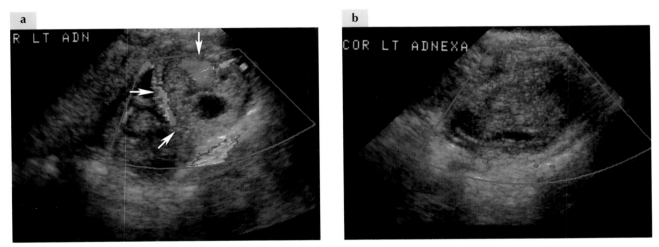

Figure 19.14 Sonographic and color Doppler follow-up of an ectopic pregnancy. (a) Transvaginal color Doppler image of a left adnexal ectopic pregnancy shows prominent blood flow around the margins of the adnexal ring (arrows). This patient was managed expectantly, with close clinical and sonographic follow-up, due to a co-existent intrauterine triplet gestation and multiple prior adnexal surgeries. (b) Follow-up scan 5 days later shows interval disappearance of the prominent vascularity. The patient's symptoms resolved without treatment, and the triplet intrauterine gestation had a successful outcome.

correlate with non-viable tissue or an involuting ectopic pregnancy.[44–46] Such patients may be appropriate candidates for non-surgical treatment, such as systemic or directly injected methotrexate, or even for expectant management. In these patients, continued absence of flow at color Doppler follow-up can provide clinical reassurance (*Fig. 19.14*).[47]

Color Doppler sonography may supply useful information in a patient in whom a cervical ectopic pregnancy is suspected. In this unusual form of

ectopic pregnancy, implantation occurs within the cervical canal, leaving the patient at high risk for hemorrhage as the gestation progresses. The diagnosis of cervical ectopic pregnancy can be difficult at gestational ages under 6 weeks, when the lack of cardiac activity may cause confusion between a true cervical ectopic and a spontaneous abortion passing through the cervical canal. With the addition of color Doppler, flow can sometimes be demonstrated within the trophoblastic ring of a cervical pregnancy (*Fig. 19.15*). No flow is seen in the rim of an aborting sac (*Fig. 19.16*).

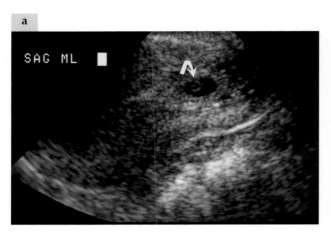
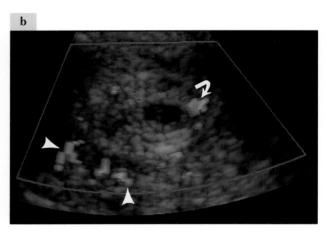

Figure 19.15 Cervical ectopic pregnancy. (a) Sagittal transvaginal sonogram of the uterus shows a well formed cervical gestational sac (arrow) containing a yolk sac. (b) Magnified color Doppler image of the gestational sac demonstrates vascularity within the echogenic wall of the sac (arrow), as well as within the cervix itself (arrowheads).

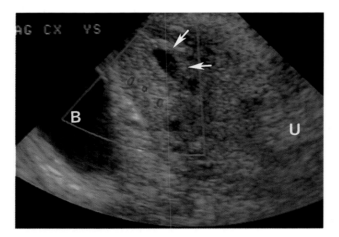

Figure 19.16 Spontaneous abortion-in-progress. An irregularly shaped gestational sac (arrows) with tiny yolk sac is seen within the cervical canal of a retroverted uterus (U, uterus; B, bladder). A trace amount of flow is seen with color Doppler within the cervical wall; however, none is found around the gestational sac.

Transvaginal sonography alone has a proven high sensitivity and specificity for the diagnosis of ectopic pregnancy. The addition of color or pulsed Doppler imaging to transvaginal sonography for the diagnosis of ectopic pregnancy does not improve diagnostic accuracy, and therefore Doppler imaging should not be considered a necessity in the evaluation of ectopic pregnancy.

In conclusion, Doppler interrogation in the first trimester is primarily a research tool. In most first trimester patients, color and pulsed Doppler are not essential nor even indicated. However, a growing understanding of the physiology of early pregnancy will continue to spur additional investigation into the blood supply of the first trimester.

REFERENCES

1. AIUM. *AIUM Official Statement on Clinical Safety.* Laurel, MD: AIUM, 1998.
2. Dillon E, Taylor K. Doppler ultrasound in the female pelvis and first trimester of pregnancy. In: Taylor KJW, Strandness DE, ed. *Duplex Doppler Ultrasound: Clinics in Diagnostic Ultrasound* vol 26. New York: Churchill Livingstone, 1989:93–116.
3. Shulman H, Fleischer A, Farmakides G, Bracero L, Rochelson B, Grunfeld L. Development of uterine artery compliance in pregnancy as detected by Doppler ultrasound. *Am J Obstet Gynecol* 1986; **155**:1031–1036.
4. Coppens M, Loquet P, Kollen M, De Neubourg F, Buytaert P. Longitudinal evaluation of uteroplacental and umbilical blood flow changes in normal early pregnancy. *Ultrasound Obstet Gynecol* 1996; **7**:114–121.
5. Jauniaux E. Intervillous circulation in the first trimester. The phantom of the color Doppler obstetric opera. *Ultrasound Obstet Gynecol* 1996; **8**:73–76.

6. Hustin J, Schaaps J. Echographic and anatomic studies of the maternotrophoblastic border during the first trimester of pregnancy. *Am J Obstet Gynecol* 1987; **157**:162–168.

7. Umaoka Y, Noda Y, Narimoto K, Mori T. Effects of oxygen toxicity on early development of mouse embryos. *Mol Reprod Dev* 1992; **31**:28–33.

8. Jauniaux E, Jurkovic D, Campbell S. In vivo investigations of the anatomy and the physiology of early human placental circulations. *Ultrasound Obstet Gynecol* 1991; **1**:435–445.

9. Jaffe RJE, Hustin J. Maternal circulation in the first-trimester human placenta—Myth or reality? *Am J Obstet Gynecol* 1997; **176**:695–705.

10. Jaffe R, Woods JR. Color Doppler imaging and in vivo assessment of the anatomy and physiology of the early uteroplacental circulation. *Fertil Steril* 1993; **60**:293–297.

11. Jauniaux E, Jurkovic D, Campbell S. Doppler ultrasonographic features of the developing placental circulation: correlation with anatomic findings. *Am J Obstet Gynecol* 1992; **166**:585–587.

12. Meuris S, Nagy A-M, Delogne-Desnoeck J, Jurkovic D, Jauniaux E. Temporal relationship between the human chorionic gonadotrophin peak and the establishment of intervillous blood flow in early pregnancy. *Human Reprod* 1995; **10**:947–950.

13. Merce L, Barco M, Bau S. Color Doppler sonographic assessment of placental circulation in the first trimester of normal pregnancy. *J Ultrasound Med* 1996; **15**:135–142.

14. Valentin L, Sladkevicius P, Laurini R, Soderberg H, Marsal K. Uteroplacental and luteal circulation in normal first-trimester pregnancies: Doppler ultrasonographic and morphologic study. *Am J Obstet Gynecol* 1996; **174**:768–775.

15. Merce LT, Barco MJ, de la Fuente F. Doppler velocimetry measured in retrochorionic space and uterine arteries during early human pregnancy. *Acta Obstet Gynecol Scand* 1989; **68**:603–607.

16. Kurjak A, Kupesic S, Kos M, Latin V, Zudenigo D. Early hemodynamics studied by transvaginal color Doppler. *Prenat Neonat Med* 1996; **1**:1–12.

17. Arduini D, Rizzo D, Romanini C. Doppler ultrasonography in early pregnancy does not predict adverse pregnancy outcome. *Ultrasound Obstet Gynecol* 1991; **1**:180–185.

18. Simpson N, Nimrod C, De Vermiette R, Leblanc C, Fournier J. Sonographic evaluation of intervillous flow in early pregnancy: use of echo-enhancemcnt agents. *Ultrasound Obstet Gynecol* 1998; **11**:204–208.

19. Emerson D, Cartier M, Altieri L *et al.* Diagnostic efficacy of endovaginal color doppler flow imaging in an ectopic pregnancy screening program. *Radiology* 1992; **183**:413–420.

20. Parvey H, Dubinsky T, Johnston D, Maklad N. The chorionic rim and low-impedance intrauterine arterial flow in the diagnosis of early intrauterine pregnancy: evaluation of efficacy. *Am J Roentgenol* 1996; **167**:1479–1485.

21. Dillon E, Feyock A, Taylor K. Pseudogestational sacs: Doppler US differentiation from normal or abnormal intrauterine pregnancies. *Radiology* 1990; **176**:359–364.

22. Kurjak A, Zalud I, Predamic M, Kupesic S. Transvaginal color and pulsed Doppler study of uterine blood flow in the first and early second trimesters of pregnancy: normal versus abnormal. *J Ultrasound Med* 1994; **13**:43–47.

23. Jaffe R, Warsof S. Color Doppler imaging in the assessment of uteroplacental blood flow in abnormal first trimester intrauterine pregnancies: an attempt to define etiologic mechanisms. *J Ultrasound Med* 1992; **11**:41–44.

24. Jauniaux E, Zaidi J, Jurkovic D, Campbell S, Hustin J. Comparison of colour Doppler features and pathological findings in complicated early pregnancy. *Human Reprod* 1994; **9**:2432–2437.

25. Benson C, Doubilet P, Cooney M, Frates M, David V, Hornstein M. Early singleton pregnancy outcome: effects of maternal age and mode of conception. *Radiology* 1997; **203**:399–403.

26. Frates M, Benson C, Doubilet P. Pregnancy outcome after a first trimester sonogram demonstrating fetal cardiac activity. *J Ultrasound Med* 1993; **12**:383–386.

27. Frates M, Doubilet P, Brown D *et al.* Role of Doppler ultrasonography in the prediction of pregnancy outcome in women with recurrent spontaneous abortion. *J Ultrasound Med* 1996; **15**:557–562.

28. Jaffe R, Dorgan A, Abramowicz JS. Color Doppler imaging of the uteroplacental circulation in the first trimester: value in predicting pregnancy failure or complication. *Am J Roentgenol* 1995; **164**:1255–1258.

29. Csapo A, Pulkkinen M, Sauvage J, Wiest W. The significance of the human corpus luteum in pregnancy maintenance. *Am J Obstet Gynecol* 1972; **112**:1061–1067.

30. Glock JL, Blackman JA, Badger GJ, Brumsted JR. Prognostic significance of morphologic changes of the corpus luteum by transvaginal ultrasound in early pregnancy monitoring. *Obstet Gynecol* 1995; **85**:37–41.

31. Frates M, Durfee S, Doubilet P *et al.* Sonographic and Doppler characteristics of the corpus luteum: can they predict pregnancy outcome? *J Ultrasound Med* 1998; **17**:54 (abstract).

32. Salim A, Zalud I, Farmakides G, Schulman H, Kurjak A, Latin V. Corpus luteum blood flow in normal and abnormal early pregnancy: evaluation with transvaginal color and pulsed Doppler sonography. *J Ultrasound Med* 1994; **13**:971–975.

33. Alcazar JL, Laparte C, Lopez-Garcia G. Corpus luteum blood flow in abnormal early pregnancy. *J Ultrasound Med* 1996; **15**:645–649.

34. Cotran R, Kumar V, Robbins SL. Female genital tract. In *Robbins Pathologic Basis of Disease*. Philadelphia: Saunders, 1989:1174–1178.

35. Berkowitz RS, Goldstein DP. Chorionic tumors. *N Engl J Med* 1996; **335**:1740–1748.

36. Green CL, Angtuaco TL, Shab HR, Parmley TH. Gestational trophoblastic disease: a spectrum of radiologic diagnosis. *RadioGraphics* 1996; **16**:1371–1384.

37. Taylor KJW, Schwartz PE, Kohorn EI. Gestational trophoblastic neoplasia: diagnosis with Doppler US. *Radiology* 1987; **165**:445–448.

38. Jaffe R. Investigation of abnormal first-trimester gestations by color Doppler imaging. *J Clin Ultrasound* 1993; **21**:521–526.

39. Pellerito J, Taylor K, Quedens-Case C *et al*. Ectopic pregnancy: evaluation with endovaginal color flow imaging. *Radiology* 1992; **183**:407–411.

40. Cacciatore B, Stenman U, Ylostalo P. Diagnosis of ectopic pregnancy by vaginal ultrasonography in combination with a discriminatory serum hCG of 1000 IU/l [IRP]. *Br J Obstet Gynecol* 1990; **97**:904–908.

41. Rempen A. Vaginal sonography in ectopic pregnancy. *J Ultrasound Med* 1988; **7**:381–387.

42. Brown D, Doubilet P. Transvaginal sonography for diagnosing ectopic pregnancy: positivity criteria and performance characteristics. *J Ultrasound Med* 1994; **13**:259–266.

43. Cacciatore B. Can the status of tubal pregnancy be predicted with transvaginal sonography? A prospective comparison of sonographic, surgical and serum hCG findings. *Radiology* 1990; **177**:481–484.

44. Kurjak A, Zalud I, Schulman H. Ectopic pregnancy: transvaginal color Doppler of trophoblastic flow in questionable adnexa. *J Ultrasound Med* 1991; **10**:685–689.

45. Tekay A, Joupilla P. Color Doppler flow as an indicator of trophoblastic activity in tubal pregnancies detected by transvaginal ultrasound. *Obstet Gynecol* 1992; **80**:995–999.

46. Kemp B, Funk A, Hauptmann S, Rath W. Doppler sonographic criteria for viability in symptomless ectopic pregnancies. *Lancet* 1997; **349**:1220–1221.

47. Tekay A, Martikainen H, Keikkinen H, Kivela A, Jouppila P. Disappearance of the trophoblastic blood flow in tubal pregnancy after methotrexate injection. *J Ultrasound Med* 1993; **12**:615–618.

Index

Page numbers in *italics* indicate figures (when separated from their discussion in the main text).